FLUOROPYRIMIDINES
in Cancer Therapy

Acknowledgment

The Symposium was organized under sponsorship of the
Japanese Foundation for Multidisciplinary Treatment
of Cancer.
Publication of this proceedings has been supported by
Taiho Pharmaceutical Co., Ltd.

FLUOROPYRIMIDINES
in Cancer Therapy

Proceedings of the International Symposium on
Fluoropyrimidines, Nagoya, Japan, November 3-5, 1983

Editors:

Kiyoji Kimura, Nagoya
Setsuro Fujii, Osaka
Makoto Ogawa, Tokyo
Gerald P. Bodey, Houston
Pierre Alberto, Geneva

 1984
Excerpta Medica, Amsterdam - New York - Oxford

International Congress Series No. 647
ISBN 0 444 80612 1

Library of Congress Cataloging in Publication Data

International Symposium on Fluoropyrimidines (1983 :
    Nagoya-Shi, Japan)
    Fluoropyrimidines in cancer therapy.
    (International congress series ; no. 647)
    Includes bibliographies.
    1. Fluoropyrimidines--Therapeutic use--Congresses.
2. Cancer--Chemotherapy--Evaluation--Congresses.
3. Fluorouracil--Analogs--Testing--Congresses. I. Kimura,
Kiyoji. II. Title. III. Series. [DNLM: 1. Neoplasms--
drug therapy--congresses. 2. Pyrimidines--therapeutic
use--congresses. W3 EX89 no. 647 / QZ 267 I61f 1983]
RC271.F55I58 1983   616.99'4061   84-13770
ISBN 0-444-80612-1 (U.S.)

Published by:

Elsevier Science Publishers B.V.
P.O. Box 211
1000 AE Amsterdam
The Netherlands

Sole distributors for the USA and Canada:

Elsevier Science Publishing Company Inc.
52 Vanderbilt Avenue
New York, NY 10017
USA

Printed in The Netherlands

PREFACE

The development of 5-fluorouracil was an important event in the history of cancer chemotherapy. It represented one of the few instances when an antitumor agent was synthesized, based upon biochemical rationale. Dr. Charles Heidelberger and his colleagues selected the biosynthetic pathway for thymine, a pyrimidine base unique to DNA, as a critical point for chemotherapeutic intervention. They reasoned that the substitution of fluorine for hydrogen in the 5 position of uracil or deoxyuridine might alter DNA synthesis profoundly via the thymidylate synthetic pathway. They synthesized 5-fluorouracil and, subsequently, 5-fluorodeoxuridine as possible antitumor agents. 5-Fluorouracil was the first antitumor agent with substantial activity against some adenocarcinomas. Although its activity against some of the most common adenocarcinomas, such as hepatoma, colorectal carcinoma and bronchogenic carcinoma, is only marginal, it remains an important component of many therapeutic regimens.

A great deal of progress has been made in our understanding of the activity of 5-fluorouracil during the past 25 years since it was introduced. Although it has been shown that the drug does interfere with the synthesis of thymidylic acid, its biochemical effects on DNA and RNA synthesis are far more complex than originally hypothesized. The discovery of the antitumor activity of 5-fluorouracil gave impetus to the synthesis of other pyrimidine analogues with potentially useful biological properties. The utility of 5-fluorouracil has been expanded by the use of new delivery systems such as intra-hepatic infusions and implantable continuous infusion pumps. Also new analogues, such as tegafur, have been introduced into our armamentarium.

This symposium on fluoropyrimidines has brought together an outstanding group of laboratory and clinical investigators from all over the world. They have contributed extensively to our knowledge about the mechanisms of action, the pharmacokinetics and the clinical applications of fluoropyrimidines. Hopefully, the information presented in these proceedings will lead to a greater interest in this group of compounds and further advances in the treatment of malignant diseases.

Kiyoji Kimura
Setsuro Fujii
Makoto Ogawa
Gerald P. Bodey
Pierre Alberto

CONTRIBUTORS

Osahiko ABE
(461) (511)

Department of General Surgery, School of Medicine, Keio University, 35 Shinano-machi, Shinjuku-ku, Tokyo 160 Japan

Reto ABELE
(175)

Division of Oncology, Geneva University Hospital, Rue Micheli-du-Crest 24, 1211 Geneva 4 Switzerland

Peter AEBERHARD
(534)

Department of Surgery, Kantonsspital, Aarau CH-5000 Switzerland

James D. AHLGREN
(321)

Division of Medical Oncology, Vincent T. Lombardi Cancer Research Center, Georgetown University School of Medicine, 3800 Reservoir Road, N.W., Washington, D.C. 20007 USA

Pierre ALBERTO
(175) (431)

Division of Oncology, Geneva University Hospital, Rue Micheli-du-Crest 24, 1211 Geneva 4 Switzerland

Baha'Uddin M. ARAFAH
(407) (471)

Department of Medicine, Case Western Reserve University School of Medicine, 2074 Abington Road, Cleveland, Ohio 44106 USA

Claude AUBERT
(108)

Laboratory of Pharmacokinetics, Faculty of Pharmacy, INSERM SC 16, 27 Blv. Jean Moulin 13385 Marseille Cedex 05 France

Agop Y. BEDIKIAN
(199)

Section of Infectious Diseases, Department of Developmental Therapeutics, M.D. Anderson Hospital and Tumor Institute, The University of Texas System Cancer Center, 6723 Bertner Avenue, Houston, Texas 77030 USA

John A. BENVENUTO
(57)

Department of Developmental Therapeutics, M.D. Anderson Hospital and Tumor Institute, The University of Texas System Cancer Center, 6723 Bertner Avenue, Houston, Texas 77030 USA

Joseph R. BERTINO
(251)

Section of Medical Oncology, Department of Internal Medicine, Yale University School of Medicine, 333 Cedar Street, New Haven, Connecticut 06510 USA

Numbers in parentheses indicate the pages on which authors' contributions begin.

Nadezhda G. BLOKHINA
(442)

Diagnostic Department, All-Union Cancer Research Center, USSR Academy of Medical Sciences, Kashirskoye sh. 24, Moscow 115478 USSR

George R. BLUMENSCHEIN
(392)

Department of Developmental Therapeutics M.D. Anderson Hospital and Tumor Institute, The University of Texas System Cancer Center, 6723 Bertner Avenue, Houston, Texas 77030 USA

Gerald P. BODEY
(199) (392)

Department of Internal Medicine, M.D. Anderson Hospital and Tumor Institute, The University of Texas System Cancer Center, 6723 Bertner Avenue, Houston, Texas 77030 USA

Kurt W. BRUNNER
(431)

Institute of Medical Oncology, University of Bern, Inselspital, Bern CH-3010 Switzerland

Aman U. BUZDAR
(392)

Department of Developmental Therapeutics, M.D. Anderson Hospital and Tumor Institute, The University of Texas System Cancer Center, 6723 Bertner Avenue, Houston, Texas 77030 USA

Patrick J. BYRNE
(321)

Division of Medical Oncology, Vincent T. Lombardi Cancer Research Center, Georgetown University School of Medicine, 3800 Reservoir Road, N.W., Washington, D.C. 20007 USA

Jean-Paul CANO
(108)

Laboratory of Pharmacokinetics, Faculty of Pharmacy, INSERM SC 16, 27 Blv. Jean Moulin 13385 Marseille Cedex 05 France

Francesco CAVALLI
(175) (431)

Division of Medical Oncology, Ospedale San Giovanni, Bellinzona CH-6500 Switzerland

Delia F. CHIUTEN
(57)

Department of Developmental Therapeutics, M.D. Anderson Hospital and Tumor Institute, The University of Texas System Cancer Center, 6723 Bertner Avenue, Houston, Texas 77030 USA

Harold O. DOUGLASS, Jr.
(497)

Department of Surgical Oncology, Roswell Park Memorial Institute, 666 Elm Street, Buffalo, New York 14263 USA

Rudolf EGELI
(534)

Surgical Oncology, Department of Surgery, Geneva University Hospital, Rue Micheli-du-Crest 24, 1211 Geneva 4

Yousry M. EL SAYED
(3)

Department of Pharmacy, School of Pharmacy, University of California San Francisco, San Francisco, California 94143 USA

Kohji ENOMOTO
(461)

Department of General Surgery, School of Medicine, Keio University, 35 Shinano-machi, Shinjuku-ku, Tokyo 160 Japan

Gholam-Rezah FARROKH
(280)

Medical Clinic, University of Cologne, Joseph-Stelzmannstrasse 9, 5000 Cologne 41, Federal Republic of Germany

Setsuro FUJII
(20)

Division of Regulation of Macromolecular Function, Institute for Protein Research, Osaka University, 3-2 Yamada-Oka, Suita, Osaka 565 Japan

Fumiko FUJITA
(121)

Department of Oncologic Surgery, Research Institute for Microbial Diseases, Osaka University, 3-1 Yamada-Oka, Suita, Osaka 565 Japan

Hiroshi FUJITA
(93)

Department of Bacteriology, School of Dental Medicine, Tsurumi University, 2-1-3 Tsurumi, Tsurumi-ku, Yokohama 230 Japan

Masahide FUJITA
(121) (359)

Department of Oncologic Surgery, Research Institute for Microbial Diseases, Osaka University, 3-1 Yamada-Oka, Suita, Osaka 565 Japan

August M. GARIN
(70)

Clinical Pharmacology Department, All-Union Cancer Research Center, USSR Academy of Medical Sciences, Kashirskoye sh. 24, Moscow 115478 USSR

Nahida H. GORDON
(471)

Department of Surgery, Case Western Reserve University School of Medicine, 2074 Abington Road, Cleveland, Ohio 44106 USA

Yasuhiro HARA
(80)

Department of Gastroenterology, National Kyushu Cancer Center, 595 Notame, Minami-ku, Fukuoka 815 Japan

Takao HATTORI
(511)

Department of Surgery, Research Institute for Nuclear Medicine and Biology, Hiroshima University, 1-2-3 Kasumi, Minami-ku, Hiroshima 734 Japan

E. Douglas HOLYOKE
(497)

Department of Surgical Oncology, Roswell Park Memorial Institute, 666 Elm Street, Buffalo, New York 14263 USA

Noboru HORIKOSHI
(379)

Division of Clinical Chemotherapy, Cancer Chemotherapy Center, Japanese Foundation for Cancer Research, 1-37-1 Kami-Ikebukuro, Toshima-ku, Tokyo 170 Japan

Tadashi HORIUCHI
(311)

Department of Internal Medicine, National Nagoya Hospital, 4-1-1 Sannomaru, Naka-ku, Nagoya 460 Japan

Gabriel N. HORTOBAGYI
(199) (392)

Department of Developmental Therapeutics, M.D. Anderson Hospital and Tumor Institute, The University of Texas System Cancer Center, 6723 Bertner Avenue, Houston, Texas 77030 USA

Akio HOSHI
(34)

Pharmacology Division, National Cancer Center Research Institute, 5-1-1 Tsukiji, Chuo-ku, Tokyo 104 Japan

Charles A. HUBAY
(471)

Case Western Reserve University School of Medicine, 2074 Abington Road, Cleveland, Ohio 44106 USA

Tadashi IKEDA
(461)

Department of General Surgery, School of Medicine, Keio University, 35 Shinano-machi, Shinjuku-ku, Tokyo 160 Japan

Kazuhiro IKENAKA
(20)

Division of Regulation of Macromolecular Function, Institute for Protein Research, Osaka University, 3-2 Yamada-Oka, Suita, Osaka 565 Japan

Athanassios ILIADIS
(108)

Laboratory of Pharmacokinetics, Faculty of Pharmacy, INSERM SC 16, 27 Blv. Jean Moulin 13385 Marseille Cedex 05 France

Jiro INAGAKI
(379)

Division of Clinical Chemotherapy, Cancer Chemotherapy Center, Japanese Foundation for Cancer Research, 1-37-1 Kami-Ikebukuro, Toshima-ku, Tokyo 170 Japan

Kiyoshi INOKUCHI
(511)

Department of Surgery, Kyushu University School of Medicine, 3-1-1 Maidashi, Higashi-ku, Fukuoka 812 Japan

Katsuhiro INOUE
(379)

Division of Clinical Chemotherapy, Cancer Chemotherapy Center, Japanese Foundation for Cancer Research, 1-37-1 Kami-Ikebukuro, Toshima-ku, Tokyo 170 Japan

Tsuguhiko IZUMI
(229)

Department of Internal Medicine, Juntendo University School of Medicine, 3-1-3 Hongo, Bunkyo-ku Tokyo 113 Japan

Charles JACQUET
(108)

Laboratory of Pharmacokinetics, Faculty of Pharmacy, INSERM SC 16, 27 Blv. Jean Moulin 13385 Marseille Cedex 05 France

Tamaki KAJITANI
(484)

Japanese Foundation for Multidisciplinary Treatment of Cancer, Cancer Institute Hospital, Japanese Foundation for Cancer Research, 1-37-1 Kami-Ikebukuro, Toshima-ku, Tokyo 170 Japan

Toshiki KAMANO
(229)

First Department of Surgery, Juntendo University School of Medicine, 3-1-3 Hongo, Bunkyo-ku, Tokyo 113 Japan

Takao KANKO
(330)

Department of Internal Medicine and Clinical Oncology, Cancer Institute Hospital, Japanese Foundation for Cancer Research, 1-37-1 Kami-Ikebukuro, Toshima-ku, Tokyo 170 Japan

Kimiyuki KATO
(549)

Third Department of Surgery, Aichi Cancer Center Hospital, 81-1159 Kanokoden, Tashiro-cho, Chikusa-ku, Nagoya 464 Japan

Tomoyuki KATO
(549)

Third Department of Surgery, Aichi Cancer Center Hospital, 81-1159 Kanokoden, Tashiro-cho, Chikusa-ku, Nagoya 464 Japan

Yasuhiko KIMOTO
(359)

Department of Oncologic Surgery, Research Institute for Microbial Diseases, Osaka University, 3-1 Yamada-Oka, Suita, Osaka 565 Japan

Kiyoji KIMURA
(147) (186) (311)

National Nagoya Hospital, 4-1-1 Sannomaru, Naka-ku, Nagoya 460 Japan

Hans O. KLEIN
(280)

Department of Internal Medicine, Medical Clinic, University of Cologne, Joseph-Stelzmann Strasse 9, 5000 Cologne 41, Federal Republic of Germany

Junichi KOH
(461)

Department of General Surgery, School of Medicine, Keio University, 35 Shinano-machi, Shinjuku-ku, Tokyo 160 Japan

Chihiro KONDA
(217)

Hematology Division, Department of Internal Medicine, National Cancer Center Hospital, 5-1-1 Tsukiji, Chuo-ku, Tokyo 104 Japan

Akiro KONO
(80)

Research Institute, National Kyushu Cancer Center, 595 Notame, Minami-ku, Fukuoka 815 Japan

Hiroki KOYAMA
(420)

Department of Surgery, The Center for Adult Diseases, Osaka, 1-3-3 Nakamichi, Higashinari-ku, Osaka 537 Japan

Yoshiyuki KOYAMA
(161)

National Medical Center Hospital, 1-21-1 Toyama, Shinjuku-ku, Tokyo 162 Japan

Tetsuro KUBOTA
(461)

Department of Surgery, Kitasato Institute Hospital, 1-15-1 Kitasato Sagamihara 228 Japan

Keijiro KUNO
(484)

Department of Surgery, Cancer Institute Hospital, Japanese Foundation for Cancer Research, 1-37-1 Kami-Ikebukuro, Toshima-ku, Tokyo 170 Japan

Minoru KURIHARA
(229)

Department of Internal Medicine, Toyosu Hospital, Showa University, 4-1-18 Toyosu, Kooto-ku, Tokyo 135 Japan

Urban LAFFER
(534)

Department of Surgery, University Hospital, Basel CH-4031 Switzerland

Sewa S. LEGHA
(392)

Department of Developmental Therapeutics, M.D. Anderson Hospital and Tumor Institute, The University of Texas System Cancer Center, 6723 Bertner Avenue, Houston, Texas 77030 USA

Tamara G. LOBOVA
(70)

Clinical Pharmacology Department, All-Union Cancer Research Center, USSR Academy of Medical Sciences, Kashirskoye sh. 24, Moscow 115478 USSR

Ti Li LOO
(57)

Pharmacology Section, Department of Chemotherapy Research, M.D. Anderson Hospital and Tumor Institute, The University of Texas System Cancer Center, 6723 Bertner Avenue, Houston, Texas 77030 USA

Fardil F. MAMEDOV
(70)

Clinical Pharmacology Department, All-Union Cancer Research Center, USSR Academy of Medical Sciences, Kashirskoye sh. 24, Moscow 115478 USSR

James S. MARSHALL
(407) (471)

Department of Endocrinology, Case Western Reserve University School of Medicine, 2074 Abington Road, Cleveland, Ohio 44106 USA

Sebastiano MARTINOLI
(534)

Department of Surgery, Hospital Civico, Lugano CH-6904 Switzerland

William L. McGUIRE
(471)

Department of Medicine and Oncology, University of Texas Health Science Center at San Antonio, Texas 78284 USA

Bernadette MERMILLOD
(175) (431) (534)

SAKK Operations Office, 62 Rue de Carouge, Geneva 1205 Switzerland

Urs F. METZGER
(534)

Division of Surgical Oncology, Department of Surgery, Zurich University Hospital, Zurich CH-8091 Switzerland

Ljudmila M. MIKHAILOVA
(47)

Laboratory of Pharmacology and Toxicology, All-Union Cancer Research Center, USSR Academy of Medical Sciences, Kashirskoye sh. 24, Moscow 115478 USSR

Antonius A. MILLER
(57)

Department of Developmental Therapeutics, M.D. Anderson Hospital and Tumor Institute, The University of Texas System Cancer Center, 6723 Bertner Avenue, Houston, Texas 77030 USA

Enrico MINI
(251)

Section of Medical Oncology, Department of Internal Medicine, Yale University School of Medicine, 333 Cedar Street, New Haven, Connecticut 06510 USA

Keiichi MIYASAKA
(229)

Department of Radiology, Showa University 1-5-8 Hatanodai, Shinagawa-ku, Tokyo 142 Japan

Rüdiger MOHR
(280)

Department of Internal Medicine, Medical Clinic, University of Cologne, Joseph-Stelzmann Strasse 9, 5000 Cologne 41, Federal Republic of Germany

E. Colleen MOORE
(57)

Department of Developmental Therapeutics, M.D. Anderson Hospital and Tumor Institute, The University of Texas System Cancer Center, 6723 Bertner Avenue, Houston, Texas 77030 USA

Toshifusa NAKAJIMA
(484)

Department of Surgery, Cancer Institute Hospital, Japanese Foundation for Cancer Research, 1-37-1 Kami-Ikebukuro, Toshima-ku, Tokyo 170 Japan

Yosuke NAKANO
(121) (359)

Department of Oncologic Surgery, Research Institute for Microbial Diseases, Osaka University, 3-1 Yamada-Oka, Suita, Osaka 565 Japan

Isao NAKAO
(330)

Department of Internal Medicine and Clinical Oncology, Cancer Institute Hospital, Japanese Foundation for Cancer Research, 1-37-1 Kami-Ikebukuro, Toshima-ku, Tokyo 170 Japan

John R. NEEFE
(321)

Division of Medical Oncology, Vincent T. Lombardi Cancer Research Center, Georgetown University School of Medicine, 3800 Reservoir Road, N.W., Washington, D.C. 20007 USA

Ichiro NISHI
(330)

Department of Internal Medicine and Clinical Oncology, Cancer Institute Hospital, Japanese Foundation for Cancer Research, 1-37-1 Kami-Ikebukuro, Toshima-ku, Tokyo 170 Japan

Michael J. O'CONNELL
(350) (524)

Department of Medical Oncology, Mayo Clinic, Rochester, Minnesota 55905 USA

Hans OERKERMANN
(280)

Department of Internal Medicine, Medical Clinic, University of Cologne, Joseph-Stelzmann Strasse 9, 5000 Cologne 41, Federal Republic of Germany

Makoto OGAWA
(379)

Division of Clinical Chemotherapy, Cancer Chemotherapy Center, Japanese Foundation for Cancer Research, 1-37-1 Kami-Ikebukuro, Toshima-ku, Tokyo 170 Japan

Nobuya OGAWA
(511)

Department of Pharmacology, Ehime University School of Medicine, Ooaza-Shizukawa, Shigenobu-cho, Onsen-gun, Ehime 791-02 Japan

Yasuhiko OHASHI
(330)

Departments of Internal Medicine and Clinical Oncology, Cancer Institute Hospital, Japanese Foundation for Cancer Research, 1-37-1 Kami-Ikebukuro, Toshima-ku, Tokyo 170 Japan

Jun OHTA
(359)

Department of Oncologic Surgery, Research Institute for Microbial Diseases, Osaka University, 3-1 Yamada-Oka, Suita, Osaka 565 Japan

Kazuo OTA
(186) (261)

Department of Medical Oncology, Aichi Cancer Center Hospital, 81-1159 Kanokoden, Tashiro-cho, Chikusa-ku, Nagoya 464 Japan

Olof H. PEARSON
(407) (471)

Department of Endocrinology, Case Western Reserve University School of Medicine, 2074 Abington Road, Cleveland, Ohio 44106 USA

Wolfgang SADÉE
(3)

Department of Pharmacy, School of Pharmacy, University of California San Francisco, San Francisco, California 94143 USA

Tatuo SAITO
(330)

Departments of Internal Medicine and Clinical Oncology, Cancer Institute Hospital, Japanese Foundation for Cancer Research, 1-37-1 Kami-Ikebukuro, Toshima-ku, Tokyo 170 Japan

Tsuneo SASAKI
(269)

Department of Clinical Chemotherapy, Tokyo Metropolitan Komagome Hospital, 3-18-22 Hon-Komagome, Bunkyo-ku, Tokyo 113 Japan

Yozo SASAKI
(229)

Department of Internal Medicine, Juntendo University School of Medicine, 3-1-3 Hongo, Bunkyo-ku Tokyo 113 Japan

Philip S. SCHEIN
(321)

Smith Kline & French Laboratories, 1500 Spring Garden Street, P.O. Box 7929, Philadelphia PA 19101 USA

Rudolf SCHROEDER
(534)

Department of Surgery, University Hospital, Bern CH-3010 Switzerland

Volker SCHULZ
(280)

Medical Clinic, University of Cologne, Joseph-Stelzmann Strasse 9, 5000 Cologne 41, Federal Republic of Germany

Tetsuhiko SHIRASAKA
(20)

Division of Regulation of Macromolecular Function, Institute for Protein Research, Osaka University, 3-2 Yamada-Oka, Suita, Osaka 565 Japan

Frederick P. SMITH
(320)

Division of Medical Oncology, Vincent T. Lombardi Cancer Research Center, Georgetown University School of Medicine, 3800 Reservoir Road, N.W., Washington, D.C. 20007 USA

Alberto SOBRERO
(251)

Section of Medical Oncology, Department of Internal Medicine, Yale University School of Medicine, 333 Cedar Street, New Haven, Connecticut 06510 USA

Jean-Pierre SOMMADOSSI
(108)

Laboratory of Pharmacokinetics, Faculty of Pharmacy, INSERM SC 16, 27 Blv. Jean Moulin 13385 Marseille Cedex 05 France

C. Paul SPEARS
(12)

Department of Medicine, University of Southern California, School of Medicine, 1303 N. Mission Road, Los Angeles, California 90033 USA and Oncology-Hematology Unit, The Hospital of the Good Samaritan, 616 South Witmer Street, Los Angeles, California 90017 USA

Shoji SUGA
(147) (311)

Section of Gastroenterology, National Nagoya Hospital, 4-1-1 Sannomaru, Naka-ku, Nagoya 460 Japan

Nikolai I. SUSLOV
(47)

Laboratory of Pharmacology and Toxicology, All-Union Cancer Research Center, USSR Academy of Medical Sciences, Kashirskoye sh. 24, Moscow 115478 USSR

Anatol B. SYRKIN
(47)

Laboratory of Pharmacology and Toxicology, All-Union Cancer Research Center, USSR Academy of Medical Sciences, Kashirskoye sh. 24, Moscow 115478 USSR

Tetsuo TAGUCHI
(121) (359) (511)

Department of Oncologic Surgery, Research Institute for Microbial Diseases, Osaka University, 3-1 Yamada-Oka, Suita, Osaka 565 Japan

Kunio TAKAGI
(484)

Department of Surgery, Cancer Institute Hospital, Japanese Foundation for Cancer Research, 1-37-1 Kami-Ikebukuro, Toshima-ku, Tokyo 170 Japan

Martin H.N. TATTERSALL
(297)

Ludwig Institute for Cancer Research, University of Sydney, Sydney, N.S.W. 2006 Australia

Tokyo Cancer Chemotherapy Cooperative Study Group
(242)

Department of Internal Medicine, Teikyo University School of Medicine, 74 Mizonokuchi, Takatsu-ku, Kawasaki 213 Japan

Nobuhisa UEDA
(359)

Department of Oncologic Surgery, Research Institute for Microbial Diseases, Osaka University, 3-1 Yamada-Oka, Suita, Osaka 565 Japan

Masao USUGANE
(359)

Department of Oncologic Surgery, Research Institute for Microbial Diseases, Osaka University, 3-1 Yamada-Oka, Suita, Osaka 565 Japan

Manuel VALDIVIESO
(199)

Department of Developmental Therapeutics, M.D. Anderson Hospital and Tumor Institute, The University of Texas System Cancer Center, 6723 Bertner Avenue, Houston, Texas 77030 USA

Tatijana A. VORONINA
(47)

Laboratory of Pharmacology of Psychotropic Drugs, Institute of Pharmacology, USSR Academy of Medical Sciences, Baltiyskaj ul. 6, Moscow, USSR

Tomio WADA
(420)

Department of Surgery, The Center for Adult Diseases, Osaka, 1-3-3 Nakamichi, Higashinari-ku, Osaka 537 Japan

Walter WEBER
(175)

Department of Oncology, Kantonsspital, Basel, Switzerland

Premaratne Dias WICKRAMANAYAKE
(280)

Department of Internal Medicine, Medical Clinic, University of Cologne, Joseph-Stelzmann Strasse 9, 5000 Cologne 41, Federal Republic of Germany

Paul V. WOOLLEY, III
(320)

Division of Medical Oncology, Vincent T. Lombardi Cancer Research Center, Georgetown University School of Medicine, 3800 Reservoir Road, N.W., Washington, D.C. 20007 USA

Tadashi YOKOYAMA
(330)

Departments of Internal Medicine and Clinical Oncology, Cancer Institute Hospital, Japanese Foundation for Cancer Research, 1-37-1 Kami-Ikebukuro, Toshima-ku, Tokyo 170 Japan

Yasuhisa YOKOYAMA
(311)

Yokoyama Hospital, 3-14-4 Chiyoda, Naka-ku, Nagoya 460 Japan

Yuichi YOSHIDA
(311)

Department of Internal Medicine, National Nagoya Hospital, 4-1-1 Sannomaru, Naka-ku, Nagoya 460 Japan

CONTENTS

VI. Surgical Adjuvant Chemotherapy

EXPERIMENTAL ASPECTS

Fluoropyrimidines in Cancer Therapy
K. Kimura, S. Fujii, M. Ogawa, G.P. Bodey, P. Alberto, eds.

MECHANISM OF METABOLIC ACTIVATION OF TEGAFUR*

Wolfgang Sadée and Yousry M. El Sayed

1. INTRODUCTION

Tegafur (Ftorafur, [R,S-1-(tetrahydro-2-furanyl-5-fluoro-uracil]) represents one of the many 5-fluorouracil (FUra) prodrugs that have been synthesized in an attempt to obtain more efficacious fluoropyrimidine anticancer agents. Tegafur is active against several adenocarcinomas with rather mild myelotoxicity, while its CNS toxicity is more pronounced than that of FUra (review: 1). In view of FUra's rapid disappearance from the blood circulation, most prodrugs were designed to release FUra slowly over a protracted time period, thus, mimicking slow FUra infusion. The prolonged presence of FUra in blood plasma yields superior therapeutic results under selected disease conditions. Tegafur counts among the FUra prodrugs with a slow release mechanism.

One might therefore surmise that tegafur is clinically equiv-alent to slow FUra infusions. However, there is a major systematic difference between slow FUra i.v. infusion and the slow release of FUra from its prodrugs: FUra is produced from prodrugs in those tissues containing the suitable enzymes for prodrug activation,

* Supported by USPHS grant CA 27866 from the National Cancer Institute, Bethesda, Maryland, U.S.A.

rather than directly in the systemic circulation. Consequently the question arises as to whether FUra which undergoes rapid intracellular metabolism can reach the systemic circulation to be distributed throughout the body after metabolic activation. Measurements of FUra plasma levels after tegafur administration in patients provided the answer. After resolving analytical difficulties with the chemical decomposition of tegafur and its metabolites to yield artificially elevated FUra levels in vitro (2), we have demonstrated that FUra plasma levels after tegafur administration were much below those expected after an equitoxic FUra infusion (Fig. 1) (3).

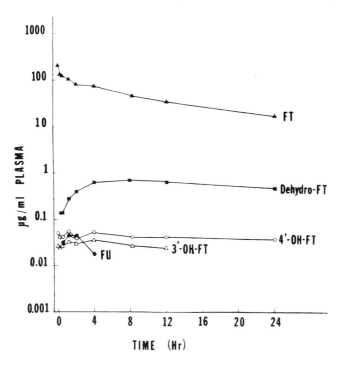

FIGURE 1   Plasma concentration-time curves of tegafur (FT) and its metabolites, i.e., FUra (FU), 4'-OH-FT, and dehydro-FT, in a patient given tegafur (2 g/sq m i.v.) infused over 30 min. Zero time refers to the end of infusion. (Taken from (2).)

It was concluded that FUra fails to redistribute throughout the body after metabolic activation, which is clearly different from direct FUra infusions.

Given these circumstances, it is important to recognize that i. the target toxicity of the prodrug is dependent upon the tissue distribution of the activating enzymes, and ii. that measurements of FUra levels in the systemic circulation do not reveal the degree of prodrug activation in individual tissues. We have therefore studied in detail the mechanism of the enzymatic conversion of Ftorafur to 5-fluorouracil. Multiple activation pathways were identified. Design of more selective prodrugs should be directed towards FUra analogs that are activated by single selected target enzymes.

2.   MATERIALS AND METHODS

Tissue Homogenate Preparations and In Vitro Incubations. Male Dutch rabbits were stunned and decapitated. The liver, brain, and small intestine were excised and rinsed in ice-cold isotonic (1.15%) KCl. Each organ tissue was homogenized in (1:2) (wt/vol) ice-cold 0.01 M potassium/sodium phosphate buffer (pH 7.4)-1.15% KCl using a Potter-Elvehjem teflon pestle homogenizer. The homogenates were centrifuged at 10,000 g for 20 min at 0-4° to yield the 10,000 g supernatant fraction. The supernatant fractions were recentrifuged at 100,000 g for 1 hr at 0.4°. The 100,000 g supernatant fraction may be used immediately or frozen at -20° until use.

Several experiments were carried out with dialyzed 100,000 g liver homogenates. The dialysis tubes containing the homogenates were incubated in 200 volumes of 100 mM tris buffer pH 7.4 for 5 hrs at 4°C. A high concentration of tris buffer was chosen to accel-erate solute exchange; moreover, the buffer was replaced every hour.

All in vitro incubations were carried out at pH 7.4 at 37° for 1 hr. Final concentration of all preparations was standardized to 1 g tissue (wet weight) per 2 ml incubation mixture. Chemical reagents and cofactors were added at the concentrations indicated. The concentrations of NADPH and NADH were 1 mM each. When incuba-tions were performed for more than one hour, additional amounts of NADPH and NADH were added every hour (yielding concentration incre-ments of 1 mM each) in order to prevent cofactor depletion. Higher concentrations of NADPH and NADH failed to increase the rate of product formation. The rate of GBL/GHB formation from ftorafur was linear over at least 4 hrs. (See also (4) for details.)

Gas Chromatographic Assay for GBL/GHB, 4-Hydroxybutanal and 1,4-Butanediol. GBL/GHB, 4-hydroxybutanal, and 1,4-butanediol were measured by the previously published GC assay of GBL/GHB (5) with the following modifications (4). The column, injector and detector temperatures were 145, 190, 210°, respectively. GC retention times for GBL, 4-hydroxybutanal and 1,4-butanediol were 3.2, 1.5, 9.5 min, respectively.

HPLC Assay of 5-Fluorouracil. 5-Fluorouracil was measured in the in vitro incubates with an HPLC assay using prepurification of extracts by column chromatography for sufficient sensitivity (100 ng/ml) (4). The column chromatography afforded separation of 5-fluorouracil from the endogenous interferences present in the tissue homogenates.

3. RESULTS AND DISCUSSION

Lack of redistribution of FUra that is generated from tegafur
in vivo suggested that metabolic activation in target tissues represents a determinant of tegafur toxicity and efficacy. It has been
suggested that the liver is the primary site of metabolism, and the
hepatic microsomal cytochrome P-450 could represent the enzyme
responsible for tegafur activation (e.g., 6). Indeed, we have shown
that this metabolic pathway proceeds via C-5' oxidation to give FUra
and succinaldehyde (7) (Fig. 2). However, this activation pathway
can hardly explain the clinical antitumor effects and toxicity of
tegafur directed against tissues which are largely devoid of the
activating P-450 enzymes.

Further potential activation pathways include dehydrogenation
of tegafur to dehydro-tegafur (dehydro-FT (Fig. 1)) (2,3) followed
by spontaneous or enzymatic decomposition to FUra. Moreover,
stereoselective hydroxylation of tegafur to β,D-4'-hydroxytegafur
followed by thymidine phosphorylase catalyzed cleavage to FUra was
found to occur (1). However, none of these pathways appeared to be
responsible for a significant part of tegafur activation in vivo.

The discovery of γ-butyrolactone as a major tegafur metabolite
in vivo and in 100,000 g supernatants of rabbit liver homogenates
(5) suggested that an important activation pathway may be mediated
by soluble enzymes of target tissues. Figure 2 depicts the
enzymatic-chemical pathways that can lead to γ-butyrolactone as the
endproduct. Both 4-hydroxybutanal and succinaldehyde rapidly
convert to γ-butyrolactone (GBL). Lack of any external cofactor
requirement made the activation pathway by direct C-2' oxidation

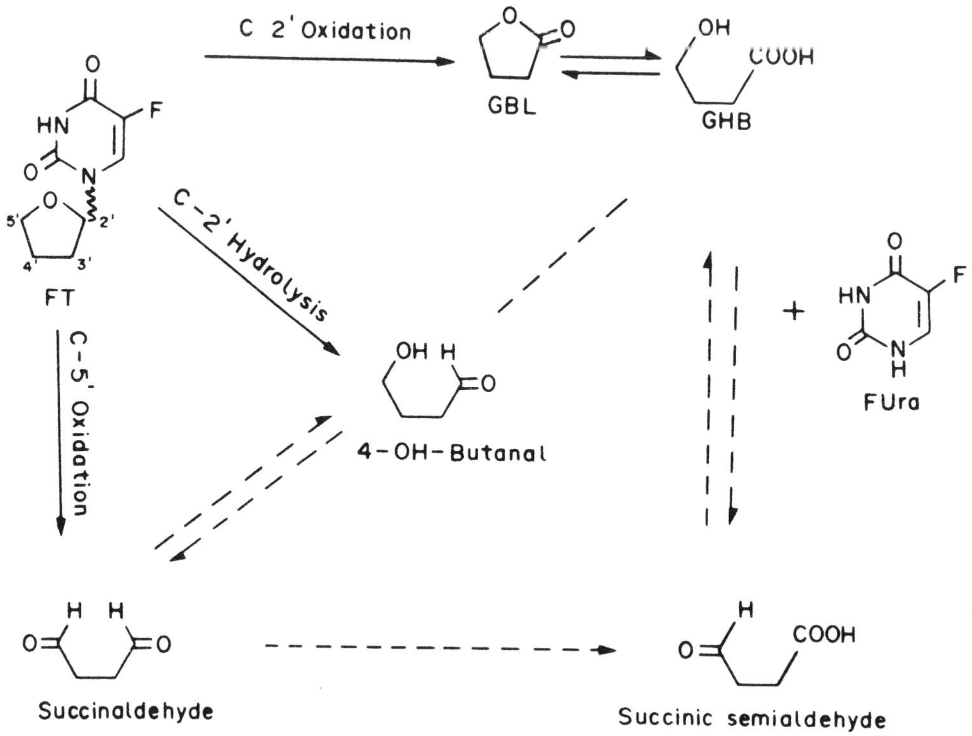

FIGURE 2   Three possible activation pathways of ftorafur that lead to 5-fluorouracil and the expected products of the tetrahydrofuran moiety.   Potential interconversion among these products is also indicated.   FT: tegafur; GBL: γ-butyrolactone; GHB: γ-hydroxybutyric acid.

unlikely. Moreover, hydrazine had no effect on γ-butyrolactone formation from tegafur, although it blocked succinaldehyde conversion to γ-butyrolactone by > 80% (4). This rules out the C-5' oxidation pathway. In contrast, the addition of alcohol dehydrogenase and NADH to the 100,000 g supernatants of rabbit liver largely inhibited the formation of γ-butyrolactone from both tegafur and

8

4-hydroxybutanal (4). We therefore conclude that metabolic activation of tegafur to 5-fluorouracil proceeds _via_ hydrolytic cleavage of the N-1-C-2' bond (although enzymatic phosphorolysis of the N-1-C-2' bond cannot be excluded as an alternative mechanism (8)). It is most significant that this pathway was also detectable in rabbit brain and intestines (4), major target organs of tegafur toxicity.

In conclusion, these results demonstrate that tegafur is activated to 5-fluorouracil by the soluble enzymes of target tissues _via_ cleavage of the N-1-C-2' bond (Fig. 3).

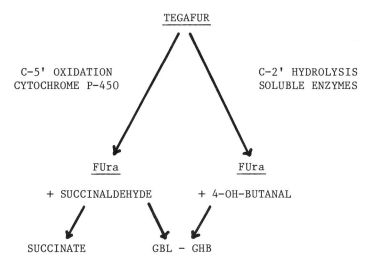

FIGURE 3   The two major activation pathways of tegafur to 5-fluorouracil. Note that the two pathways attack at different sites of the ftorafur moiety. While only a fraction of the generated succinaldehyde is converted to γ-buturolactone, 4-hydroxybutanal yields γ-butyrolactone quantitatively. (For abbreviations see legend, Fig. 2.)

9

The other major metabolic activation pathway, i.e., tegafur oxidation at C-5' by a cytochrome P-450 mediated mechanism, leads to 5-
fluorouracil and succinaldehyde (Chart 5). Since cytochrome P-450
is mainly localized in the liver, with lower levels in the g.i.
tract and much lower levels in the brain, and since 5-fluorouracil
is not redistributed via the circulation (2), it is possible
that the soluble enzyme pathway is responsible for part of the organ
toxicity as well as for the antitumor effects of tegafur. Other
previously reported activation pathways are unlikely to contribute
significantly to the tegafur effects. Further development of prodrugs related to tegafur should, therefore, be directed towards
separating the microsomal (C-5') and soluble enzymes (C-2') activation pathways of the tetrahydrofuran ring moiety. Moreover, assay
of the soluble activation pathway of tegafur may serve as a predic-
tor of the antitumor efficacy of the drug.

REFERENCES

1. Au JL, Sadée W (1981) The pharmacology of ftorafur (R,S-1-
    (tetrahydro-2-furanyl)-5-fluorouracil). In: Recent Result in
    Cancer Research, Vol. 76 (eds) Carter SK, Sakurai Y and Umezawa
    H. Berlin-Heidelberg-New York, pp. 100-114.

2. Au JL, Sadée W (1979) 5-Fluorouracil concentration in human
    plasma following R,S-1-(tetrahydro-2-furanyl)-5-fluorouracil
    (Ftorafur) administration. Cancer Res 39: 4289-4290.

3. Au JL, Wu AT, Friedman MA, Sadée W (1979) Pharmacokinetics and
    metabolism of ftorafur in man. Cancer Treat Rep 63: 343-350.

4. El Sayed YM, Sadée W (1983) Metabolic activation of ftorafur
    [R,S-1-(tetrahydro-2-furanyl)-5-fluorouracil] to 5-fluorouracil
    by soluble enzymes. Cancer Res, in press.

5. Au JL, Sadée W (1980) Activation of ftorafur [R,S-1-(tetrahy-
    dro-2-furanyl)-5-fluorouracil] to 5-fluorouracil and γ-butyro-
    lactone. Cancer Res 40: 2814-2819.

6. Fujita H, Kimura K (1973) In vivo distribution and metabolism
    of N-1-(tetrahydrofuran-2-yl)-5-fluorouracil (FT-207). Progr
    Chemother Vol 3, Proc VIII Int. Congr. Chemother. Hell. Soc.
    Chemother. Athens pp 159-164.

7. El Sayed YM, Sadée W (1982) Metabolic activation of ftorafur
    [R,S-1-(tetrahydro-2-furanyl)-5-fluorouracil]: the microsomal
    oxidative pathway. Biochem Pharmacol 31: 3006-3008.

8. Kono K, Hara Y, Matsushima Y (1981) Enzymatic formation of 5-
    fluorouracil from 1-(tetrahydro-2-furanyl)-5-fluorouracil
    (Tegafur) in human tumor tissues. Chem Pharm Bull 29: 1486-
    1488.

© 1984 Elsevier Science Publishers B.V.
Fluoropyrimidines in Cancer Therapy
K. Kimura, S. Fujii, M. Ogawa, G.P. Bodey, P. Alberto, eds.

THYMIDYLATE SYNTHETASE INHIBITION IN PEYTON ADENOCARCINOMA XENOGRAFTS FOLLOWING BOLUS 5-FLUOROURACIL

C. Paul Spears

1. INTRODUCTION

An improved method of assay of thymidylate synthetase (TS) levels in tissues following in vivo exposure to 5-FUra has provided evidence (1) that tumor responsiveness correlates with a drastic reduction in the level of free, native TS, designated TS_f. Measurement of TS_f is done by titration of enzyme binding sites with tritiated 5-fluorodeoxyuridylate (FdUMP), with correction for exchange labeling into endogenous FdUMP-folate-TS, ternary complex-bound enzyme (TS_b).

Recent study of single biopsy specimens of human gastrointestinal tumors (2) has indicated that marked and rapid reduction in TS_f after intravenous bolus 5-FUra also occurs in the clinical situation. Although the single biopsies gave kinetically useful information, it would be desirable to be able to fully determine the intracellular pharmacokinetics of FdUMP formation and loss and TS_f inhibition in human tumors. For example, ineffective TS_f inhibition could result from either inadequate peak FdUMP levels or excessive accumulation of deoxyuridylate (dUMP), which events may occur at different time intervals after 5-FUra exposure; and accurate determination of peak FdUMP levels may require rapid sampling at early time points. The feasibility of serial, repeated biopsy for study of intracellular pharmacokinetics is suggested by the present investigation of human colorectal adenocarcinoma xenografts in nude mice.

2.   MATERIALS AND METHODS

Female nude mice, weighing 25-30 g, bearing subcutaneous Peyton adenocarcinoma xenografts in the posterior thoracic area, were obtained from Dr. Beppino Giovanella of the Stehlin Foundation for Cancer Research, Houston, Texas. Peyton 1^O tumor was derived from the initial colectomy specimen of a patient whose subsequent metastatic recurrence showed a complete response to single-agent, intermittent i.v. bolus 5-FUra. A later relapse on 5-FUra treatment was the source of Peyton 2^O tumor. The tumors were studied at the 10th-15th transplant generations. Growth inhibition studies at earlier transplant generations indicated that the Peyton 1^O and 2^O tumors showed 5-FUra sensitivity and resistance, respectively, to i.p. drug (B. Giovanella, personal communication). The tumors had volume doubling times of 3-5 days and were 2-4 g in size at the time of study. Under sterile conditions, mice were restrained in the prone position, and under local lidocaine anesthesia a 2-cm incision was made 1-2 cm medial to the tumor. Tumors, attached to overlying skin, were easily exposed by gentle blunt dissection from the thoracic wall. By use of a 5 x 5 mm biopsy forceps, samples were taken prior to, and at various times after i.p. 5-FUra, 80 mg/kg. Biopsies were taken at points in the tumors most distant from integument, away from major blood vessels. The biopsies averaged 74 ± 20 mg in size. Estimated overall blood losses were consistently less than 0.5 ml. Incisions were closed in between time points with steristrip tape.

The biopsies were either stored at -80° or processed immediately, by homogenization and sonication in a 10-fold excess of Tris buffer containing phosphatase inhibitors (1,3). Assay of TS_f and TS_{tot} ($TS_f + TS_b$) was done on the 10,000 x g supernatants using charcoal isolation of protein-bound 6-[^{3}H]FdUMP (1). Acetic acid extracts of the crude sonicates were taken for

13

separation of dUMP and FdUMP. The assay for FdUMP was by isotope dilution of [^{3}H]FdUMP subsequently bound to bacterial TS enzyme (3). Conversion of dUMP to [^{14}C]thymidylate was done by use of [^{14}C]CHO condensed with tetrahydropteroylmonoglutamate, with subsequent isolation by DEAE-ammonium formate chromatography (3).

3. RESULTS

The intracellular pharmacokinetics of FdUMP formation and its loss, of TS$_f$ inhibition and reactive changes in dUMP levels, in Peyton 1° and Peyton 2° tumors following i.p. 5-FUra are presented in Figs. 1-3. The results of the 80 mg/kg dose of 5-FUra represent the average ($\pm$ S.D.) of values in 3 mice for each tumor line.

Peak FdUMP levels in Peyton 1° tumor were found at the earliest time point studied, 1 h after 5-FUra (80 mg/kg), and showed an exponential decline through 7 h with a half-life of about 2.5 h (Fig. 1). In contrast, peak FdUMP did not occur until 2 h after 5-FUra administration in Peyton 2° tumor, and

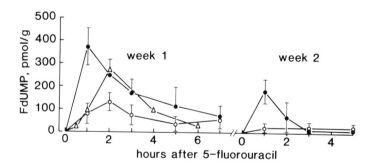

Figure 1.   Intracellular pharmacokinetics of FdUMP, obtained by serial biopsy, in Peyton colon adenocarcinoma xenografts in nude mice treated with i.p. 5-FUra, 80 mg/kg (1° tumor, [●]; 2° tumor, [O]), or 200 mg/kg (2° tumor, [△]).

was only one-third of the maximal value of the 1° tumor. The effect of increasing the dose of 5-FUra to 200 mg/kg was studied in one mouse bearing Peyton 2° tumor. The increase in peak FdUMP, to 270 pmole/g, over that formed following the lower dose was proportional to the increase in dose. The timing of maximal FdUMP level, and the values at 5-7 h were similar for the two dose levels. A second dose of 5-FUra, 80 mg/kg i.p., given at one week, resulted in substantially lower FdUMP levels in both tumor lines. The relatively more rapid rate of FdUMP formation in the 1° tumor was again observed.

The differences between Peyton 1° and 2° tumors in FdUMP levels resulted in corresponding differences in TS_f inhibition, Fig. 2. Pretreatment TS_f levels averaged 6.7 and 8.8 pmole/g in 1° and 2° tumors, respectively.

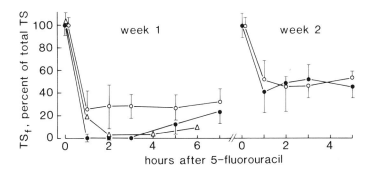

Figure 2.   Kinetics of TS_f inhibition in Peyton 1° and 2° tumors treated with 5-FUra. Symbols are the same as in Fig. 1.

TS_{tot} levels were similar to pretreatment TS_f values throughout the experimental period in both tumors. After 5-FUra treatment, however, TS_f was undetectable (<0.05 pmole/g) in Peyton 1° tumor at 1-3 h, but did not drop below 2 pmole/g in Peyton 2° tumor through 7 h. Greater TS_f inhibition occurred in 2^O tumor with the 200 mg/kg dose of 5 FUra. In this instance, maximal TS_f inhibition did not appear to occur until 2 h, corresponding to the time of delayed peak FdUMP formation.

In the second week, incomplete TS_f inhibition was found in both tumor lines. Pretreatment TS_f averaged 7.2 pmole/g in the two tumor lines. Of interest is that both the peak level of FdUMP and the degree of TS_f inhibition in Peyton 1^O tumor were similar to the results of the initial, first week 5-FUra dose on 2^O tumor. The latter also showed decreased FdUMP formation over the values from the first dose of 5-FUra, associated with lessened TS_f inhibition.

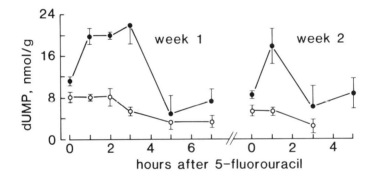

Figure 3.   Response of dUMP levels in Peyton 1^O (●) and 2^O (O) tumor xenografts to TS_f inhibition following 5-FUra, 80 mg/kg.

Figure 3 shows the results of dUMP assay. Although the Peyton 1^O and 2^O tumors had similar pretreatment levels, only 1^O tumor showed a rise in dUMP, to nearly twice baseline at 3 h. This probably was a result of effective TS_f inhibition, resulting in accumulation of the normal substrate. Less dUMP accumulation was seen in 1^O tumor following the second dose of 5-FUra given a week later, in keeping with the reduced TS_f inhibition at this time.

4. DISCUSSION

Determination of the intracellular pharmacokinetics of TS_f inhibition that results from 5-FUra treatment of human tumors may be useful for deciding which patients should receive further 5-FUra therapy, for establishing a mechanism of therapeutic effect of 5-FUra in patients who respond to 5-FUra, and for identification of mechanisms of resistance that could be overcome by biochemical modulation with other agents such as methotrexate (4) or folates (5). Conceptual obstacles to study of intracellular pharmacokinetics include concerns about heterogeneity within and between tumor metastases, and of the effects of a biopsy on the metabolic integrity of the remaining tumor nodule.

A purpose of this investigation, using large human tumor xenografts, was to gauge the feasibility of serial forceps biopsy as a surgical approach to obtaining intracellular pharmacokinetic data. In this regard, the most important conclusion of this study is that clearly characteristic profiles of FdUMP formation, TS_f inhibition, and dUMP accumulation occurred in the Peyton 1° and 2° colonic adenocarcinoma xenografts. Biologic variation among samples from the same tumor line, at the 50-100 mg size range, did not appear to be a problem for study of intracellular pharmacokinetics up to 7 h. It is not possible, however, to exclude effects of heterogeneity (base vs. surface of the tumors) or of instrumentation on the lowered FdUMP formation that occurred with the second dose of 5-FUra.

The greater TS_f inhibition in Peyton 1° than in 2° tumor was a result of higher levels of FdUMP, which also formed more rapidly in 1° tumor. In support of this are the observations that less FdUMP formation occurred on the second dose of 5-FUra, accompanied by less TS_f inhibition in both 1° and 2° tumors; and that administration of a higher initial dose of 5-FUra to 2°

tumor resulted in increased FdUMP levels and greater TS_f inhibition. The relatively higher FdUMP level in 1° tumor at 1 h resulted in a more favorable FdUMP/dUMP ratio (0.04) at this early time point, which likely contributed to more effective TS_f inhibition (2). It is interesting that the duration of TS_f inhibition to less than 1 pmole/g in 1° tumor was only about 3 h. The rise in dUMP in this tumor in response to TS_f inhibition may have labilized ternary-complex, FdUMP-bound enzyme.

The Peyton 1° and 2° adenocarcinomas derived from tumors that were likely to have been clinically sensitive and resistant, respectively, to intermittent bolus 5-FUra, and had shown these differences at earlier transplant generations in nude mice. The differences these tumors showed in TS_f inhibition could account for their variation in responsiveness to 5-FUra. A decrease in TS_f to just 2 pmole/g tissue, in Peyton 2° tumor, probably is inadequate to effectively halt DNA synthesis. For example, if the growth fraction of a tumor is 25%, the S-phase 20 h, and the DNA content 4 mg/g, then TS enzyme at only 1 pmole/g tissue (assuming a specific activity of 0.24 nmole thymidylate production/min per pmole TS) could still synthesize enough thymidylate to maintain growth.

Thus, resistance to the therapeutic effects of 5-FUra in the patient from whom the Peyton tumors were obtained could have resulted from a decrease in FdUMP formation. This explanation is best supported by the differences observed in intracellular pharmacokinetics of TS_f inhibition in Peyton 1° and 2° tumors on initial exposure to 5-FUra. The finding of a decrease in FdUMP levels in the Peyton tumors after the second dose of 5-FUra, one week after the first, also suggests that selection for tumor cells with lower levels of activating enzymes may have occurred.

REFERENCES

1. Spears CP, Shahinian AH, Moran RG, et al. (1982) In vivo kinetics of thymidylate synthetase inhibition in 5-fluorouracil-sensitive and -resistant colon adenocarcinomas. Cancer Res 42: 450-456.

2. Spears CP, Gustavsson B, Berne M, et al. (1982) Thymidylate synthetase (TS) inhibition by 5-fluorouracil (5-FU) treatment of human gastro-intestinal malignancies: dUMP/FdUMP ratio as a determinant. Proc Amer Assoc Cancer Res 24: 133.

3. Moran RG, Spears CP, and Heidelberger C. (1979) Biochemical determinants of tumor sensitivity to 5-fluorouracil: ultrasensitive methods for the determination of 5-fluoro-2'-deoxyuridylate, 2'-deoxyuridylate, and thymidylate synthetase. Proc Natl Acad Sci USA 76: 1456-1460.

4. Bertino JR, Mini E, and Fernandes DJ. (1983) Sequential methotrexate and 5-fluorouracil: mechanisms of synergy. Semin Oncol 10: 2-5.

5. Houghton JA, Maroda SJ, Phillips JO, et al. (1981) Biochemical determinants of responsiveness to 5-fluorouracil and its derivatives in xenografts of human colorectal adenocarcinomas in mice. Cancer Res 41: 144-149.

© 1984 Elsevier Science Publishers B.V.
Fluoropyrimidines in Cancer Therapy
K. Kimura, S. Fujii, M. Ogawa, G.P. Bodey, P. Alberto, eds.

ATTEMPT ON ENHANCEMENT OF ANTITUMOR ACTIVITY OF MASKED FLUOROPYRIMIDINES

Setsuro Fujii, Kazuhiro Ikenaka and Tetsuhiko Shirasaka

1. INTRODUCTION

Tegafur is a cytostatic synthesized by Dr. Hiller group (1). We studied the mechanism of action of tegafur in terms of cytostatics, and reported in 1977 that tegafur is converted to 5-FU via liver microsome (P450) (2). This study led to oral administration of tegafur.

Recently Sadee et al. described that tegafur is activated to 5-FU also via cytosol other than liver microsome (3).

In future, it must be studied in detail that significance of activation to 5-FU via cytosol in the cytostatic action of tegafur and mode of action of its activation.

During proceeding of pharmacokinetics of tegafur, many investigators and clinicians who had been studying tegafur requested us any idea or divices capable of more 5-FU release in order to obtain better antitumor effect.

We have been making every effort to enhance the antitumor activity of tegafur and finally are successful in this purpose by the combination of tegafur and uracil.

2. MATERIALS AND METHODS

Yoshida sarcoma and sarcoma-180 cells were maintained by intraperitoneal transfer in Donryu strain rats and ICR mice, respectively. Solid-type sarcoma-180 was obtained by subcutaneous injection of 2×10^7 ascites cells into the back of mice on day 0. Drugs suspended in 5% acacia were administered orally once a day for 7 consecutive days, starting 24 hr after tumor implantation, i.e. on day 1. Control mice were given 5% acacia alone in the same way. On day 10, mice were killed and their tumors were removed and weighed. The antitumor activity of a combination of tegafur and uracil, thymine, thymidine was expressed as the mean weight of tumor in trated mice to that in control mice.

Assay of degradation and phosphorylation of 5-FU were performed as previously described (4-7). FdUMP binding dTMP synthetase activity was determined by method of Heidelberger et al (8).

3. RESULTS AND DISCUSSION

Effect of uracil on growth inhibition of St. aureus 209P and HeLa cells by 5-FU

5-FU is an antagonist of uracil, therefore 5-FU degradation is probably inhibited by uracil. But it is rather problem that 5-FU undergoes phosphorylation to exhibite antitumor activities.

As metioned previously, 5-FU itself hasn't antitumor effect, the phosphorylated products from 5-FU disturbe

21

metabolism of RNA of DNA synthesis, especially FdUMP inhibits dTMP synthetase resulted in decrease tumor growth.
Therefore, the purpose is not attained, if uracil inhibits
phosphorylation of 5-FU.

The following our experience is the reason why we
chose uracil as inhibitor of 5-FU degradation.

Fig. 1 shows influence of uracil on 5-FU growth inhibition to St. aureus and HeLa cells. When 0.2 μg/ml of
5-FU was added to the medium of St. aureus, the growth of
cells was suppressed by approximately 30%. When uracil
was added at 1, 10, 100 and 1,000 times each of 5-FU
level under the same condition. The addition of uracil
at 100 times of 5-FU attained to 0% of growth inhibiton.

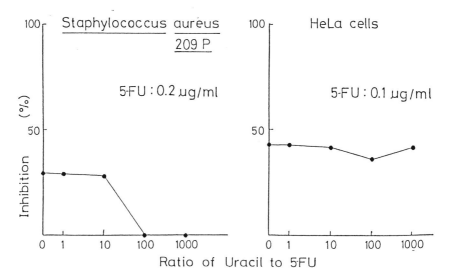

Fig. 1. Effect of uracil of growth inhibition of Staph-
lococcus aureus 209P and HeLa cells by 5-FU.

On the other hand, such phenomenon was not observed

in the case of HeLa cells. Uracil at 1,000 times the concentration of 5-FU didn't influence upon inhibition of HeLa
cells by 5-FU. At that time we wondered the phenomenon in
the case of HeLa cells experiment, but we didn't make effort to reveal the cause further. When we began to
attempt of enhancement of antitumor effect of tegafur,
we reminded this experiment suggesting that in tumor cells,
phosphorylation of 5-FU is not inhibited by uracil in some
conditions. Probably, if so, uracil will inhibit the degradation and dose not affect the phosphorylation of 5-FU.

The effect of uracil of metabolism of 5-FU

Then the studies of the influence of uracil of 5-FU
phosphorylation in Yoshida sarcoma and its degradation in
rat liver slice employing ^{14}C-5-FU were carried out.

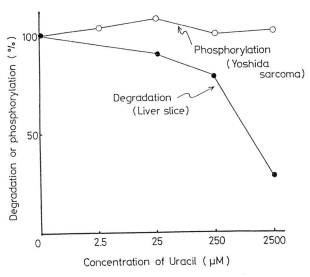

Fig. 2. Effect of uracil on metabolism of 5-FU in intact
Yoshida sarcoma cell and liver slice (5-FU:2.5µM)

As shown in Fig.2, even if addition of uracil at 1,000 times concentration in this conditions, as expected, didn't influence upon 5-FU phosphorylation. On the other hand, 5-Fu degradation was inhibited in proportion to increase in uracil concentration employing low level of 5-FU as substrate.

Km and V max values the enzymes involved in metabolism of 5-FU

In order to clarify this phenomenon from view point of enzymology. 5-FU undergoes phosphorylation by 2 pathways. Phosphorylation is catalyzed by uracil ribosyltransferase and phosphoribosyltransferase each other, while the degradation is brought about by dihydrouracil dehydrogenase. The Km and V max values of DHU dehydrogenase, uracil ribosyltransferase, and pyrimidine 5' phosphoribosyltransferase were measured with uracil of 5-FU as a substrate. As shown in Fig. 3, the Km and V max values for degradation of 5-FU and uracil (DHU dehydrogenase) were 4.0×10^{-5}M and 0.51, and 1.0×10^{-5}M and 0.22, respectively; the Km and V max values for phosphorylation of 5-FU and uracil (uracil ribosyltransferase) were 5.6×10^{-5}M and 1.2, and 4.5×10^{-4}M and 10 (with Rib1P and ATP), and 6.3×10^{-4}M and 10, and 9.1×10^{-3}M and 26 (with PPRibP), respectively. The Km value of DHU dehydrogenase was apparently lower than those of the phosphorylating enzymes, indicating that 5-FU and uracil tend to be used in the degradation pathway, but that this pathway is soon saturated (low V max value).

24

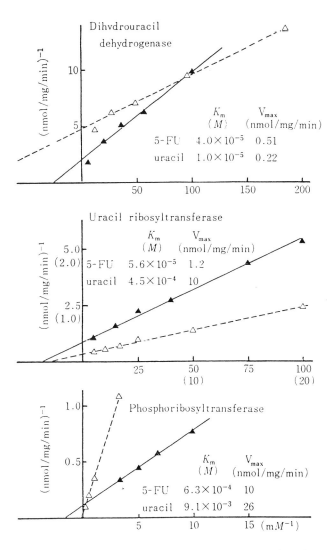

Fig. 3.   Km and V max values (▲——▲:5-FU, △---△:uracil)

On the other hand, the pathways for phosphorylation have
a large capacity so that inhibition of 5-FU phosphorylation by uracil is slight.   The result explains well that
uracil is easy to inhibit 5-FU degradation and is hard to
inhibit 5-FU phosphorylation in low level of 5-FU.

From these data, we considered that the antitumor

effect of tegafur might be enhanced by combination of tegafur and uracil. Then we performed the antitumor experiment of combination of uracil and tegafur.

Antitumor activity of oral coadministration of tegafur with uracil on sarcoma-180

The results are shown in Fig. 4. A vertical axis shows T/C, and horizontal axis shows tegafur dosage.

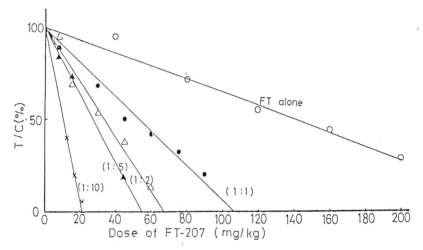

Fig.4. Antitumor activity of oral coadministration of FT-207 with uracil on sarcoma-180

When tegafur alone, 140 mg/kg is necessary to inhibit tumor growth by 50%, figures such as 1:1, 1:2, 1:5 and 1:10 in parenthesis show molar numbers of tegafur versus uracil. Figures of each column present T/C under each combination. Clearly, increased uracil to tegafur produced increased antitumor effect. For example, when the ratio was 1:10, 10mg of tegafur was needed to obtain 50% T/C, and in other words, antitumor effect was about 14 times high in the combination ratio of 1:10 as compared with tegafur alone

The effect of uracil, uridine, thymine and thymidine
on antitumor activity and body weight change of tegafur
on Sarcoma 180

The combination effect of thymidine, thymine, uridine
with tegafur   at ratio of 2:1 were presented in Fig.5.

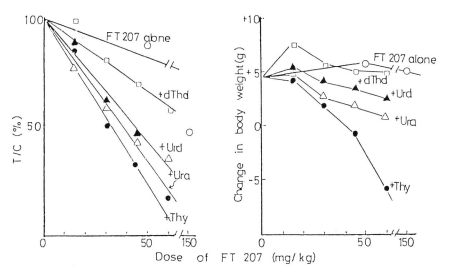

Dose of FT 207 (mg/ kg)

Fig. 5. Effect of uracil, uridine, thymine and thymidine
on antitumor activity and body weight change of tegafur
on sarcoma-180

Each case showed combined effect. The most favorable effect
was obtained with thymine. But this combination also influenced most on change in body weight. To summarize
these results, the combination of tegafur and uracil produced high antitumor effect and low toxicity as compared
with other combinations.

<u>5-FU levels in blood, tumor and various organs after</u>

<u>oral administration of uracil and tegafur</u>

We noticed another interesting fact in the combination
of tegafur and uracil. It concerns with various tissue
levels of 5-FU.

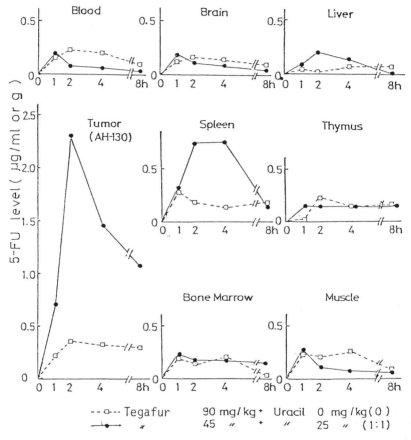

Fig.6.   5-FU levels in blood, tumor and various organs
after oral administration of uracil and tegafur (ratio 1:1)

Fig.6 showed time-course change in various tissue level
of 5-FU in AH-130 tumor bearing rats received tegafur
alone at 90 mg/kg and the combination of 45 mg/kg of
tegafur and 25 mg/kg of uracil (molar ratio is 1:1).

Tegafur alone showed no remarkable changes in various tissue level of 5-FU. For instance, 5-FU levels were 0.25 μg/ml or 0.25μg/g for blood, tumor tissue and bone marrow, respectively. However, the combination of tegafur and uracil produced high level of 5-FU only in tumor tissues as compared with other tissues. But only exception was the spleen, where 5-FU level was high. 5-FU level was about 0.2 μg/ml or /g in blood or tissues, that is, about 10 times high as compared with other tissues. Many clinicians advised us that idea; cytostatics produced high concentration in tumor tissues and low in blood and other tissues. According to their advice, 5-FU level must be less than 0.025 μg/ml in the blood and more than from 0.08 μg/g to 0.1 μg/g in tumor tissues.

Ratio of 5-FU levels in tumor and blood after coadministration of tegafur and uracil to AH-130-bearing rats

In oder to determine the most favorable ratio of tegafur and uracil to make the most difference of 5-FU level between the blood and tumor. Tegafur at 3 mg/kg or 7.5 mg/kg nearly equivalent to clinical dosage was orally administered to AH-130 tumor-bearing rats in combination with various dosage of uracil. Results were shown in Fig. 7. This study revealed that when the ratio of tegafur to uracil was around 1:4, the greatest difference occurred between the blood and tumor tissues.

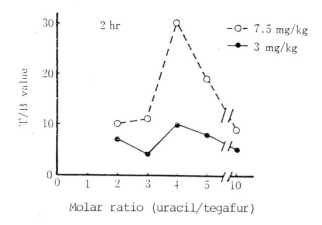

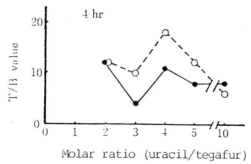

Fig. 7. Ratio of 5-FU concentration in the tumor and blood of AH-130-bearing rats after coadministration of tegafur and uracil

5-FU level in blood, normal and tumor tissues (clinical data)

To confirm this ratio clinically, we asked trials to Prof. Taguchi of Osaka University, Dr. Kimura of National Nagoya Hospital and Prof. Yamamoto of Kansai Medical College. They also revealed this ratio was favorable. Fig. 8 summarized the ratio of 1:4 in clinical trials. Tegafur and uracil at the ratio of 1:4 was administered orally to patients before surgery, and 5 FU levels in blood, tumor tissues and tumor-adjacent tissues were determined. Blood level of 5-FU less than 0.025 μg/ml was obtained in 28 patients, about 65% of 43 patients. Tumor level of 5-FU more than 0.1 μg/mg was available in 18 patients, about 42%, and more than 0.08 μg/mg, about 60%, respectively.

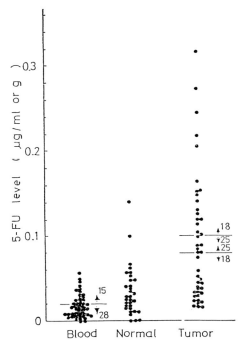

Fig. 8. 5-FU level in blood, normal and tumor tissues (clinical data)

The effect of 5-FU, tegafur and combination of tega-fur and uracil (ratio 1:4) on dTMP synthetase activities of sarcoma 180

Solid-type tumor of sarcoma-180 was prepared as describ-ed above and on the 12th day, 20 mg/kg of 5-FU, 30 mg or 120 mg/kg of tegafur and combination of 30 mg/kg of

tegafur and uracil (ratio 1:4) were administered orally
to tumor-bearing mice. The dTMP synthetase activities in
tumor tissues were determined according to method of
Heidelberger et al. (8) at 4 and 24 hrs after administration of the drugs.

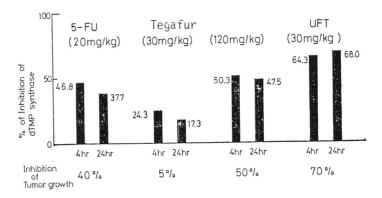

Fig. 9. Effect of 5-FU, Tegafur and UFT (tegafur:uracil,
1:4) on dTMP synthetase activities of sarcoma-180

As shown in Fig. 9, in all cases, total enzyme activities were not changed and percent of inhibition of dTMP
synthetase were calculated. Each drug showed antitumor
activity such as 40%, 5%, 50% and 70% for T/C in other experience as described in Fig. 3. Inhibition rate to dTMP
synthetase was not differed remarkably between 4 and 24
hrs. Combination of tegafur and uracil (ratio 1:4) e-
quivalent to tegafur dosage exhibited clear cut-high inhibitory activity as compared with tegafur alone.

REFERENCES

1. Hiller SA, Zhuk RA, Lidak MY (1967) Analogues of
    pyrimidine nucleosides. 1. N_1-(α-Furanydyl) deriva-
    tives of natural pyrimidine bases and their antimeta-
    bolites. Dokl Akad Nauk SSSR 176: 332-335.

2. Toide H, Akiyoshi H, Minato Y, Okuda H, Fujii S.
    (1977) Comparative studies on the metabolism of 2-
    (tetrahydrofuryl)-5-fluorouracil and 5-fluorouracil.
    Gann 68: 553-560.

3. El Sayed YM, Sadee W. (1983) Metabolic activation of
    R,S-(tetrahydro-2-furanyl)-5-fluorouracil (Ftorafur)
    to 5-fluorouracil by soluble enzymes. Cancer Res 43:
    4039-4044.

4. Fujii S, Ikenaka K, Fukushima M, Shirasaka T. (1978)
    Effect of uracil and its derivatives on antitumor
    activity of 5-fluorouracil and 1-(2-tetrahydrouracil)
    -5-fluorouracil. Gann 69: 763-772.

5. Fujii S, Kitano S, Ikenaka K, Shirasaka T. (1979)
    Effect of coadministration of uracil or cytosine on
    the antitumor activity of clinical doses of 1-(2-
    Tetrahydrouracil)-5-fluorouracil and level of 5-
    fluorouracil in rodents. Gann 70: 209-214.

6. Ikenaka K, Shirasaka T, Kitano S, Fujii S. (1979)
    Effect of uracil on metabolism of 5-fluorouracil in
    vitro. Gann 70: 353-359.

7. Fujii S, Kitano S, Ikenaka K, Fukushima M, Nakamura
    H, Maehara, Y, Shirasaka T. (1980) Effect of co-
    administration of thymine or thymidine on the anti-
    tumor activity of 1-(2-tetrahydrouracil)-5-fluoro-
    uracil and 5-fluorouracil. Gann 71: 100-106.

8. Spears CP, Shahinian AH, Moran RG, Heidelberger C,
    Corbett TH. (1982) In vivo kinetics of thymidylate
    synthetase inhibition in 5-fluorouracil-sensitive
    and -resistant murine colon adenocarcinomas. Cancer
    Res 42: 450-456.

© 1984 Elsevier Science Publishers B.V.
Fluoropyrimidines in Cancer Therapy
K. Kimura, S. Fujii, M. Ogawa, G.P. Bodey, P. Alberto, eds.

1-HEXYLCARBAMOYL-5-FLUOROURACIL,
A MASKED FORM OF 5-FLUOROURACIL

Akio Hoshi

1. INTRODUCTION

5-Fluorouracil shows a broad, strong antitumor effect
on various cancers, especially gastrointestinal cancer by
parenteral administration(1). However, phlebitis and arte-
ritis occur during treatment of cancer(1). Tegafur: 1-(2-
tetrahydrofuryl)-5-fluorouracil is the first fluoropyrimidine showing strong therapeutic effect on cancers by
oral administration(2). Tegafur shows minimal gastrointestinal toxicity(3), while 5-fluorouracil at the effective dose shows a severe toxicity by oral administration
(4).

Experimentally, oral tegafur is not so active against
ascites form of sarcoma 180, though the tumor itself is
sensitive to 5-fluorouracil. It means low liberation of
5-fluorouracil in ascites fluid or low distribution into
ascites fluid of 5-fluorouracil derived from tegafur in
plasma. More active derivatives of 5-fluorouracil in oral
use than tegafur is sought to improve therapeutic effect
and 1-hexylcarbamoyl-5-fluorouracil(HCFU) is finally
selected as the best compound for internal use.

2. CHEMISTRY

The chemical structure of 1-hexylcarbamoyl-5-fluoro-uracil(HCFU) is shown in Fig.1. The compound is synthesized with 5-fluorouracil and hexylisocyanate in pyridine (5) and its molecular weight is 257.26. This compound is freely soluble in dimethylformamide, chloroform, acetone and ethylacetate and is sparingly soluble in methanol and ethanol and is practically insoluble in water(6).

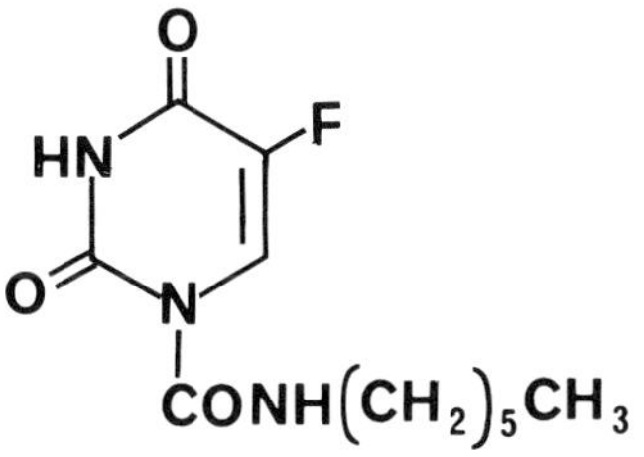

FIGURE I   Chemical structure of HCFU

This compound can be quantitatively determined by high performance liquid chromatography or non aqueous titration (in dimethylformamide) with sodium methoxide. HCFU in aqueous solution is stable at below pH 4 but it is unstable at alkaline condition and liberates gradually 5-fluorouracil. The half-life of HCFU in aqueous solution (at 20°C) at pH 7.5 is 67.2 minutes(6).

3. ANTITUMOR ACTIVITY

The antitumor activity of 1-alkylcarbamoyl derivatives of 5-fluorouracil is first found in the L1210 leukemia

35

system by oral administration(7) and relationship between chemical structure and antitumor effects is examined(8). Antitumor effect of the derivatives is also examined in a variety of murine tumor systems(9,10) and 1-hexylcarbamoyl-5-fluorouracil(HCFU) is finally selected as the best compound(11). The maximum effects of HCFU on experimental tumors as well as that of 5-fluorouracil(5-FU) and tegafur are shown in Table 1.

TABLE 1 Maximum antitumor effects at maximum torelated doses of HCFU, 5-FU and tegafur (po)

Tumor	HCFU		5-FU		Tegafur	
	MaxILS (%)	Maximum growth inhibition (%)	MaxILS (%)	Maximum growth inhibition (%)	MaxILS (%)	Maximum growth inhibition (%)
S180A		91		47		32
EAC		87		72		49
NFS		100		90		90
Ca755		92		27		56
L1210	53		50		31	
C1498	64		49		53	
LLC	100	96	33	86	69	98
B16	38	75	9	74	26	56
Colon26	199		86		-	
Colon38	123		40		-	

HCFU is more effective than the rest compounds against various tumors. HCFU is also effective on slow growing tumors such as Lewis lung carcinoma, B16 melanoma(10,12), Colon 26 and Colon 38(13). In Colon 38, tumor-free survivors are observed on Day 100 by only HCFU treatment. HCFU is also effective on a spontaneous mammary adenocarcinoma of mice and local recurrence is delayed and life-span is increased by oral HCFU in various treatment schedules(14). Lung metastases of sc tumors are decreased by HCFU in the mammary adenocarcinoma(14) and Lewis lung carcinoma(12). Effect of HCFU by long-term oral administration is slightly affected by the schedule of administration(14). Antitumor effect of HCFU on Adenocarcinoma 755 is dependent on the total dose but not on the amount of single dose or schedule of administration (Table 2).

4. PHARMACOKINETICS OF HCFU

Highest concentration of radioactivity in plasma is shown 15 min after oral administration of labeled HCFU [6-^{14}C] similar to that after 5-FU and it is retained for a long period in mice(15), rats and rabbits(16). Radioactivity derived from HCFU is excreted in urine and it is 70, 84, 72 and 67% of dose in mice(17), rats, rabbits and dogs(16), respectively. Radioactivity detected in feces of any animals within 72 hours is less than 3% of dose. It means good absorption of HCFU from gastrointestinal tract. By determination of residual radioactivity in

TABLE 2. No schedule dependency of antitumor effect of HCFU in adenocarcinoma 755 system

Treatment schedule	Total Dose (mg/kg)	Growth inhibition[a] (%)
Day 1 once	1000	88
	500	56
Day 1 and 5 q4d	2000	95[b]
	1000	92
	500	56
Day 1,3 and 5 q2d	2000	100
	1000	84
	500	64
Day 1 through 5 daily	2000	100[b]
	1000	83
	500	56
Day 1 through 5 q12h/24h	2000	100
	1000	92
	500	60
Day 1 through 5 q8h/24h	2000	100
	1000	83
	500	60

a) Evaluated on Day 12.
b) One out of six mice is died from drug toxicity.

various parts of gastrointestinal tract, absorption site of HCFU is found to be duodenum and small intestine similar to that of 5-FU(17).

5-FU is the active form liberated from HCFU and is detected in plasma and tissues of animals in high concentration. For example, plasma level of 5-FU is one-half that of HCFU 15 minutes after oral HCFU administration at 50 mg/kg in mice and 5-FU is still detected in plasma 180 minutes after dosage with HCFU, while 5-FU is no longer detected in plasma 60 minutes after dosage with 5-FU(18). Degradation products of 5-FU are detected in high concentration after 5-FU, but these products are very low after HCFU administration but hydrophobic metabolites are detected. These are penultimate oxidation products and a β-oxidation product after terminal oxidation of the side chain of HCFU(16,18). Proportion of metabolites of HCFU are different from species to species of animals (Table 3).

TABLE 3   Metabolites in plasma one hour after oral HCFU administration

Species	Dose	HCFU	Terminal oxidation products[a]	Penultimate oxidation products[b]	5-FU
	(mg/kg)		(μg/ml)		
Mice	50	6.0	0.3[c]	10.4[c]	5.0[c]
Rats	10	0.2	0.8	0.1	0.2
Rabbits	10	2.5	3.2	4.7	0.3
Dogs	10	1.4	0.3	1.0	0.4

a) 1-(5-carboxypentylcarbamoyl)- and 1-(3-carboxypropyl-carbamoyl)-5-fluorouracil.
b) 1-(5-hydroxyhexylcarbamoyl)- and 1-(5-oxohexylcarba-moyl)-5-fluorouracil.
c) In mice, the concentration is μgHCFU equivalents/ml.

Penultimate oxidation is the main pathway in mice and dogs, but terminal oxidation is that in rats and both oxidations are metabolic pathways in rabbits.

In mice bearing ascites sarcoma 180, patterns of metabolism and disposition after oral administration of HCFU resemble to those in normal mice, but elimination of HCFU and 5-FU is slower in tumor-bearing mice. 5-FU originating from HCFU is retained in plasma over 6 hours, while intact 5-FU after 5-FU administration disappeares within 2 hours. Pattern of metabolites in ascites fluid is similar to that in plasma after HCFU administration, but 5-FU is retained for a long period. In sarcoma 180 cells, the concentration of intact HCFU is low and the principal metabolites are nucleotides that are accumulated and maintained for a long period after administration of HCFU or 5-FU(19).

Pharmacokinetics of 1-alkylcarbamoyl-5-fluorouracils relating to chemical stracture is examined in tumor-bearing mice. All of the alkylcarbamoyl derivatives are absorbed rapidly as intact form through the gastrointestinal tract and distribute into ascites fluid. Area under curve (AUC) in plasma and ascites fluid decreased in order by extention of the carbon chain of the alkyl moiety. Antitumor activity of the compounds is correlated with both maximum concentration(C_{max}) and AUC values of 5-FU formed and C_{max} of total (intact form plus 5-FU formed) in ascites fluid and with both C_{max} and AUC of 5-FU formed in plasma. Alkylcarbamoyl structure is valuable for rapid

40

absorption through the gastrointestinal tract, for penetration of the blood-ascites barrier and for maintenance of 5-FU level in plasma and ascites fluid(20).

5.   MECHANISM OF ACTION

Antiproliferation activity of HCFU is one-fifth that of 5-FU against L5178Y cells in culture(21). It means good liberation of 5-FU from HCFU in physiological conditions. Distribution pattern and 5-FU concentrations in tissues of mice after HCFU are not affected by liver function, while 5-FU level after tegafur is increased by pretreatment with phenobarbital plus glutathion but decreased by carbon tetrachloride(22). It means 5-FU liberation from HCFU is not mainly depending upon liver function.

Metabolites of HCFU containing 5-fluorouracil moiety in molecules are active against L5178Y cells in culture (21). As a result, HCFU is found to be a "masked form" of 5-fluorouracil and to liberate 5-fluorouracil in tumor tissues and plasma.

6.   TOXICITY

Subacute and chronic toxicity of HCFU are similar to those of 5-FU and tegafur in rats(23) and dogs(24). In a Phase I study, pollakisuria syndrome is found as a side-effect of HCFU(25). Cause and mechanism of the action are examined. 1-(5-Carboxypentylcarbamoyl)-5-fluorouracil which is a metabolite of HCFU causes acceleration of bladder movement in cats, rabbits and rats and the metabo

lites stimulates the micturition reflux center in the

brain stem(26). Another side-effect of HCFU in clinic is

a hot sensation around the face and trunk(25). The cause

of the action is the same metabolite or HCFU itself and

they affect the neuron activity of preoptic area in hypo-

thalamus of rats(27). These side effects are specific to

HCFU.

7.   FUTURE DIRECTIONS

To eliminate the specific side-effects, antitumor ef-

fect of new derivatives of 5-fluorouracil containing nor-

mal amino acids, cyclic alkylamine and aromatic alkyl-

amines instead of alkylamine in the side chain of HCFU is

examined(28). Further, antitumor effect of the metabolites

of HCFU,that arc found in plasma and urine after oral

HCFU, is examined. These metabolites are more active than

HCFU against L5178Y cells in culture, but they are toxic

to mice by both oral and parenteral administrations(21).

Antitumor effect of the derivatives of 5-fluorouracil

that contain no nitrogen in the side chain is also exam-

ined and several 1-acyloxymethyl derivatives of 5-fluoro-

uracil are found to be active against L1210 leukemia(29).

But no better derivative is obtained than HCFU.

Future direction to improve the therapeutic effect of

5-fluorouracil is synthesis of "masked form"s of various

derivatives containing 5-fluorouracil moiety, which are

not only nucleobases but also nucleosides and nucleotides as shown in Fig. 2.

Among them, ditoluoylester of 5-fluoro-deoxyuridine shows higher therapeutic ratio in L1210 system(30) and hexadecylester of 5-fluorouridine 5'-monophosphate shows no cross resistance in 5-fluorouridine-resistant L5178Y cells(31).

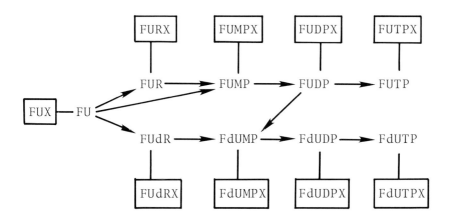

FIGURE 2   Possible masked forms of 5-fluorouracil
             derivatives

REFERENCES

1. Carter SK, Glatstein E, Livingston RB ed.(1982)
    "Principles of Cancer Treatment" McGraw-Hill Inc.,
    New York.

2. Konda C, Niitani H, Sakauchi N et al. (1973) Chemo-
    therapy of cancer with oral administration of N_1-(2-
    furanidyl)-5-fluorouracil. Gan no Rinsho 19: 495-499.

3. Fujimoto S, Akao T, Itoh B et al. (1976) Follow-up
    studies of the gastrointestinal cancer patients treat-
    ed by the extended oral 5-FU and FT-207 as an adju-
    vant to surgical treatment. Gan no Rinsho 22: 471-477.

4. Hahn RG, Moertel CG, Schutt AJ et al. (1975) A double-
    blind comparison of intensive couse 5-fluorouracil by
    oral vs. intravenous route in the treatment of colo-
    rectal carcinoma. Cancer 35: 1031-1035.

5. Ozaki S, Ike Y, Mizuno H et al. (1977) 5-Fluorouracil
    derivatives. I. The synthesis of 1-carbamoyl-5-fluoro-
    uracils. Bull Chem Soc Jpn 50: 2406-2412.

6. Miura T, Uchiyama T, Takahashi M et al. (1980) Physi-
    co-chemical properties and stabilities of 1-hexyl-
    carbamoyl-5-fluorouracil(HCFU). Iyakuhin Kenkyu 11:
    73-81.

7. Hoshi A, Iigo M, Yoshida M et al. (1975) Antitumor
    activity of carbamoyl derivatives of 5-fluorouracil
    by oral administration. Gann 66: 673-674.

8. Hoshi A, Iigo M, Nakamura A et al. (1978) Antitumor
    activity of alkylcarbamoyl derivatives of 5-fluoro-
    uracil against L1210 leukemia. Chem Pharm Bull (Tokyo)
    26: 161-165.

9. Iigo M, Hoshi A, Nakamura A et al. (1978) Antitumor
    activity of 1-alkylcarbamoyl derivatives of 5-fluoro-
    uracil in a variety of mouse tumors. Cancer Chemother
    Pharmacol 1: 203-208.

10. Iigo M, Hoshi A, Nakamura A et al. (1979) Antineoplas-
    tic effect of orally administered 1-alkylcarbamoyl
    derivatives of 5-fluorouracil on sc implanted Lewis
    lung carcinoma and B16 melanoma. Cancer Treat Rep 63:
    1895-1899.

11. Hoshi A, Iigo M, Nakamura A et al. (1976) Antitumor
    activity of 1-hexylcarbamoyl-5-fluorouracil in a
    variety of experimental tumors. Gann 67: 725-731.

12. Iigo M, Hoshi A, Nakamura A et al. (1978) Antitumor
    activity of 1-hexylcarbamoyl-5-fluorouracil in Lewis
    lung carcinoma and B16 melanoma. J Pharm Dyn 1: 49-54.

13. Tsuruo T, Iida H, Naganuma K et al. (1980) Inhibition
    of murine colon adenocarcinomas and Lewis lung carci-
    noma by 1-hexylcarbamoyl-5-fluorouracil. Cancer
    Chemother Pharmacol 4: 83-87.

14. Tokuzen T, Iigo M, Hoshi A et al (1980) Effect of
    1-hexylcarbamoyl-5-fluorouracil on spontaneous mammary
    adenocarcinoma of mice. Gann 71: 724-728.

15. Iigo M, Nakamura A, Kuretani K et al. (1979) Distribution of 1-hexylcarbamoyl-5-fluorouracil and 5-fluorouracil by oral administration in mice. J Pharm Dyn 2: 5-11.

16. Kobari T, Iguro Y, Ujiie A et al. (1981) Metabolism of 1-hexylcarbamoyl-5-fluorouracil(HCFU), a new antitumor agent in rats, rabbits and dogs. Xenobiotica 11: 57-62.

17. Iigo M, Nakamura A, Kuretani K et al. (1981) Excretion of 1-hexylcarbamoyl-5-fluorouracil in urine of mice. J Pharm Dyn 4: 490-496.

18. Iigo M, Nakamura A, Kuretani K et al. (1980) Metabolic fate of 1-hexylcarbamoyl-5-fluorouracil after oral administration in mice. Xenobiotica 10: 847-854.

19. Iigo M, Kuretani K, Hoshi A (1981) Metabolic fate of 1-hexylcarbamoyl-5-fluorouracil and 5-fluorouracil in mice bearing ascites sarcoma 180. J Natl Cancer Inst 66: 345-349.

20. Iigo M, Hoshi A, Kuretani K (1980) Pharmacokinetics of 1-alkylcarbamoyl-5-fluorouracils in plasma and ascites fluid after oral administration in mice. Cancer Chemother Pharmacol 4: 189-193.

21. Hoshi A, Yoshida M, Inomata M et al. (1980) Antitumor activity of metabolites of 1-hexylcarbamoyl-5-fluorouracil and related compounds against L1210 leukemia in vivo and L5178Y lymphoma cells in vitro. J Pharm Dyn 3: 478-481.

22. Fujita H, Ogawa K (1981) In vivo distribution and activation of 1-hexylcarbamoyl-5-fluorouracil(HCFU). Rinsho Yakuri 12: 233-243.

23. Ishimura K, Toizumi S, Inoue H et al. (1979) Toxicological study on 1-hexylcarbamoyl-5-fluorouracil(HCFU) (1) Subacute and chronic toxicity studies in rats. Oyo Yakuri 17: 575-595.

24. Ishimura K, Toizumi S, Neda K et al. (1979) Toxicological study on 1-hexylcarbamoyl-5-fluorouracil(HCFU) (2) Subacute and chronic toxicity studies in dogs. Oyo Yakuri 17: 597-615.

25. Koyama Y, Koyama Y (1980) Phase I study of a new antitumor drug, 1-hexylcarbamoyl-5-fluorouracil(HCFU), administered orally: An HCFU clinical study group report. Cancer Treat Rep 64: 861-867.

26. Horikomi K, Ozeki K, Mitsushima T et al. (1980) Effects of 1-hexylcarbamoyl-5-fluorouracil(HCFU) and its metabolites on bladder movement. Rinsho Yakuri 11: 27-36.

27. Horikomi K, Muramoto K, Araki K et al. (1980) Effect of 1-hexylcarbamoyl-5-fluorouracil(HCFU) on hypothalamic neurons in the rat. Rinsho Yakuri 11: 17-25.

28. Iigo M, Hoshi A, Inomata M et al. (1981) Antitumor activity of alkoxycarbonylalkylcarbamoyl-5-fluorouracil derivatives by oral administration. J Pharm Dyn 4: 203-210.

29. Hoshi A, Inomata M, Kanzawa F et al. (1982) Antitumor activity of acyloxymethyl derivatives of 5-fluorouracil against L1210 leukemia. J Pharm Dyn 5: 208-212.

30. Kanzawa F, Hoshi A, Kuretani K et al. (1981) Antitumor activity of 3',5'-diesters of 5-fluoro-2'-deoxyuridine against murine leukemia L1210 cells. Cancer Chemother Pharmacol 6: 19-23.

31. Kanzawa F, Hoshi A, Kuretani K (1979) Antitumor activity of alkylesters of 1-β-D-ribofuranosyl-5-fluorouracil-5'-phosphate against murine lymphoma L5178Y resistant to 1-β-D-ribofuranosyl-5-fluorouracil. Bull Cancer (Paris) 66: 497-501.

© 1984 Elsevier Science Publishers B.V.
Fluoropyrimidines in Cancer Therapy
K. Kimura, S. Fujii, M. Ogawa, G.P. Bodey, P. Alberto, eds.

INTERACTION OF ANTITUMOR AGENTS TEGAFUR AND 5-FLUOROURACIL WITH PSYCHOTROPIC AGENTS AMINAZINE AND PHENAZEPAM

Anatol B. Syrkin, Tatijana A. Voronina
Ljudmila M. Mikhailova and Nikolai I. Suslov

1. INTRODUCTION

In chemotherapy of oncologic patients together with antitumor drugs agents for treatment of concomitant diseases and antitumor therapy complications are utilized. Significant place in palliative therapy of oncologic patients belongs to psychotropic agents.

Psychotropic agents may influence significantly therapy results of oncologic patients. At the same time utilization of antitumor drugs together with psychotropic agents may also change activity of the latter.

Aminazine - is a well-known psychotropic agent, belonging to phenothiazine derivative. Phenazepam - is a new original tranquilizer of benzodiazepin structure, synthesized and studied in the USSR. Structural formula is presented in Figure 1.

Among pharmacologic characteristics of phenazepam dominant position has tranquilizing effect which is supplemented with hypnotic and anticonvulsive effect. The agent has also sedative and myorelaxation effect. Phenazepam is utilized for therapy of various neurotic and neurosis

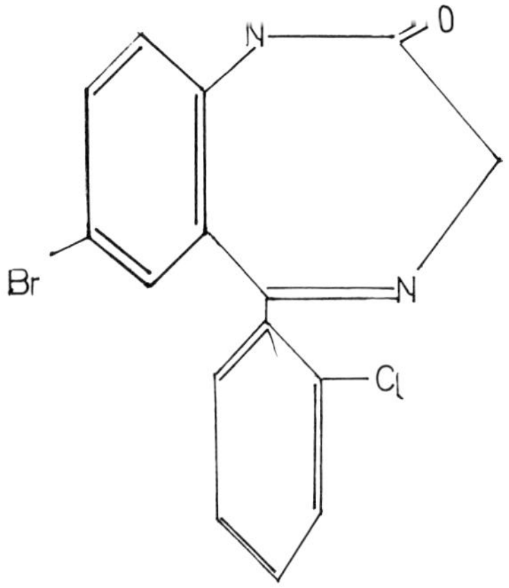

Figure 1. Phenazepam (7-brom-5-(O-chlorphenil)-1,2-dihydro -1,4-benzodiazepin-2ON)

states. By its pharmacologic characteristics it surpasses diazepam and nitrazepam.

Study results of influence of psychotropic agents aminazine and phenazepam on toxicity and antitumor activity of tegafur (TF) and 5-Fluorouracil (5-FU), study of their psychotropic activity and TF and 5-FU influence on aminazine and phenazepam psychotropic activity are presented in this paper.

2. MATERIALS AND METHODS

The study was carried out in 2836 mice SHK line, $C_{57}B1/6_j$, F_1 hybrids ($C_{57}B1/6_j$xCBA) of both sexes and in 84 female rats. TF and 5-FU were administered intravenously; aminazine - subcutaneously; phenazepam - per os. Antitumor and psychotropic agents were applicated simultaneously.

Acute toxicity was estimated by change of LD dose. Subacute toxicity was estimated by change of leukocyte number in mouse blood. The drug was administered 5 times, daily, at doses: TF - 160 mg/kg; 5-FU - 20 mg/kg; aminazine - 4 mg/kg; phenazepam - 2 mg/kg.

Under studyung antitumor activity 4 transplanted mouse tumors, differ by their biologic characteristics were used: "La" hemocytoblastosis, ELD line of ascites Ehrlich cancer, mammary gland adenocarcinoma 755 (AC-755) and Lewis lung carcinoma (LL). "La" hemocytoblastosis was transplanted intraperitonealy with suspension of spleen cells at amount of 10^6 of cells on a mouse. Therapy was initiated 24 hours post transplantation. TF was administered at 80-320 mg/kg doses; 5-FU - 10-40 mg/kg. Therapy results were evaluated by duration of life. AC-755 was transplanted subcutaneously into axilary cavity with suspension of tumor tissue in 1:10 solution at 0,3 ml on a mouse. LL was transplanted intramuscularly as a suspension in 1:10 solution at 0,5 ml on a mouse. Therapy was initiated post 48 hours. ELD was transplanted intraperitonealy at 0,1 ml of 7 day ascites on a mouse; therapy was initiated 24 hours post transplantation. Criterion for evaluation was percentage of tumor growth inhibition by their average diameter for AC-755 and LL; by average number of tumor cells for ELD.

Classic techniques for studying psychotropic activity were used (1, 2, 3, 4). Results were analyzed statistically, utilizing checking method of zero hypothesis with the use of X^2 criterion and Student-Fisher method.

3. RESULTS

3.1. Influence of psychotropic agents on TF and 5-FU
toxicity.

Table 1. LD_{50} for Tegafur, 5-Fluorouracil and Their Combinations with Aminazine and Phenazepam

Psychotropic agent	LD_{50} in mg/kg	
	TF	5-FU
-	950 (826 ÷ 1092)	320 (258 ÷ 397)
Aminazine	650 (586 ÷ 720)	280 (244 ÷ 320)
Phenazepam	740 (625 ÷ 851)	215 (192 ÷ 241)

Table 1 demonstrates that aminazine increases TF toxicity and does not influence 5-FU toxicity. Phenazepam increases TF and 5-FU toxicity, however increase of TF toxicity is less marked than in combined utilization of TF and
aminazine. In administration of TF together with aminazine
rise in mouse death in the result of neurotoxicity from
36,1% to 54,8% (P < 0,01) was observed; mouse death in
neurotoxic phase, receiving TF in combination with phenazepam, was only 26%. In five administrations aminazine intensified TF toxicity and did not influence 5-FU toxicity.
Thus, in mouse group, receiving TF in combination with
aminazine, leukocyte number was 3 times less than in mice,
receiving TF alone; besides, 44% of animals died, as in
other groups no death was observed. In combined application of aminazine and 5-FU aminazine did not change leuko-

50

penic effect of 5 FU itself. Phenazepam did not change TF
toxicity and slightly increased 5-FU toxicity.

3.2. Aminazine and phenazepam influence on antitumor acti-
     vity.

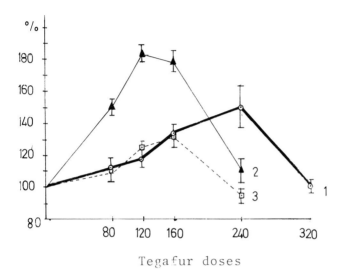

Figure 2. Median of life duration of "La" mice in adminis-
          tration of TF and its combinations with aminazi-
          ne and phenazepam (in % to control; 1 - TF; 2 -
          TF + aminazine; 3 - TF + phenazepam)

It is seen from Fig. 2 and 3 that aminazine prolonged
life duration of "La" mice, treated with TF and 5-FU, by
increasing dosages of antitumor agents up to a certain level. Further increasing dosages resulted in mouse death
from toxicity. Aminazine and phenazepam did not influence
life duration of "La" mice.

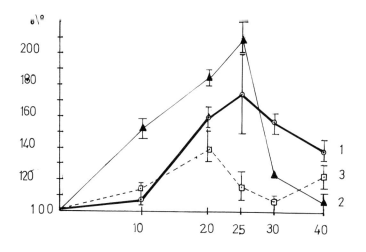

5-Fluorouracil doses

Figure 3. Median of life duration of "La" mice in administration of 5-FU and its combinations with aminazine and phenazepam (in % to control; 1 - 5-FU;
2 - 5-FU + aminazine; 3 - 5-FU + phenazepam)

It is seen from Table 2 that aminazine and phenazepam
increase inhibitory TF amd 5-FU influence on ELD growth
and do not influence LL. Phenazepam relaxes 5-FU influence
on AC-755 and aminazine decreases TF effect on this tumor.

3.3. Results of psychopharmacologic experiments.

It was found that 5-FU does not have psychotropic activity and does not change pharmacologic effect of aminazine and phenazepam. TF has marked influence on the central nervous system. At 30 mg/kg dose it caused increase of
aggressiveness, emotional reaction and motor activity of

Table 2. Influence of TF and 5-FU and their combinations with aminazine and phenazepam on growth of transplanted AC-755, LL and ELD tumors

Antitumor agent	Psychotropic agent	Tumor growth inhibition (in %)		
		ELD	LL	AC-755
5-Fluorouracil	-	39,0±6,3	55,2±4,2	57,3±11,5
	Aminazine	60,4±16,0	46,6±4,7	46,7±9,2
	Phenazepam	60,9±21,2	42,3±9,1	22,2±11,9
Tegafur	-	37,5±6,6	28,8±9,8	52,9±8,7
	Aminazine	73,4±10,9	45,3±8,0	30,7±9,3
	Phenazepam	71,2±15,5	35,6±5,6	46,5±14,0
-	Aminazine	30,6±23,8	9,2-±8,1	35,0±7,5
	Phenazepam	8,5±29,8	11,0±6,7	5,4±17,6

mice in an open field. Under increasing a dose up to 80 mg/kg suppressive effect was developed. At 120 mg/kg dose TF caused decrease of motor activity, aggressiveness and temperature. Decrease of animal activity under increasing TF dose was not developed simultaneously by all indices. Break of movement coordination by turning rot test was developed beginning with 400 mg/kg dose (ED_{50}=500 mg/kg). TF did not develop anticonvulsive activity relating to maximum electrospastic attack.

Under studying combined TF application with aminazine and phenazepam 3 dosages were used - 30, 120, 430 mg/kg. Aminazine was administered at 1 mg/kg dose, except series of aggressive behaviour where 2 mg/kg dose was utilized.

Phenazepam was administered at 1 mg/kg dose.

In combined aminazine and TF utilization at 30 mg/kg activating TF effect was completely eliminated. Besides, effects of TF and aminazine combination did not differ significantly from aminazine alone effects.

Under simultaneous TF administration at 120 mg/kg dose and aminazine significant intensification of sedative characteristics of aminazine was observed; its influence on coordination of movements and anticonvulsive effect was intensified, clear mutual intensification of hypothermal effect of these agents was observed. In combined administration of aminazine and TF at 430 mg/kg severe suppression of mouse activity by all indices was observed.

Simultaneous administration of TF at 30 mg/kg and phenazepam resulted in complete elimination of aggressiveness and decrease of motor activity. Emotional reactions, significantly increased in the result of TF administration, under its combined application with phenazepam decreased, maintaining close to control level.

Under administration of TF at 120 mg/kg in combination with phenazepam complete elimination of aggressiveness was also observed. Emotional reactions happened to be close to control level, sedative characteristics of the agents intensified. Influence of the drug combination on motor activity and coordination of movements did not differ from phenazepam alone effect.

Increasing TF dose up to 430 mg/kg mutual intension of

myorelaxant quality of both drugs and increasing of anti-convulsive phenazepam effect were observed.

4. DISCUSSION

In result of conducted studies it was ascertained that aminazine intensifies TF toxicity both in a single and multiple administration, besides cytotoxic and neurotoxic drug characteristics increased. Aminazine effects 5-FU toxicity. Phenazepam increases TF and 5-FU toxicity, administered only at high toxic doses.

Phenazepam and aminazine have diversed influence on TF and 5-FU antitumor activity, that may be accounted for difference in biological features of studied tumors.

TF has two-phase influence on CNS functions. At low doses it has activating influence; at high - suppressive. Aminazine and phenazepam at low doses eliminate activating TF influence on CNS; besides, aminazine provokes deep suppression of activity which significantly intensifies with increasing TF doses. Phenazepam, successfully eliminating stimulating effect of TF low doses, normalizes animal's behaviour. Tranquilizing phenazepam effect is maintained. Phenazepam is expedient to be evaluated in oncologic clinic as more adequate than aminazine psychotropic agent.

REFERENCES

1. Tedeschi R. et al. (1959) Effect of various centrally acting drugs on fighting behaviour of mice. J.Pharmacol. expther. 125:28-34.

2. Brady J.V., Nauta W.J.H. (1953) Subcortical mechanisms in emotional behavioral affective changes following septal forebrain lessions in the albino rat. J. Comperative and phisiol. psychol. 46: 339-349.

3. Dunham N.W., Miy T.S. (1957) A note on a simple apparatus for detecting neurological deficit in rats. J. Am. Pharm Ass. 46: 203-209.

4. Toman J.E.P., Ewinyard E.A., Goodman L.S. (1946) Properties of maximal seizures and their alteration by anticonvulsant drugs and other agents. J. Neurophysiol. 8: 231-239.

Fluoropyrimidines in Cancer Therapy
K. Kimura, S. Fujii, M. Ogawa, G.P. Bodey, P. Alberto, eds.

BIOCHEMICAL AND PHARMACOKINETIC STUDIES OF A NEW 5-FLUOROURACIL COMBINATION

Ti Li Loo, John A. Benvenuto, Delia F. Chiuten
Antonius A. Miller and E. Colleen Moore

1. INTRODUCTION

Undoubtedly the inhibition of thymidylate synthetase is the primary but not the sole mechanism of anticancer action of 5-fluorouracil (5-FU). 5-FU is randomly incorporated into a variety of RNA; however, how much does this incorporation contribute to the tumor inhibition property of 5-FU remains unclear. Nevertheless, conceivably the incorporation of 5-FU into RNA plays a significant role in the mode of cytotoxic action of this agent, especially in tumors resistant to 5-FU because of the insensitivity of their cellular thymidylate synthetase to the inhibition by 5-fluoro-2'-deoxyuridylate (FdUMP), an active anabolite of 5-FU.

To improve the therapeutic efficacy of 5-FU, a number of combinations with other agents have been proposed and tried, including the triple combination of 5-FU with N-(phosphonacetyl-L-aspartate (PALA) and thymidine (TdR), the subject matter of this presentation. The rationale of the combination deserves a brief discussion. In experimental systems the natural metabolite TdR at high doses has shown antitumor activity (1,2) presumably on account

57

of its ready stepwise conversion in vivo to TdR triphosphate (dTTP) that exerts feedback inhibition on ribonucleotide reductase and ultimately on DNA synthesis. In a
limited trial in patients with advanced cancer, TdR alone
seems to have minimal but definitive activity when administered by continuous intravenous (iv) infusion (3).
Subsequently it was reasoned that in combination with
5-FU, the excess exogenous TdR administered may circumvent
the inhibition of DNA synthesis by FdUMP so that the incorporation of 5-FU into RNA becomes a predominant con-
tributing factor to the cytotoxicity of this agent. The
combination appears to have synergistic antitumor effect
(4,5). Some objective antitumor responses in advanced
colorectal carcinoma were observed when TdR and 5-FU were
administered by continuous infusion (6).

An ingeniously designed antimetabolite and the first
transition state analogue that has reached clinical trials
as an anticancer agent, PALA inhibits an early step of
pyrimidine ribonucleotide de novo biosynthesis. This
inhibition of L-aspartate carbamoyltransferase (ACTase)
by PALA reduces intracellular concentrations of pyrimidine
ribonucleotides. Hence, in combination with 5-FU, PALA is
also expected to enhance the incorporation of 5-FU into
RNA in response to its decrease of uridine triphosphate
(UTP) concentration in cells. Clinically, the combination of 5-FU with PALA seems to be promising (7), and
further investigation is in progress in the U.S.

The present clinical, biochemical, and pharmacokinetic study was therefore undertaken to ascertain the possible synergistic antitumor effects of 5-FU in a triple combination with TdR and PALA based on the above rationale.

2. MATERIALS AND METHODS

2.1. Patients

Patients with histophathological evidence of adeno-carcinoma, mostly colorectal, and a life expectancy of at least 8 weeks, were eligible for the triple drug combination trial; the results of 28 of them were considered evaluable. Response was evaluated according to standard criteria. In the pharmacological study, PALA at 1 g/m^2 was administered intravenously (iv) over 1 h. on day 1. To 11 patients, 30 g. of TdR as a total dose together with 5-FU (150-300 mg/m^2) was infused simultaneously over 3 h. at different sites, while to another 4 patients TdR was infused in 3 h. followed immediately with 5-FU over 1 h. Blood was sampled at intervals; urine was collected as voided.

2.2. Drugs, Chemical, and Reagents

5-FU, PALA, and TdR were provided by the Drug Development Branch of the National Cancer Institute, U.S. Public Health Service. 5-Fluoro-2'-deoxyuridine (FUdR), pyrimidine ribonucleosides and ribonucleotides were supplied by Sigma Chemical Co., St. Louis, MO. All other

chemicals and reagents were purchased from regular
sources.

2.3. Chromatographic Analysis

The quantitative analysis for 5-FU, its metabolites,
pyrimidine ribonucleosides and ribonucleotides by high
performance liquid chromatography (HPLC) in blood, urine,
and tumor tissues follows our previously described procedures (8).

2.4. ACTase Assay

The enzymatic assay for ACTase has also been reported
previously (9).

2.5. Pharmacokinetic Analysis

The results of plasma 5-FU, FUdR, TdR, and thymine
(Thy) concentrations _versus_ time determinations were
subjected to standard nonlinear regression analysis to
enable the computation of pharmacokinetic parameters.

3.   RESULTS

3.1. Pharmacokinetics of 5-FU, TdR, and Their Metabolites

The clearance curves of 5-FU, FUdR, TdR, and Thy from
the plasma of a patient after a dose of PALA followed by
5-FU simultaneously with TdR are shown in Fig. 1.
Compared with our past experience with iv administration
of 5-FU alone at a similar dose, the plasma 5-FU concentrations were not only consistently higher but also persisted longer. More important, in our experience FUdR
was never detectable in the plasma after 5-FU administra-

tion; however, with the simultaneous administration of TdR, it became measurable at significant concentrations for at least 6 h. Also, plasma concentrations of TdR and Thy derived therefrom were very high. Not shown in Fig. 1 was the plasma concentration of uracil (U) which was lower than that of 5-FU 15 min. after drug administration but higher at 60 min. In fact, this was observed in most of the patients studied, namely, plasma U exceeded 5-FU in concentration in 1-2 h. usually. The average pertinent pharmacokinetic parameters of TdR and 5-FU as well as those of the derived Thy and FUdR in the 2 groups of 11 and 4 patients are listed in Table 1. Plasma half-life of TdR in the terminal (β) phase was 2.6 h. in the simultaneous study and 1.6 h. in the sequential study; these may be compared with 1.7 h. previously reported when TdR was given alone at 75 g/m^2 as a 24-h. iv infusion (10). Strikingly, the plasma half-life of 5-FU was 7.5 h. in the simultaneous study and 6.8 h. in the sequential study, nearly 15 times greater than that estimated from the published work in which 5-FU was administered alone (11). Because of wide variations, no significant differences in the pharmacokinetic parameters were apparent between the simultaneous and the sequential study; that is, pharmaco-kinetically, there was little advantage of one schedule over the other.

As for the urinary excretion of TdR, Thy, 5-FU, and FUdR in the simultaneous study, on average the 24 h.

TABLE 1   Average Pharmacokinetic Parameters, PALA-5-FU-TdR

	$t_{\frac{1}{2}\beta}$ h.	CL 1/h.	V 1	Urinary Excretions,% in 24 h.
Simultaneous 5-FU-TdR				
n=11				
TdR	2.6	68.7	257.7	16.1
Thy	4.3			3.5
5-FU	7.5	10.5	113.6	13.2
FUdR	1.3			12.8
Sequential 5-FU-TdR				
n=4				
TdR	1.6	37.7	87.0	ND
Thy	5.0			ND
5-FU	6.8	5.1	50.0	ND
FUdR	3.7			ND

ND = Not Done

cumulative excretion of 5-FU was 13% of the dose as the unchanged drug, surprisingly with an additional 13% as FUdR. Hitherto we have never detected FUdR in the urine or plasma of patients treated with 5-FU. During the same period, 16% of the administered TdR was in the urine unchanged, with another 4% as Thy (Table 1). In other words, the 24-h. cumulative excretion of 5-FU was similar to that estimated from the results reported by Clarkson et al. who gave the drug alone iv (11). But the excretion of TdR and Thy was greatly diminished when compared with the results of the study of TdR administered at high dose by iv infusion (10).

3.2. Biochemical Studies

Serial tumor species were obtained from each of 2 patients with metastatic lung cancer by punch or needle biopsy, 1 before and 4 after therapy. As shown in Fig. 2, after PALA cellular ACTase activity was maximally depressed to 20-30% of pretreatment values. This inhibition lasted for at least 52 h. after PALA therapy. These results are in agreement with our previous findings (9).

Tumor pyrimidine concentrations also diminished together with the decrease of ACTase activity (Fig. 3). But they returned to the baseline values after the 5-FU and TdR administration, especially with U concentration which actually surpassed dramatically the pretreatment value. Likewise, tumor pyrimidine ribonucleotides also decreased concentration in response to PALA (Fig. 4). They similarly returned to the pretreatment concentrations 1 day after the 5-FU and TdR administration. Unfortunately, the tumor tissue specimens were too small to permit the quantitative assay of cellular pyrimidine deoxyribonucleotides and 5-FU incorporation into RNA.

3.3. Clinical Responses

Of the 28 evaluable patients entered into this study, 1 complete and 1 minor (decrease in liver metastasis) responses were elicited from 2 patients with colorectal adenocarcinoma. Disease stabilization of 8 to 16 weeks in duration was seen in 5 patients with colo-

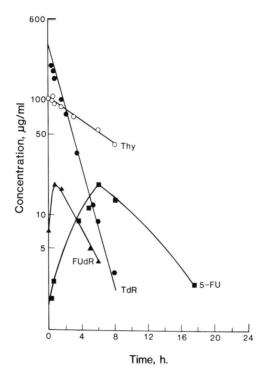

FIGURE 1 Plasma clearance of TdR, Thy, 5-FU and FUdR after 1 g PALA, 30 g TdR, 150 mg/m^2 5-FU.

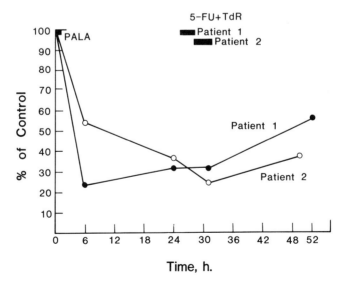

FIGURE 2 Tumor actase activity.

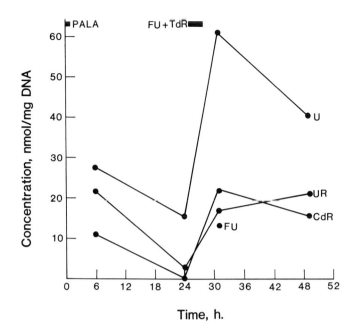

FIGURE 3   Tumor pyrimidines after PALA-5-FU-TdR

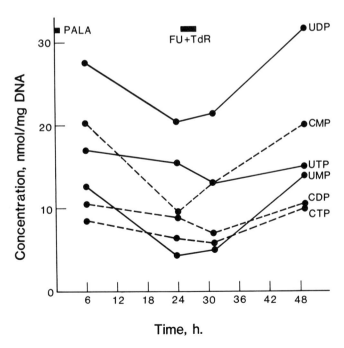

FIGURE 4   Tumor pyrimidine nucleotides after PALA-5-FU-TdR.

65

rectal, 2 with gastric, and 1 with lung cancer. However, the patient who experienced a complete remission had prior surgery and nitrosourea therapy for Dukes D adeno-carcinoma of the colon; recurrence of the disease was limited to the liver. After 3 courses of the triple combination therapy, computer-assisted tomographic scan revealed no liver metastasis. The duration of the response was 24 weeks from the initiation of the treat-ment but 9 weeks after complete remission was achieved.

Dose-limiting toxicities were mostly gastrointes-tinal and confined to the central nervous system, includ-ing nausea, vomiting, and mucositis; central nervous system atology usually occurred after TdR. Dose-related leukopenia and neutropenia were mild at doses below 250 mg/m^2 but pronounced with increasing 5-FU dose. Drug-caused death was absent.

4. DISCUSSION

The triple PALA-5-FU-TdR combination protocol is designed to produce synergism among these agents by hopefully shunting the 5-FU preferentially into RNA and additionally by inhibiting the de novo biosynthesis of pyrimidines with PALA. Unfortunately, based on our studies the triple combination did not appear to be par-ticularly effective, and certainly not superior to 5-FU alone, or in combination with PALA or TdR. But it must be emphasized that this trial was conducted in a relatively small population of patients with advanced malignancies.

However, certain biochemical and pharmacokinetic

findings from the present investigation are worthy of comments. Our previous observation (8) that PALA only exerts marginal influence on the biochemical and pharmacokinetic effects of 5-FU in beagle dogs has been confirmed in patients. On the other hand, pharmacokinetically TdR and 5-FU interact appreciably as expected. In another study in dogs we reported (12) that TdR prolonged the plasma half-life of 5-FU from about 40 min. to 60 min., and markedly elevated the concentration of FUdR in the plasma. Moreover, as a result of TdR administration, in 5 h. the urinary excretion of 5-FU was increased by 50% while the catabolism of 5-FU to carbon dioxide and other degradative products was reduced 10-fold. Again, most of these observations find support from the present clinical investigation. In man, TdR also prolonged the plasma half-life of 5-FU, in fact, much more so than in the dog. Although the urinary excretion of 5-FU was not apparently increased by TdR co-administration in man, considerable amounts of FUdR were found in the urine; in other words, the excretion of total fluoropyrimidines was increased. These findings are readily explained by the inhibition of 5-FU catabolism by the Thy derived from the large excess of exogenous TdR administered. Moreover, the deoxyribose phosphate generated from the phosphorolysis of TdR would greatly facilitate the conversion of 5-FU to sizable quantities of FUdR. Clearly, the inhibition of pyrimidine degradation by Thy was also responsible for the high U concentrations in the plasma of patients receiving the 5-FU-TdR therapy. In combination with 5-FU, the urinary excretion of TdR and the Thy derived from it was far less than that when TdR only was administered. Possibly in the renal mechanisms for the excretion of pyrimidines, fluoropyrimidines are better substrates than the natural metabolites.

In response to PALA inhibition of ACTase, pyrimidine concentrations in tumor tissues showed significant decreases (Fig. 3 and 4). But after 5-FU and TdR, they returned to the pretreatment values at varying rates; actually, U and UDP concentrations considerably exceeded the pretreatment values. Some of the increases could probably be accounted for by Thy inhibition of pyrimidine catabolism. Regrettably, we were unable to determine whether the incorporation of 5-FU into tumor RNA was really enhanced after the 3-drug combination therapy.

We did not anticipate any significant schedule-related differences in the pharmacokinetics of 5-FU and TdR; none was observed.

In summary, the combination of 5-FU with PALA and TdR is a novel approach to enhance the efficacy of those agents. But biochemically and pharmacokinetically the net effect seems to be merely the suppression of 5-FU catabolism by the Thy derived from the exogenous TdR. Clinically, no synergism among the 3 agents was apparent thus far.

REFERENCES

1. Martin DS, Stolfi, RL, Sawyer RC, et al. (1980) An Overview of thymidine. Cancer 45: 1117-1128.

2. Lee SS, Giovanella BC, Stehlin JS, Jr., et al. (1979) Regression of human tumors established in nude mice after continuous infusion of thymidine. Cancer Res 38: 2928-2933.

3. Chiuten DF, Wiernik PH, Zaharko DS, and Edwards L. (1979) Clinical phase I-II and pharmacokinetic study of high-dose thymidine (NSC-21548) given by continuous IV infusion. Cancer Res 40: 818-822.

4. Santelli G and Valeriote F. (1978) In vivo enhancement of 5-fluorouracil cytotoxicity to AKR leukemia cells by thymidine in mice. J NCI 61: 843-847.

5. Woodstock W and Spiegelman S. (1978) Enhancement of 5-fluorouracil chemotherapy with emphasis on the use of excess thymidine. Cancer Bull 30: 219-224.

6. Vogel SJ, Presant CA, Ratkin GA, and Klahr C. (1979) Phase I study of thymidine plus 5-fluorouracil infusions in advanced colorectal carcinoma. Cancer Treat Rep 63: 1-5.

7. Casper ES, Yale K, Williams LJ, et al. (1983) Phase I and clinical pharmacological evaluation of biochemical modulations of 5-fluorouracil with N-(phosphonacetyl)-L-aspartic acid. Cancer Res 43: 2324-2329.

8. Miller AA, Moore EC, Hulbert RB, et al. (1983) Pharmacological and biochemical interactions of N-(phosphonacetyl)-L-aspartate and 5-fluorouracil in beagles. Cancer Res 43: 2565-2570.

9. Loo TL, Friedman J, Moore EC, et al. (1980) Pharmacological disposition of N-(phosphonacetyl)-L-aspartate in humans. Cancer Res 40: 86-90.

10. Zaharko DS, Bolten BJ, Chiuten DF, and Wiernik PH. (1979) Pharmacokinetic studies during phase I trials of high-dose thymidine infusions. Cancer Res 39: 4777-4781.

11. Clarkson B, O'Connor A, Winston LaR, and Hutchinson D. (1964) The physiological disposition of 5-fluorouracil and 5-fluoro-2'-deoxyuridine in man. Clin Pharmac Ther 5: 581-610.

12. Cooley J, Furlong NB, Jr., and Loo TL. (1979) Pharmacokinetics of 5-fluorouracil in combination with thymidine in the dog. Proc Am Assoc Cancer Res 20: 161.

© 1984 Elsevier Science Publishers B.V.
Fluoropyrimidines in Cancer Therapy
K. Kimura, S. Fujii, M. Ogawa, G.P. Bodey, P. Alberto, eds.

MODIFICATION OF TOXIC AND ANTITUMOR ACTIVITY OF 5-FLUOROURACIL

August M. Garin, Fardil F. Mamedov and Tamara G. Lobova

There has been accumulated tremendous experience of the use of 5-FU in many countries. A desire to administer maximum tolerated doses of antimetabolite during monotherapy is widely recognized. The drug is used until there appear side-effects that are sometimes very serious. Response observed in some cases is usually of short duration. Oncologists seem never to forget that this treatment is incomplete. If one could administer one more drug, if it were possible to increase, the total dosage, the antitumour effect might possibly be more significant. Detailed biochemical knowledge of 5-FU and its outstanding effectiveness for patients with tumours of digestive tract were the reasons for intensive research of modification of toxic and antitumour activity of this agent. The aim of this research was to decrease toxicity, to increase and expand the effectiveness of fluoropirimidines.

6-Azauridine (Figure 1), synthesized in Czechoslovakia and the USA in the 1950s and later on given up by clinicians because of its ineffectiveness, though it was not very toxic, attracted our attention for the following reasons: in the process of metabolism 6-azauridine accumu-

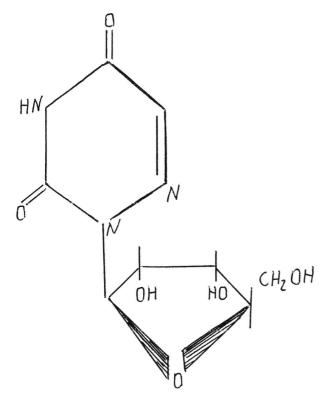

Figure 1   6-Azauridine

lates orotidylate decarboxylase. In the functional
complex this enzyme is associated with orotate phosphoribosyltransferase that is necessary as one of the means of
the bioactivation of fluorouracil. Change in the activity
of one of the enzymes is followed by the change in the
activity of the other in the same direction.

The hypothesis of the antagonism between 5-FU and
6-azauridine was subjected to experimental testing. The
results are presented in the series of tables.

Table 1

Toxicity for mice BALB/c(without tumours)		
Dosage mg/kg		Number of animals
6-Azauridine	5-FU	death/total
-	130	0/20
-	250	17/20
468	250	0/20
-	390	10/10
737	390	0/20

As is seen from Table, 6-azauridine protected mice from death, even when LD-100 FU was administered, 6-azauridine being administered 4 hours before the injection of 5-FU.

Table 2 shows the decrease of 5-FU toxicity for mice hybrids F_1(CBA-C_{57}Bl) without tumours under the influence of 6-azauridine.

Table 2

Toxicity 5-FU + 6-Azauridine		
Dosage mg/kg		Death from/total number
6-Azauridine	5-FU	toxicity of animals
-	250	6/8
-	500	8/8
-	700	8/8
736	700	5/9
1471	700	3/8
3678	-	0/5

Even when superlethal doses are administered the toxicity of 5-FU is decreased.

Table 3 shows how 6-azauridine protects animals with tumours from toxicity.

Table 3

Toxicity 5-FU + 6-Azauridine for mice BDF_1 with L-1210		
Dosage mg/kg		Death from /total number
6-Azauridine	5-FU	toxicity of animals
-	312	2/6
2940	312	0/6
-	390	3/6
2940	390	0/6
-	610	6/6
2940	610	0/6
2940	-	0/6

Frequency of diarrhoea, a typical side-effects of the toxicity of 5-FU is shown on table 4.

Table 4

Rate of diarrhoea (5-FU+6-Azauridine) for mice F_1 (CBA-C_{57}b1) without tumours		
Dosage mg/kg		Number of / total number
6-Azauridine	5-FU	mice with / of mice diarrhoea
-	250	2/8
-	500	6/8
-	700	7/8
245	700	4/9
736	700	0/9
2207	700	0/8
3678	-	0/5

Most effective protection of mucous membrane of the intestines was observed in cases when the dose of 6-azauridine was twice as small or equal to that of 5-FU (in mM).

Table 5

| Hematological toxicity 5-FU + 6-Azauridine for mice BALB/c AKATOL | | |

| Dosage mg/kg | | Weight of spleen in mg |
6-Azau	5-FU	
–	–	437 (control)
–	390	83
737	390	410
	610	55
1154	610	257
	763	48
1449	763	216
	954	46
1792	954	255
1792	–	284

Weight of the spleen was chosen as a criterion of the degree of the hematological protection. The data are presented on table 5.

Hematological protection is quite evident.

Unfortunately, the results of the therapeutic experiments are far from being very good. 6-Azauridine decreased antitumour effect.

The results of the administration of the combination of the above-said drugs to mice with L-1210 are shown on table 6.

Table 6

Survival of mice BDF$_1$ with L-1210 due to the 5-FU
+ 6-Azau therapy

Dosage mg/kg		Increase of survival
6-Azau	5-FU	% to control
-	200	141
2942	312	70
2942	390	84
2942	610	94
2942	-	32

In one of the experiments with Akatol tumour we increased survival without toxicity.

Table 7

Survival for mice BALB/c with AKATOL tumor

6-Azauridine	5-FU	Death from toxicity	Survival after injection in days
-	-	-	42
-	200	6/6	12
-	250	7/7	9
-	390	7/7	9
736	390	0/7	55
1790	-	0/7	47

We also appreciated the fashionable idea of the modification of the action of 5-Fu with the help of allopuri-

nol. The methods we used are presented below:

Method 1. 5-FU-daily,i.v. bolus 500 mg/m^2 not more than
for 10 days; allopurinol - 200 mg 4 times a day
orally. The first dose should be taken 24 hours
before the administration of 5-FU and continued
to the end of the course.

Method 2. 5-FU in drops in the course of 6 hours (during
6 hours) (3 day running) in doses 1,3 - 2,2
g/m^2. Allopurinol - 800 mg (200 mg 4 times a
day), starting a day before the administration
of 5-FU and continuing during the course of the
5-FU administration.

12 patients had 31 courses of treatment according to
method 1 (table 8). Mean duration of the course - 7.2
days, the mean total dose of 5-FU - 6.6 g.

Table 8

Method 1. 5-FU + Allopurinol

Number of courses	Nausea and vomiting	Diarrhoea	Stomatitis	Leucopenia	Thrombopenia
31	8(25.8%)	7(22.6%)	1(3.2%)	4(16%)	1(4%)

Diarrhoea and stomatitis are less often observed than
usual. As to leucopenia it was rather often observed,
leucopenia less 2000 was registered 4 times in 16%.

55 patients had 117 courses of treatment according to
method 2. Course doses varied from 7 to 13.5 gr. The data
on toxicity are presented on table 9.

Table 9

Method 2. Allopurinol + 5-FU toxicity in %.

Total number of courses	Nausea and vomiting	Diarrhoea	Stomatitis	Leucopenia	Thrombopenia
117	29	3.4	1	8.2	6.8

Nausea and vomiting were quite moderate. Diarrhoea and stomatitis were seldom observed though 5-FU doses were quite high. Leucopenia was of reversible character. Method 2 is quite safe.

The therapy results are presented on table 10 and 11.

Table 10

Results of treatment of stomach cancer with
5-FU + Allopurinol (method 1)

Total No of patients	Evaluated	Objective response	Stabilization	Progression
12	10	3	3	5

Duration of objective remissions - 3.9 months, stabilization - 3 months.

Objective response was observed in the treatment of the patient with lung metastases of hypernephroma. For over a year there has been observed stabilization of the process in the patient with carcinoid of mediastinum. The

objective effect observed in the cases of stomach cancer
is rentgenologically documented. Its duration is not more
than four months.

Table 11

Results of the treatment of patients with

5-FU + Allopurinol (Method 2)

Type of tumour	Total number of pts	Evaluated	Objective response	Stabili-zation	Progression
Stomach	14	13	3	5	5
Colon	13	10	-	4	6
Breast	4	4	1	-	3
Kidney	13	13	1	3	9
Carcinoid	3	3	-	1	2
Liver	2	2	-	1	1
Head and neck tumours	2	2			2
Lung	4	4			4

In general it should be noted that the above mentioned
methods make it possible to increase single and total doses
of 5-FU and to decrease toxicity which is especially
essential for weakened patients.

Search for new conditions and tumours in which the
administration of modificators that change the cytotoxic
action of 5-FU is a challenge for the future.

REFERENCES

1. Townsend LB, Cheng CC. (1974) Design of pyrimidine nucleosides as cytotoxic agents. In: Antineoplastic and Immunosuppressive Agents. 1. (eds) AC Sartorelli and DG Johns. p. 127.

2. Preobrazhenskaya MN, Garin AM, Lobova TG, Lichinicer MR, Mamedov FF. (1981) Antagonism 6-azauridina i 5-ftoruracila. Khimiko-Farmacevticheski Zhurnal 9: s.18-19.

3. Fox RM, Woods RL, Tattersall MHN, Brode GW. (1979) Allopurinol modulation of high-dose fluorouracil toxicity. Cancer Treat Rev 6: 143-147.

© 1984 Elsevier Science Publishers B.V.
Fluoropyrimidines in Cancer Therapy
K. Kimura, S. Fujii, M. Ogawa, G.P. Bodey, P. Alberto, eds.

ENZYMATIC CONVERSION OF 5'-DEOXY-5-FLUOROURIDINE (5'-DFUR) AND TEGAFUR TO 5-FLUOROURACIL (5-FU) IN HUMAN TUMOR TISSUE

Yasuhiro Hara and Akira Kono

1. INTRODUCTION

Recently there have been many reports on the derivatives of fluoropyrimidines. The authors have investigated 5'-deoxy-5-fluorouridine (5'-DFUR) and 1-(tetrahydro-2-furanyl)-5-fluorouracil (tegafur) which are comfirmed to be activated by enzymes in human tumors. These two drugs were investigated from various aspects concerning their activation in human tumors and the results obtained are reported.

2. MATERIALS AND METHODS

1) 5'-DFUR

(a) The conversion of 5'-DFUR to 5-FU in the tissue of various organs of human malignant tumors

The conversion from 5'-DFUR to 5-FU in malignant tumor tissues of the stomach, colon, lung, uterus, ovary, as well as in the adjacent normal tissue were investigated using surgical specimens.

(b) Enzymes involved in the conversion of 5'-DFUR to 5-FU in human and experimental tumors

The formation of thymine, uracil and 5-FU from thymidine, uridine and 5'-DFUR as the substrates was observed using mouse sarcoma-180, guinea pig line 10 tumors and human pulmonary carcinoma. Effects on the formation of thymine, 5-FU and uracil were investigated using 1-(2-deoxy-β-D-glucopyranosyl)-thymine (GPT), a specific inhibitor of uridine phosphorylase.

(c) Serum and tissue concentrations of 5'-DFUR and 5-FU in clinical cases after 5'-DFUR administration

After intravenous administration of 500 mg of 5'-DFUR to patients with cervical, ovarian, hepatic or pancreatic carcinoma, the concentrations of 5'-DFUR and 5-FU in the tumor tissues obtained by surgery or biopsies, and the concentration in the blood collected at the same time were measured.

Then, the concentrations of 5'-DFUR and 5-FU in tumor tissues obtained surgically from patients with cervical cancer when 600 mg of 5'-DFUR was administered orally, and those in the blood obtained at the same time were measured. The concentrations of 5'-DFUR and 5-FU in tumor tissue obtained from surgical specimens and in normal tissue adjacent to the tumors in gastric cancer patients given 400 mg of 5'-DFUR orally were also measured.

2) Tegafur

(a) Kinetic study of 5-FU formation

The in vitro conversion of tegafur to 5-FU was observed using partially purified thymidine phosphrylase. The 5-FU formation during the various incubation time in a 5×10^{-3}M tegafur solution with or without the enzyme was observed.

(b) Tegafur concentration effect on 5-FU formation

By raising the tegafur concentration, the formation of 5-FU was investigated.

(c) Tegafur and 5-FU concentrations in the specimens obtained at autopsy

The concentrations of tegafur and 5-FU in the blood and normal and tumor tissues in various organs which were obtained at autopsies were measured in eight cases of long-term administration of 800 mg/day of tegafur continuously, during intravenous hyperalimentation.

3) Method of partial purification of thymidine phosphorylase from human malignant tumors

The purification was performed by the procedures shown in Table 1.

4) Calculation of the Km values by thymidine phosphorylase

The formation of thymine, 5-FU or uracil was observed with thymidine, 5'-DFUR, tegafur or uridine as substrates, and the Km values in each reaction were calculated using the partially purified thymidine phosphorylase.

5) 5-FU level in the blood and tumors after intravenous administration of 5-FU to patients with cervical cancer

When 250 mg of 5-FU was administered intravenously to patients with cancer of the uterine cervix, the concentrations of 5-FU in the tumor tissue and blood were measured in surgical or biopsy specimens.

All measurements of pyrimidine bases and its derivatives were performed by means of high-speed liquid chromatography.

3. RESULTS

1) 5'-DFUR

(a) The conversion of 5'-DFUR to 5-FU in the tissue of various organs of human malignant tumors

The conversion of 5'-DFUR to 5-FU in tumor tissue and in its adjacent normal tissue is shown in Fig. 1. The conversion in tumor tissue was several times higher than that in normal tissue.

(b) Enzymes involved in the conversion of 5'-DFUR to 5-FU in human and experimental tumors

As shown in Fig. 2, the conversion of 5'-DFUR to 5-FU in human malignant tumors seems to be catalyzed by thymidine phosphorylase; while in animal experimental tumors, it is considered to be catalyzed by uridine phosphorylase.

(c) The serum and tissue concentration of 5-FU in patient administered 5'-DFUR

In patients with uterine cervical cancer or ovarian cancer given 500 mg of 5'-DFUR intravenously, the concentration of 5'-DFUR was higher in the serum than in tumor tissue, but the 5-FU concentration was higher in the tumor tissues than in the serum as shown in Fig. 3. The same results were also shown in the specimens from liver and pancreatic cancer patients.

In patients with uterine cancer given 600 mg of 5'-DFUR orally, the concentration of 5'-DFUR in the serum was also higher than in the tissue, but the

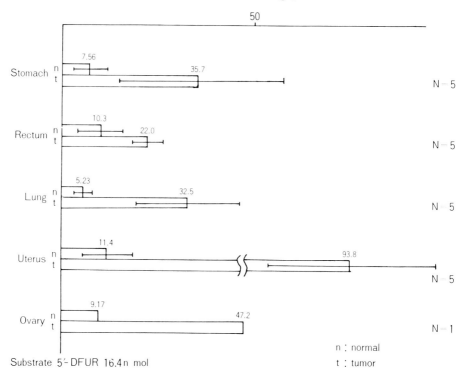

(n mol 5-FU formed/mg protein/hr.)

Substrate 5'-DFUR 16.4 n mol

n : normal
t : tumor

Fig 1 Rate of Conversion of 5'-DFUR to 5-FU

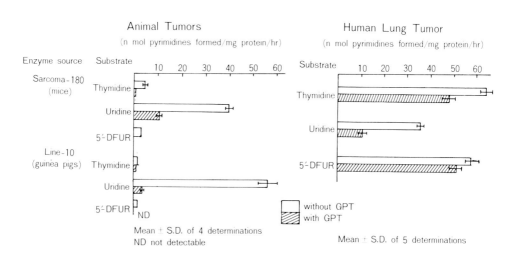

Fig 2 Pyrimidine Nucleosides Phosphorylase Activity

concentration of 5-FU was clearly higher in the tumor tissues than in the serum. Unlike the case of intravenous administration of 5'-DFUR, the concentration of 5-FU was maintained for a long time in the tumor.

The concentration of 5'-DFUR in the tumor and normal tissues of patients with gastric cancer administered 400 mg of 5'-DFUR orally did not show any constant trends, but the concentration of 5-FU was definitely much higher in the tumor tissue than in the normal tissue (Fig. 4).

2) Tegafur

(a) Kinetic study of 5-FU formation

The formation of 5-FU increased with time in the mixture without enzyme, but when the enzyme was added, the formation of 5-FU was further increased. It indicates that this enzyme plays a role in the formation of 5-FU from tegafur.

(b) Tegafur concentration effect on 5-FU formation

The results are shown in Fig. 5. In the left part of the figure, A; with enzyme and B; without enzyme, C which represents A - B (A minus B) shows the true reaction catalyzed by the enzyme itself. C shows the Micaelis curve, and the same results are shown on the linear curve of Lineweaver and Burk (right of the Fig. 5).

(c) Tegafur and 5-FU concentrations in the blood and normal and tumor tissue of autopsy cases

The results of typical case are shown in Fig. 6. The level of tegafur was higher in the normal and tumor

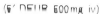
(5'-DFUR 500mg iv)

Ovarian Ca.

Uterine Ca.

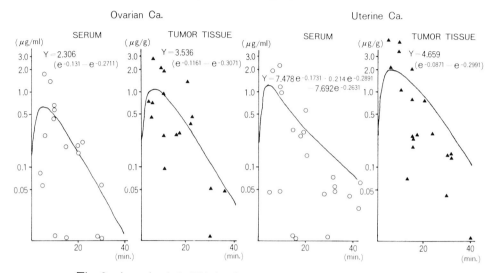

Fig 3   Level of 5-FU in Serum and Tumor Tissues

(5'-DFUR 400mg po)
Gastric Ca.

☐ normal tissue
▨ tumor tissue

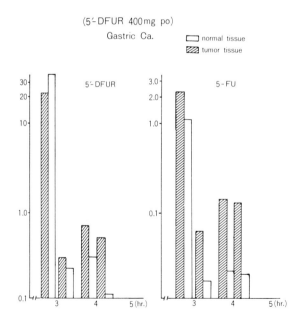

Fig 4   Levels of 5'-DFUR and 5-FU in Normal and
Tumor Tissues

86

tissues than in the blood, but there was no particular difference in the level between the normal and tumor tissues. However, 5-FU concentration was higher in the normal and tumor tissues than in the blood, and that in the tumor tissue was higher than that in the normal tissue.

3) Partial purification of thymidine phosphorylase from human malignant tumors

Table 2 shows the specific activities of the enzyme on each purification step shown in Table 1.

4) Km values of thymidine phosphorylase

The results are shown in Table 3. The Km values for the conversion of thymidine to thymine were almost the

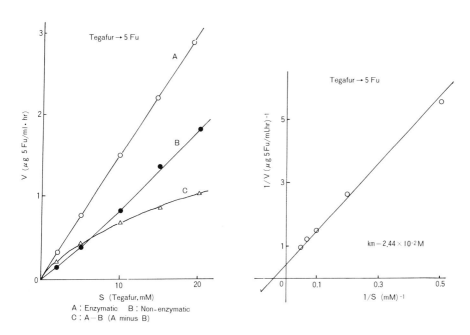

Fig 5   Relation between the concentration of the substrate (tegafur) and the 5-FU formation velocity
Linear curve of Lineweaver and Burk obtained from curve C on the left.

TABLE 1 Procedure for partial purification of thymidine
phosphorylase

Tumor
|
7% homogenate/Buffer A (10mM Tris-HCl pH 7.4)

↳↗ X 7,000 g 30 min. 4 C
|
Sup.
| 0-20% $(NH_4)_2SO_4$
↳↗ X 7,000 g 30 min. 4 C
|
Sup.
| 20-40% $(NH_4)_2SO_4$
↳↗ X 7,000 g 30 min. 4 C
|
Suspension of ppt./Buffer B (20mM (Na)-Phosphate pH 7.4)

| dialysis/Buffer B
↳↗ X 7,000 g 30 min. 4 C
|
Con A Sepharose/Buffer B
|
DEAE Sephacel/Buffer C (20mM (K)-phosphate pH 7.4)

| Buffer C (0-400mM KCl Gradient)
|
Hydroxylapatite/Buffer D (2mM (K)-phosphate pH 7.4)

TABLE 2 Purification of thymidine phosphorylase

Procedure	Activity (units)	Protein (mg)	Specific activity (units/mg)
Homogenate sup.	481,600	2,439	197
Ammonium sulfate			
20-40% ppt.	432,900	437	991
Con A-Sepharose	192,700	115	1,676
DEAE-Sephacel	126,540	11.5	11,003
Hydroxylapatite	60,444	0.81	74,622

1 unit = 1 n mole thymine/hr.ml

same for the enzyme purified from various organs, such as human gastric, liver and lung cancer. The values were also basically the same as those obtained by Nakayama et al. (1) for the conversion of thymidine to thymine by means of horse liver thymidine phosphorylase.

5) 5-FU level in the serum and tumors after intravenous administration of 5-FU to patients with uterine cervical cancer

The concentration of 5-FU was higher in the serum than in the tumor for approximately two hours after intravenous administration.

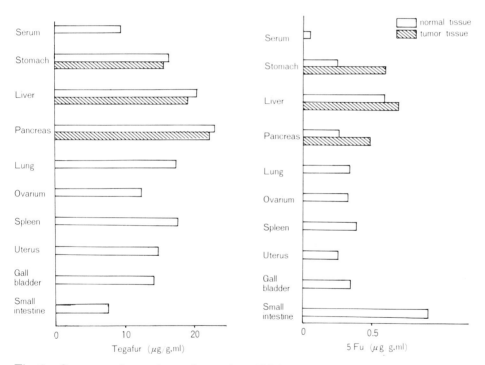

Fig 6 Concentrations of tegafur and 5-FU in the blood, normal and tumor tissue obtained at autopsy after long-term administration of tegafur [108.2 g (400-800 mg/day; 152 days), 58-year old female with gastric cancer]

TABLE 3 Km and V max values with thymidine phosphorylase

Substrate	Stomach	Human tumor Lung	Human tumor Liver	Horse Liver*
dThd	1.68×10^{-4} (826)	2.43×10^{-4}	2.53×10^{-4}	1.87×10^{-4}
5'-DFUR	1.72×10^{-3} (531)	1.69×10^{-3}	1.75×10^{-3}	
Tegafur	1.33×10^{-2} (7.02)		2.44×10^{-2}	
Urd	4.76×10^{-2} (3.47)			

Apparent Km (M) and V max (in parentheses, mol hr^{-1} (mg protein)$^{-1}$) values with thymidine phosphorylase
* C. Nakayama et al. J Med Chem 23, 962 (1980)

4. DISCUSSION

5'-DFUR, a derivative of 5-FU, was synthesized in 1979 by Cook et al. (2). It has been reported to have antitumor activity against various types of experimental cancers. It is also clear that in experimental cancer in animals, 5'-DFUR is activated in the tumors by uridine phosphorylase, and that this enzyme shows higher activity in tumors than in normal tissues (3). The authors have shown that in human malignant tumors, 5'-DFUR is activated by thymidine phosphorylase rather than uridine phosphorylase, and that this enzyme shows activity in human malignant tumors several times higher than that in normal tissues (4): Therefore, when 5'-DFUR is administered to humans, there should be higher concentration of 5-FU in the tumors than in the serum or normal tissue. This has been proven by the author using patients with uterine, ovarian, gastric, hepatic and pancreatic cancer.

Next, an attempt was made to purify thymidine phosphorylase and the purification partially succeeded. Experiments are now underway to further increase the purity and the results will be reported in the near future.

Tegafur is considered to be converted into 5-FU in the liver by detoxification enzymes involving P450 and to show antitumor activity (5). The authors have shown that tegafur is activated by thymidine phosphorylase in human tumors in addition to the activation in the liver (6,7). It has also been found that the concentration of 5-FU in the tumors of patients who are administered tegafur is higher than that in the adjacent normal tissue. Takasaki et al. (8) reported that the concentration of 5-FU was much higher in cancer foci than in normal tissue in patients with gastric cancer. The authors also found that the concentration was higher in the blood than in the tumor when 5-FU was administered to patients intravenously. This result supports the author's result that tegafur is activated by thymidine phosphorylase in tumor tissue.

REFERENCES

1. Nakayama C, Wataya Y, Meyer RB, et al. (1980) Thymidine phosphorylase substrate specificity for 5-substitued 2'-deoxyuridines. J Med Chem 23: 962-964.

2. Cook AF, Holman MJ. (1979) Fluorinated pyrimidine nucleosides 3, synthesis and antitumor activity of a series of 5'-deoxy-5-fluoropyrimidine nucleosides. J Med Chem 22: 1330-1335.

3. Ishitsuka H, Miwa M, Takemoto K, et al. (1980) Role of uridine phosphorylase for antitumor activity of 5'-deoxy-5-fluorouridine. Gann 71: 112-123.

4. Kono A, Hara Y, Sugata S, et al. (1983) Activation of 5'-deoxy-5-fluorouridine by thymidine phosphorylase in human tumors. Chem Pharm Bull 31: 175-178.

5. Fujita H, Sugiyama M, Kimura K. (1976) Pharmacokinetics of futrafur (FT207) for clinical application. In Cancer Chemotherapy II (Proceedings of the 9th International Congress of Chemotherapy London July 1975) (Hellman K. and Connors et al.) New York Plenum Press Vol. 8: 51-57.

6. Kono A, Hara Y, Matsushima Y. (1981) Enzymatic formation of 5-fluorouracil from 1-(Tetrahydro-2-furanyl)-5-fluorouracil (Tegafur) in human tumor tissues. Chem Pharm Bull 29: 1486-1488.

7. Hara Y, Sugata S, Kono A, et al. (1983) Enzymatic conversion of tegafur to 5-FU in human tumor tissues. Jpn J Cancer Chemotherapy 10: 1151-1517.

8. Takasaki T, Asado S, Kitamura Y, et al. (1981) Clinical pharmacologic investigation into continuous intravenous infusion of futrafur 1. Transfer into gastric tumor. Jpn J Cancer Chemotherapy 8: 1241-1245.

Fluoropyrimidines in Cancer Therapy
K. Kimura, S. Fujii, M. Ogawa, G.P. Bodey, P. Alberto, eds.

PHARMACOKINETIC STUDIES OF SEVERAL DERIVATIVES OF FLUOROPYRIMIDINES

Hiroshi Fujita

1. INTRODUCTION

Since 1970, we have studied the pharmacokinetics of tegafur and have observed the characteristics of its behavior in clinical applications (1,2,3,4,5,6). Oral or rectal administration of tegafur is widely utilized in cancer chemotherapy in Japan, and several new masked type derivatives of fluoropyrimidines which are considered to be more active or less toxic than tegafur have been synthesized.

The pharmacokinetics of four derivatives of 5-FU, i.e. tegafur, HCFU, 5'-DFUR and 1-phthalidyl-5-FU, and two derivatives of FUDR, i.e. FF-705 and TK-177 are described in this report.

2. ANALYTICAL METHODS

The methods for extraction and estimation of unchanged drugs and metabolites were as follows.
Tegafur: Chloroform extraction (pH 2.0), Tegafur...HPLC,

5 FU......GC MS or bioassay using St. aureus 209P

HCFU: Chloroform extraction, TLC, HCFU fraction (HCFU, CPEFU, CPRFU, etc.)...bioassay after conversion to 5-FU by NaOH treatment, 5-FU...bioassay or HPLC

5'-DFUR: Deproteination by TCA → Column chromatography → TLC, 5'-DFUR...HPLC, 5-FU...HPLC or bioassay

1-phthalidyl-5-FU: Chloroform extraction, 1-phthalidyl-5-FU...bioassay or GC-MS after conversion to 5-FU by NaOH, 5-FU...bioassay or GC-MS after ethyl acetate extraction

FF 705; Ethyl acetate extraction → TLC, FF-705 and intermediates...HPLC, FUDR, 5-FU...HPLC or bioassay

TK-117; Methylene chloride → Chloroform extraction, TK-117...HPLC, FUDR, 5-FU...GC-MS

3. RESULTS

3.1. Tegafur

Tegafur

Tegafur is a masked form of 5-FU and it becomes effective after conversion to the active form of 5-FU and anabolic products in the body. In 1970, we clarified this phenomenon by using autobiograms in which paper chromatograms of tissue emulsions of mice administered tegafur and agar plates inoculated with St. aureus 209P were combined (2,3).

The blood level of tegafur was high and decreased slowly after intravenous injection. The blood level of the active substance, 5-FU derived from tegafur was low (1/50-1/400 of tegafur), but it persisted in the blood for several hours in parallel with the tegafur curve (1).

Tegafur was absorbed well following oral or rectal administration, and the tendency for long-lasting blood levels was more pronounced than with intravenous administration (1,3,4). In many cases administered 600-800 mg of tegafur orally per day by three divided doses, the blood level of tegafur was 10-20 µg/ml and that of 5-FU was 0.02-0.05 µg/ml for several hours.

Tegafur is lipophilic and is able to pass through the GI tract or blood-brain barrier by the passive diffusion method (4).

The concentration of tegafur and its active metabolite, 5-FU, in the cerebrospinal fluid increased rapidly after oral administration of tegafur, reached the same level as that in the plasma after 3 hours, and continued thereafter for several hours in cancer patients (4).

To clarify the activation process of tegafur, in vitro and in vivo experiments were carried out (2,4).

Five hundred µg/ml of tegafur and 10% tissue homogenates from autopsied human materials were mixed and incubated at 37 °C for 2 hours, and the amount of 5-FU produced was estimated. As a result, tegafur was activated most remarkably by hepatic homogenates (about 3.4 µg/ml of 5-FU was produced), but less by other tissues, although some of the tegafur were spontaneously or enzymatically converted to 5-FU in the latter (2,4). An in vivo study of hepatic clearance test was undertaken using dogs (4). The blood level of tegafur and derived 5-FU and the blood circulation volume were measured in the hepatic artery, portal vein and hepatic vein. From these data, the amount of 5-FU in the hepatic vein, showed the highest levels at all times after administration of tegafur, and the hepatic clearance of 5-FU was calculated to be 120% on the average (4).

It has been shown that tegafur is mainly activated by P-450 in the liver microsomes (7,8). The activity of P-450 is known to be enhanced by phenobarbital, etc. and inhibited by SKF-525A, etc.

Our experiments (5,6) showed that the tissue level of 5-FU in sarcoma-180 bearing mice administering tegafur was elevated moderately by pretreatment with phenobarbital and greatly by phenobarbital and glutathione in combination, while, pretreatment with CCl_4 made it much lower. Some immunomodulators, such as anaerobic Corynebacterium and OK-432 (product of St. haemolyticus) inhibited the activity of P-450, and resulted in a decrease in the 5-FU level. However, PSK (product of Basidiomycetes) and Ge-132 (organic germanium) did not have such inhibitory action (9).

It was reported that coadministration of tegafur and uracil resulted in inhibition of the catabolism of 5-FU produced and an increase in the anticancer effects of tegafur (10). Our study (6) showed that when a large dose (100 mg/kg) of tegafur was administered to mice bearing Lewis lung carcinoma, the 5-FU level was elevated markedly in proportion to the dose of uracil added (molar ratio: 1:4 > 1:2 > 1:1) not only in the tumor tissues but also in all normal tissues. However, when a moderate dose of tegafur (20 mg/kg) was administered to mice with uracil (tegafur: uracil = 1:4), the 5-FU level in the tumor was elevated to 8.7 times higher than that when tegafur alone was administered, and the 5-FU level in the blood and many normal tissues was not greatly increased by this combination, although some elevation of 5-FU was shown in the spleen, digestive tract, kidneys and liver.

3.2. 1-Hexyl-carbamoyl-5-fluorouracil (HCFU)

HCFU

HCFU is activated into 5-FU by relatively strong natural degradation through some oxidation products, such as 1-carboxypentylcarbamoyl-5-FU (CPE-FU), 1-carboxypropylcarbamoyl-5-FU (CPR-FU), etc. (11,12).

The pharmacokinetics of HCFU following oral administration was studied using rabbits and mice bearing sarcoma 180 (12). HCFU was absorbed gradually from the gastrointestinal tract, and the HCFU fraction (HCFU+CPE-FU+CPR-FU) persisted for several hours in the body and was successively converted to 5-FU. The blood level of the HCFU fraction in rabbits reached a maximum soon after administration and decreased rapidly at first, but gradually after 3 hours. The blood level of 5-FU produced from HCFU was observed at somewhat (1.0-1.5 times) higher levels for several hours than those for the same dose of tegafur.

In sarcoma 180 bearing mice, HCFU fraction and 5-FU were distributed at a high level in the stomach, intestine, kidneys and liver, and at a low level in the brain and spleen. A moderate level of 5-FU was observed in the tumor (solid). The concentrations of HCFU fraction and 5-FU in the ascites of patients with peritonitis carcinomatosa and ascitic tumor bearing mice were high and persisted for a long time. The production of 5-FU from HCFU was not influenced by pretreatment with phenobarbital and glutathione, or CCl_4 (12).

This phenomenon indicates that the activation of HCFU is not mainly depend on liver microsomal enzyme in contrast to tegafur.

From these observations, effects of HCFU can be expected in patients with liver dysfunctions and also in patients with cancerous ascites or pleural fluids.

3.3. 5'-Deoxy-5-fluorouridine (5'-DFUR)

5'-DFUR

5'-DFUR is a masked compound of 5-FU, which is converted to 5-FU in the presence of uridine phosphorylase (mice and rats) or thymidine phosphorylase (humans) (13,14).

5'-DFUR was absorbed well from the gastrointestinal tract and showed high blood levels of 5'-DFUR and derived 5-FU following oral administration to rabbits. However, they disappeared relatively rapidly from the blood due to high urinary excretion. The maximum blood level of 5-FU produced from 5'-DFUR was higher, but decreased faster than that produced from tegafur or HCFU (15). The tissue level of 5'-DFUR in mice was high in the stomach, intestine and kidneys, and very low in the brain.

The concentration of 5-FU derived from 5'-DFUR was selectively high in various tumor tissues, such as sarcoma-180, Lewis lung carcinoma, MC-induced fibrosarcoma of mice and DMBA-induced tongue carcinoma of hamsters (15). The 5-FU level derived from 5'-DFUR in the tumors was markedly higher than that from produced tegafur and HCFU. This result might be due to the high distribution level of uridine phosphorylase in these tumor tissues (13).

The concentration of 5-FU formed from 5'-DFUR was moderate in the intestine, stomach, kidneys and lungs, and very low in the other organs, although the distribution of phosphorylase and the production of 5-FU in normal or tumor tissues varied considerably among animal species and among individuals.

The activation of 5'-DFUR to 5-FU was not influenced by pretreatment with phenobarbital or CCl_4, which indicates that the activation does not depend on the liver drug-metabolizing enzyme (15).

This pharmacokinetic behaviors of 5'-DFUR account for its high antitumor activity in a broad dosage range and its low toxicity in experimental animals.

3.4. 1-Phthalidyl-5-fluorouracil (PH-FU)

PH-FU

PH-FU is a new masked compound of 5-FU, which showed a lower toxicity and a higher antitumor activity in experimental animals than 5-FU or tegafur (16).

The blood level of PH-FU following oral administration to rabbits reached a maximum 30 minutes later, but it was considerably lower than that of tegafur, HCFU or 5'-DFUR (17).

The blood level of 5-FU derived from PH-FU reached a maximum after 30 minutes. The 5-FU level was higher than that derived from the other 5-FU derivatives, but it disappeared more rapidly (4 hours) (17).

PH-FU was detected at a low level for 6 hours in various tissues of mice bearing sarcome 180, which indicates the rapid conversion of PH-FU to 5-FU, etc. (17). The tissue level of 5-FU was high in the digestive tract and kidneys. The concentration of 5-FU in the tumor tissues was relatively high and persisted for several hours (17).

To demonstrate the activation process, 25 µg/ml of PH-FU and 10% tissue homogenates from humans and mice were mixed and incubated for 2 hours (17). The result showed that PH-FU was converted to 5-FU strongly in the liver (75%), kidneys (82%), muscle (58%), heart (67%) and testis (59%) of mice. Essentially the same results were obtained in human tissues. In conclusion, PH-FU seems to be characterized by low blood and tissue levels of unchanged drug, relatively high production of 5-FU and a short duration of the levels.

Clinical studies of PH-FU have just begun in Japan, and a suitable method of administration in accordance with the pharmacokinetics should be established.

3.5. FUdR derivatives

FF-705   TK-117

FUdR shows much stronger cytocidal activity in vitro than 5-FU. However, these two drugs were equally effective in vivo although some clinical superiority of FUDR (for example, by arterial infusion) over 5-FU was seen. This is due to the rapid metabolism of FUdR to 5-FU and rather strong urinary excretion in vivo.

To solve this problem, oral form and masked type compounds which release FUdR iu the body for a long period have been synthesized in Japan

Two FUdR derivatives are called FF-705 [3',5'-di-O-acetyl-3-(3-methyl benzoyl)-FUdR] and TK-117 [3-(3,4-methylenedioxy benzoyl)-FUdR]. FF-705 was activated to FUdR in the body through intermediates, di-or mono-acetyl FUdR or 3-methyl benzoyl FUdR. Then part of FUdR was changed to 5-FU (18,19). TK-117 was converted to FUdR and piperonylic acid without intermediates and some of the FUdR was changed to 5-FU (20).

Oral administration of FF-705 or TK-117 gave the highest blood level of FUdR among all metabolites and the 5-FU level was about 1/4-2/3 of the former (19,20). The levels of these active substances from FF-705 were not so high, but they persisted for over 8 hours. On the other hand, levels of FUdR and 5-FU derived from TK-117 in the blood were high but they disappeared relatively rapidly. Following oral administration of FF-705 or TK-117 to sarcoma 180 bearing mice (19,20), the tissue level of FUdR was high in the kidneys, digestive tract, spleen, testes and tumor, and that of 5-FU was high in the kidneys, intestine, tumor, liver and lungs. A very high concentration of FUdR was detected in the urine.

The in vitro metabolism was studied by incubating FF-705 or TK-117 with various sera or tissue homogenates (19,20). Sera of mice, rats, rabbits and humans produced FUdR from FF-705 or TK-117, but they did not produce 5-FU. Human and mouse tissue homogenates metabolized FF-705 to FUdR and then to 5-FU through intermediates. A large amount of FUdR was produced in the homogenates of the tumor, spleen, lungs and testes, and 5-FU was produced in the liver, intestine, kidneys and tumor.

In the experiment on TK-117, FUdR was produced abundantly in the homogenates of the stomach, tumor, kidneys, spleen and pancreas, and 5-FU in the liver, kidneys, intestine, tumor and lungs. In phase 1 studies of FF-705 and TK-117, fairly strong adverse effects on digestige organs, mainly diarrhea appeared in some patients, and this was the reason for the limitation of the dosage.

FF-705 and TK-117 had better antitumor activities on various animal tumors than tegafur. The establishment of a suitable administration method or a treatment method should regulate this clinical side effect, which should make them more desirable drugs.

4. DISCUSSION

The pharmacokinetics of four derivatives of 5-FU and

two derivatives of FUdR were described in this report. Among these drugs, the concentration and duration of unchanged drugs and the activation products, 5-FU or FUdR and 5-FU in the blood and tissues varied considerably. This may be caused by differences in the rate and speed of absorption from the gastrointestinal tract, the first pass effect, the rate of excretion, the process of activation, and the rate of anabolism and catabolism of 5-FU or FUdR.

The mode of activation seems to be the most important. Tegafur is mainly converted to 5-FU by P-450 in the liver, HCFU by oxidation and relatively strong natural degradation, 5'-DFUR by thymidine- or uridine-phosphorylase, and PH-FU by an enzyme or enzymes in some tissues. FF-705 and TK-117 are metabolized to FUdR in sera, and to FUdR and 5-FU in various tissues. The distribution and activity of these enzymes in the liver, kidneys, gastrointestinal tract, tumor, etc. are related to the antitumor efficacies and the side effects of these drugs.

In consideration of the mode of activation and the characteristics of the kinetics of absorption, blood and tissue levels and excretion, a suitable method of administration and suitable patients should be selected for each drug.

REFERENCES

1. Fujita H, Ogawa K, Sawabe T, et al. (1972) In vivo distribution of IV_1-(2'-tetrahydrofuryl)-5-fluorouracil (FT-207). Jpn J Cancer Clinics 18: 911-916.

2. Fujita H, Ogawa K, Sawabe T, et al. (1972) Metabolism of IV_1-(2'-tetrahydrofuryl)-5-fluorouracil (FT-207). Jpn J Cancer Clinics 18: 917-922.

3. Fujita H, Kimura K. (1974) In vivo distribution and metabolism of IV_1-(2'-tetrahydrofuryl)-5-fluorouracil (FT-207). Progress in Chemotherapy Vol. III: 159-165, Hellenic Soc of Chemother. Athens

4. Fujita H, Sugiyama M and Kimura K. (1976) Pharmacokinetics of futraful (FT-207) for clinical application. Chemotherapy Vol.8: 51-57, Plenum Publishing Corporation, New York.

5. Fujita H. (1977) Anticancer agents and glutathione. Tsurumi Univ. Dental J. 3: 1-7.

6. Fujita H, Ogawa K, Marunaka T, et al. (1980) Experimental approach to increasing the effect of futraful (FT-207) by phenobarbital, glutathione, and uracil on the basis of pharmacokinetics. Current Chemother and Infectious Dis. 1535-1536, Am Soc Microbiol, Washington DC

7. Ohira S, Maezawa S, Irinoda Y, et al. (1976) Studies on the cytochrome P-450 difference spectra induced by various anticancer drugs by liver microsomes from rats. Jpn J Cancer Chemother 3: 663-669.

8. Au JL and Sadee W. (1980) Activation of ftorafur [R,S-1-(tetrahydro-2-furanyl)-5-fluorouracil] to 5-fluorouracil and -butyrolactone. Cancer Res 40: 2814-2819.

9. Fujita H, Nakajima S. and Shimamura M. (1983) Influence of immunoaduvants on the activation of tegafur and P-450 enzymatic activities. Presented at the 6th Asia Pacific Cancer Cong, Sendai, Japan.

10. Fujii S, Ikenaka K, Fukushima M, et al. (1978) Effect of uracil and its derivatives on antitumor actvity of 5-fluorouracil and 1-(2-tetrahydrofuryl)-5-fluorouracil. Gann 69: 763-772.

11. Hoshi A, Iigo M, Nakamura A, et al. (1976) Antitumor activity of 1-hexylcarbamoyl-5-fluorouracil in a variety of experimental tumors. Gann 67: 725-731.

12. Fujita H, Ogawa K. (1981) In vivo distribution and activation of 1-hexyl-carbamoyl-5-fluorouracil (HCFU). Jpn J Clin Pharmacol Therapeutics 12: 73-83.

13. Ishitsuka H, Miwa M, Takemoto K, et al. (1980) Role of uridine phosphorylase for antitumor activity of 5'-deoxy-5-fluorouridine. Gann 71: 112-123.

14. Shirasaka T, Nagayama S, Kitano S, et al. (1981) Pyrimidine nucleoside phosphorylase in rodents and humans. Jpn J Cancer Chemother 8: 262-269.

15. Fujita H, Ogawa K, Nakagawa H, et al. (1983) Pharmacokinetics of 5'-deoxy-5-fluorouridine (5'-DFUR) by oral administration. J Jpn Soc Cancer Ther 18: 916-926.

16. Nitta K, Uehara N, Tanaka T, et al. (1983) Antitumor activity of phthalidyl 5FUS, new derivatives of 5-FU, on experimental animal tumors. Presented at 13th Int Congr Chemother, Vienna.

17. Fujita H, Takao A. (1983) Pharmacokinetics of a new 5-FU derivative, 1-phthalidyl-5-FU. Presented at 42nd Jap Cancer Cong; Proceedings of Jpn Cancer Assoc, the 42nd Annual Meeting, p.252.

18. Fujii S, Ikenaka K, Maehara Y, et al. (1981) Studies on antitumor activity and in vivo fate of the derivaties of 2'-deoxy-5-fluorouridine (FdUrd). Jpn J Cancer Chemother 8: 1548-1553.

19. Fujita H, Ogawa K, Matsubara Y, et al. (1983) Pharmacokinetics of a new FUDR derivative...FF-705. Presented at 13th Int Congr Chemother, Vienna.

20. Fujita H, Ogawa K. and Kimura K. (1983) Pharmacokinetics of a new FUDR derivative...TK-117. Presented at 31st Jpn Congr Chemother, Osaka.

© 1984 Elsevier Science Publishers B.V.
Fluoropyrimidines in Cancer Therapy
K. Kimura, S. Fujii, M. Ogawa, G.P. Bodey, P. Alberto, eds.

THE PHARMACOLOGY AND METABOLISM OF 5′-DEOXY-5-FLUOROURIDINE

Jean-Pierre Sommadossi, Claude Aubert, Charles Jacquet
Athanassios Iliadis and Jean-Paul Cano

1. INTRODUCTION

5'-Deoxy-5-fluorouridine (5'-DFUR) is a relatively new fluoropyrimidine derivative synthesized in 1976 by COOK et al (1). Its antineoplastic activity has been observed as well in a wide range of animal tumors (2,3,4) than in cultured human tumors (5), and would be dependent upon its clearage to 5-fluorouracil (5-FU) (2). In addition, 5'-DFUR exhibits a higher therapeutic index (3,6,7) and is far less immunosuppressive than other fluoropyrimidines (2,6,7).

The purpose of the present paper was to develop a new strategy in a Phase I study, in investigating the dose and the time dependency of 5'-DFUR and in elucidating the metabolic route of this novel antimetabolite in humans. Furthermore, since the unique biological properties of 5'-DFUR appear mediated by the conversion to 5-FU, and that 80 to 90 % of this compound are metabolized via a degradative pathway, studies were undertaken to investigate the metabolism of 5-FU at the cellular level, using an isolated rat hepatocyte model.

108

2. MATERIALS AND METHODS

2.1. In vivo pharmacokinetic studies

Pharmacokinetics of 5'-DFUR and its metabolites in plasma and the urinary excretion were studied following administration of 1 g to 23 g of the drug as a 30 min or 6 hr I.V. infusion, in patients randomly recruited from a Phase I clinical trial. Venous blood samples were drawn at specified times into 10 ml oxalated tubes over 4 hr or 6 hr depending of the administred dose of 5'-DFUR. The blood samples were then centrifuged for 15 min of 2400 xg and the plasma was adjusted to a pH value of 7, frozen and stored at - 20°C until analysis. Urine specimens were collected when voided spontaneously, over 24 hr after 5'-DFUR administration. Volume of specimens were recorded and aliquots (25 ml) stored at -20°C. Unmetabolized 5'-DFUR in plasma was assayed by a reversed phase high performance liquid chromatography method as described previously (8). The identical technique without solvent extraction was carried out for its determination in urine. Simultaneous determination of the two metabolites, 5-FU and 5,6-dihydrouracil (5-FUH$_2$) were performed by a gas chromatography-mass spectrometry (GC/MS) method, described in detail previously (9).

Elimination half-lives were obtained by linear regression analysis of the kinetics terminal points. Total plasmatic clearance (CL) of 5'-DFUR was assessed according to the relationship : $CL = \dfrac{DOSE}{AUC}$, where the areas under the curves were determined from experimental points using the trapezoïdal rule. The dose and the time-dependent relationship for 5'-DFUR were evaluated by two different processes :

a/ comparaison of the total clearance values

b/ appariement test point by point between two kinetics, by the mean of a linear regression analysis.

2.2. In vitro studies

Freshly isolated rat hepatocytes were obtained by a collagenase perfusion of rat liver via the hepatic foetal vein. Hepatocytes in suspension ($5x10^6$ cells/ml) were incubated at $37°C$ and pH 7.4 under 95 % O_2 5 % CO_2 in Krebs -Henseleit buffer containing 0.25 % gelatin and 10 mM glucose. Experiments were initiated with the addition of 30 uM of ^3H - 5-FU and the extracellular medium was separated from the cell pellet by a silicone oil technique (10). Analysis of the intracellular and the extracellular tritium was performed using an ion pair reversed phase chromatography, which rapidly and simultaneously resolves the unchanged 5-FU, the major hypothesized 5-FU catabolites and the 5-FU anabolites (10).

3. RESULTS

3.1. Time-dependence relationship

Fig. 1 shows the plasma concentrations of 5'-DFUR in patient 1 following 3 successive courses of 3 g of 5'-DFUR administred by I.V. infusion over 30 min.

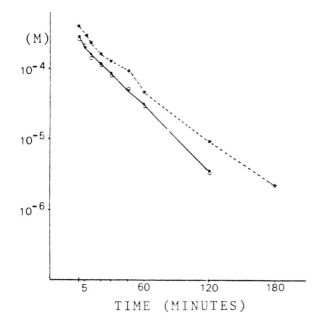

FIGURE 1. Plasma levels of 5'-DFUR following three successive courses of 3 g of 5'-DFUR, administred over 30 min.

A rapid decrease of 5'-DFUR can be observed within the
first 2 hr and the apparent half-life was 21 min. Most notable, is the significant variation of the total clearance
value between the first two courses (64.8 and 65.2 1/h)
compared to the third one (41.2 1/h). The appariement test
between the third kinetic and the first two, in which the
Y intercept of the linear regression analysis was different from 1, confirmed this time dependency by the third
administration of 5'-DFUR. These results were confirmed
in another patient who received repeated doses of 5'-DFUR
by a 30 min infusion, as illustrated in fig. 2.

3.2. Dose-dependence relationship

The dosage escalation of 5'-DFUR during this phase I

clinical trial have led us to examine the dose dependency
for 5'-DFUR.

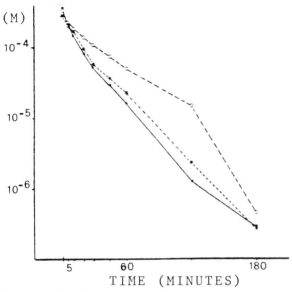

FIGURE 2 Plasma levels of 5'-DFUR following three successive courses of 4 g of 5'-DFUR, administred over 30 min.

Fig. 3 shows the disappearance of 5'-DFUR from plasma in a
patient following successive administration of 2 g and 4 g
of 5'-DFUR by a 30 min I.V. infusion.

The total clearance values, 86.07 l/h and 94.7 l/h
were not significantly different, reflecting a possible
linear process, at these doses, for 5'-DFUR. However, a
more accurate approach with an appariement test, as illustrated in fig. 3, shows that the value of the slope is different from the ratio of the administred dose indicating
a non linear process, at doses $\geqslant$ 4 g for this drug.

When doses of 5'-DFUR were increased to determine the
maximum tolerable dose in humans, a structural non linear

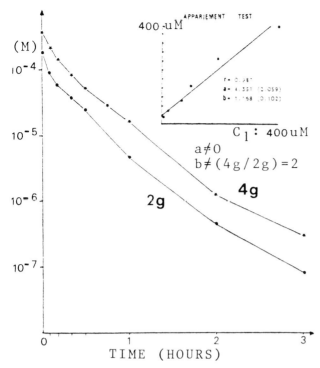

FIGURE 3   Disappearance of 5'-DFUR from the plasma in a patient who received 2 g and 4 g of 5'-DFUR over 30 min.

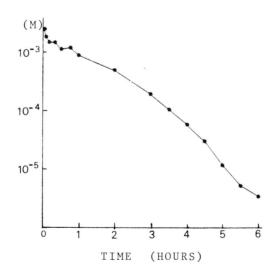

FIGURE 4   Disappearance of 5'-DFUR from the plasma in a patient who received 23 g of 5'-DFUR over 27 min.

process (i.e. a set of differential equation can't be used to describe the concentration-time of the drug) could be observed for this drug as illustrated in fig. 4. At this dose of 23 g, the kinetic of the 5'-DFUR shows a convex log plasma concentration-time curve, reflecting a critical saturable clearance process. In addition, this phenomenon was similarly observed after enhancement of the rate of infusion of 5'-DFUR (data not shown).

3.3. Metabolic studies in humans

Fig. 5a illustrates the plasma kinetics of 5'-DFUR and its metabolites, 5-FU and 5-FUH$_2$ after a short I.V. infusion of 3.4 g of 5'-DFUR.

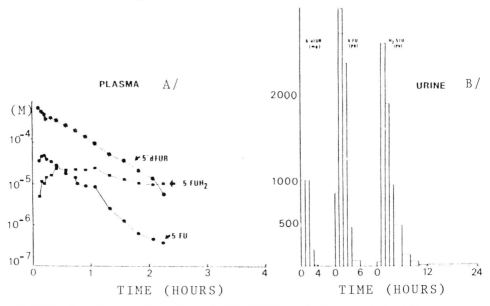

FIGURE 5 Plasma levels of 5'-DFUR and its metabolites 5-FU and 5-FUH$_2$ after a 5-min infusion of 5'-DFUR, 3.4 g (A) and urinary excretion of total 5'-DFUR and metabolites in 24-hr periods in the same patient (B).

The levels of 5-FU approximated 15 uM at the end of the infusion and 0.38 uM after 2 hr. The apparent elimination half-life of 5-FU was 17 min. In contrast, 5-FUH$_2$ reached a maximum level of 22.4 uM within 20 min which was maintained for more than 30 min and subsquently slowly declined.

The urinary excretion of the unchanged drug and its metabolites 5-FU and 5-FUH$_2$ was studied during the same course of 5'-DFUR (fig. 5b). In this patient, the cumulative elimination of unmetabolized 5'-DFUR after 4 hr represented 37.5 % of the administred dose, whereas the 2 metabolites 5-FU and 5-FUH$_2$ represented a minor fraction with 3.7 ‰ and 1.8 ‰, respectively.

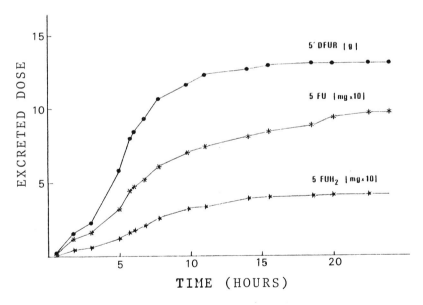

FIGURE 6   Cumulative urinary excretion of 5'-DFUR and metabolites after a 6 hr infusion of 23 g of 5'-DFUR.

115

The importance of the renal excretion was independent of the administration modalities but the data were not conclusive with respect to the dose dependence relationship. It can be seen (fig. 6) that in a patient receiving 23 g of 5'-DFUR over 6 hr, the cumulative dose of the unchanged drug was 57.2 % whereas the metabolite fractions were similarly low, being 4.2 ‰ for the 5-FU and 1.8 ‰ for the 5-FUH_2.

3.4. Metabolic studies in vitro

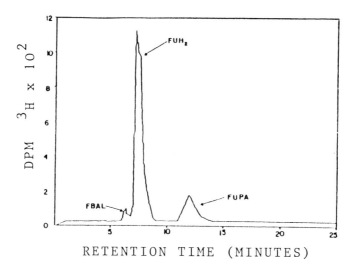

RETENTION TIME (MINUTES)

FIGURE 7 Radiochromatogram of intracellular ^{3}H after incubation of a hepatocyte suspension for 4.5 min with 30 uM ^{3}H-FU.

Exposure of 5×10^6 cells/ml to 30 uM of ^{3}H-FU resulted in a rapid and complete conversion of 5-FU to several catabolites, i.e. 5-FUH_2, α-fluoro-β-ureidopropionic acid (FUPA) and α-fluoro-β-alanine (FBAL), while formation of anabolites was insignificant (fig. 7). 5-FUH$_2$ represented the major intracellular metabolite and unmetabolized 5-FU was not detected within cells even after very short exposure as 1 min, which suggests that 5-FU is catabolized rapidly relative to membrane transport, under these conditions.

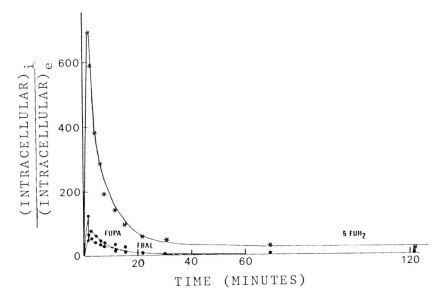

FIGURE 8   Intracellular to extracellular concentration ratio of 5-FU metabolites as a function of time.

In addition, as shown in fig. 8, a high transmembrane gradient of 700 for 5-FUH$_2$ was generated within 1 min and subsequently declined. However, a transmembrane gradient (25 fold) was still present after 2 hr of incubation. Since 5-FUH$_2$ was not bound to cellular macromolecules (10), these data suggest that the elimination of 5-FUH$_2$ (i.e. degradation and efflux from the cells) is very slowly relative to its formation, and active transport for this catabolito is possiblo as woll.

4. DISCUSSION

These studies, undertaken in humans during a Phase I clinical trial, provide pharmacokinetic and metabolic data of 5'-DFUR. The analysis of the plasma kinetics of 5'-DFUR showed striking intra-individual variations in the total plasmatic clearance by the third course of treatment, consistent with a time-dependency for this drug. The origin of this phenomenon has not still been clarified, but the fluctuations of 5'-DFUR disposition and elimination might represent a possible hypothesis. Comparison of the clearance values for 5'-DFUR following successive therapy in the same patient (fig. 3) suggested a linear relationship for doses comprised between 2 and 4 g. However, a more accurate approach, such as an appariement test indicated a net dose-dependency for 5'-DFUR. As the doses and/or the rate of infusion were increased, this non linearity was enhanced and a convex behavior for 5'-DFUR could be observed (fig. 4). The metabolism and the urinary elimination of 5'-DFUR were investigated, in order to propose a fonctionnal sheme which describes the kinetic behavior of this drug. Plasma concentrations of 5-FU represented about 6 % and the apparent elimination half-life was similar to that of 5'-DFUR. In contrast, plasma values of 5-FUH_2 remained to a steady-state level and/or slowly declined (fig. 5) so that a meaningful half-life for 5-FUH_2 could not be estimated. The in vitro data, obtained using

118

an isolated rat hepatocyte model, suggested that the accumulation of 5-FUH$_2$ _in vivo_, might result not only from a saturable process in the conversion of 5-FU to 5-FUH$_2$ but also in the degradation and/or the transport of 5-FUH$_2$. Further evidence that the two saturable mechanisms are associated alternatively, is provided by the consistency of the plasma values for 5-FUH$_2$ as the administred doses of 5'-DFUR increased (11). The renal excretion of 5'-DFUR was variable, representing during a 24-hr period, 40 to 57 % of the dose. The quantitative importance of this elimination route was found independent of the administration modalities, however further studies are needed to evaluate the role of this route in the dose and the time-dependency behavior of this drug, described in this paper. In contrast this route of elimination was pratically negligible for the 2 metabolites, 5-FU and 5-FUH$_2$.

ACKNOWLEDGEMENTS

The authors are indebted to Prof. G. MATHE and Y. CARCASSONNE who made possible the clinical applications of the 5'-DFUR and to J. COVO for his generous technical assistance. This study was supported in part by INSERM Grant N°119017 under the INSERM-NCI (France-USA), by a scientist exchange program G 50111 (France-USA Cancer program) and by a grant from the "Association pour le Développement de la Recherche sur le Cancer".

REFERENCES

1. Cook AF, Holamn MJ, Kramer MJ, et al. (1979) Fluori-
    nated pyrimidine nucleosides. Synthesis and antitu-
    mor activity of a series of 5'-deoxy-5-fluoropyrimi-
    dine nucleosides. J Med Chem 22 : 1330-1335.

2. Armstrong RD, Diasio RB (1980) Metabolism and biologi-
    cal activity of 5'-deoxy-5-fluorouridine, a novel
    fluoropyrimidine. Cancer Res 40 : 3333-3338.

3. Bollag W, Hartman HR (1980) Tumor inhibitory effects
    of a new fluorouracil derivative : 5'-deoxy-5-fluo-
    rouridine. Eur J Cancer 16 : 427-432.

4. Ishitsuka H, Masanori M, Takemoto K, et al. (1980)
    Role of uridine phosphorylase for antitumor activity
    of 5'-deoxy-5-fluorouridine. Gann 71 : 112-123.

5. Armstrong RD, Gesmonde J, Wu T, et al (1983) Cytoto-
    xic activity of 5'-deoxy-5-fluorouridine in cultured
    human tumors. Cancer Treat Rep 67 : 541-545.

6. Armstrong RD, Diasio RB (1981) Selective activation
    of 5'-deoxy-5-fluorouridine by tumor cells as a basis
    for an improved therapeutic index. Cancer Res 41 :
    4891-4894.

7. Au JLS, Rustum YM, Minowada J, et al. (1983) Differen-
    tial selectivity of 5-fluorouracil and 5'-deoxy-5-
    fluorouridine in cultured human B lymphocytes and
    mouse L1210 leukemia. Biochem Pharmacol 32 : 541-546.

8. Sommadossi JP, Cano JP (1981) Determination of a no-
    vel fluoropyrimidine, 5'-deoxy-5-fluorouridine, in
    plasma by high performance liquid chromatography.
    J Chromatogr 225 : 516-520.

9. Aubert C, Sommadossi JP, Coassolo P, et al. (1982)
    Quantitative analysis of 5-fluorouracil and 5,6-dihy-
    drouracil in plasma by gas chromatography/mass spec-
    trometry. Biomed Mass Spectrom 9 : 336-339.

10. Sommadossi JP, Gewirtz DA, Diasio RB, et al. (1982)
    Rapid catabolism of 5-fluorouracil in freshly isola-
    ted rat hepatocytes as analyzed by high performance
    liquid chromatography. J Biol. Chem 257 : 8171-8176.

11. Sommadossi JP, Aubert C, Cano JP, et al. (1983) Kine-
    tics and metabolism of a new fluoropyrimidine 5'-deo-
    xy-5-fluorouridine, in humans. Cancer Res 43 :
    930-933.

© 1984 Elsevier Science Publishers B.V.
Fluoropyrimidines in Cancer Therapy
K. Kimura, S. Fujii, M. Ogawa, G.P. Bodey, P. Alberto, eds.

EXPERIMENTAL CHEMOTHERAPY WITH FLUOROPYRIMIDINE COMPOUNDS ON HUMAN GASTROINTESTINAL AND BREAST CANCERS XENOGRAFTED TO ATHYMIC NUDE MICE

Masahide Fujita, Fumiko Fujita, Yosuke Nakano
and Tetsuo Taguchi

1. INTRODUCTION

One of the most effective use of the human cancer-nude mouse system is the application to screening for anticancer drugs, because it is expected that human cancer xenografted to nude mice would predict better the clinical effect of a drug than transplantable animal tumors. Since 1976 3 different types of human tumor have been added to the NCI screening panel in the drug development program (1,2). Besides drugs in clinical use, a lot of compound were screened in this system, and a breast cancer line, MX-1, was the most responsive to chemotherapy among the 3 tumors. This panel is limited to the use of primary screening of new drugs. A single xenograft of each type is insufficient to the secondary screening which aims to clarify the organ specificity of a drug. Different system with a set of tumors of each type should be prepared for this purpose.

In our laboratory 15 lines of human gastrointestinal and breast cancers xenografted in nude mice from surgical materials have been selected for the secondary screening

121

and a variety of drugs in clinical use or in consideration
of clinical phase trial were evaluated in this system (3).
In this paper we describe antitumor activity of three
kinds of fluoropyrimidine compounds, tegafur, UFT(uracil
plus tegafur in molar ratio of 4 to 1) and 5'-deoxy-5 flu-
orouridine(5'-DFUR), as a single-agent chemotherapy on the
human cancer-nude mouse panel.

2. MATERIALS AND METHODS

As indicated in Table 1, a total of 15 human cancer
lines(7 gastric, 3 colorectal, 2 pancreatic and 3 breast
cancers) xenografted in male or female nude mice of BALB/c
background under s.p.f. condition were used.

TABLE 1

Characteristics of Human Cancer Lines Xenografted in BALB/c-nu/nu Mice

Tumor Line	Histology	Doubling Time (Day)	Tumor Marker[*] LDH-5	CEA
Gastric Cancer				
H-55	Well diff. adenoca.	9.1±0.7	H	L
H-111	Well diff. adenoca.	4.6±0.2	H	I
H-23	Moderately diff. adenoca.	7.7±0.6	H	L
H-30	Moderately diff. adenoca.	6.4±0.4	T	H
H-106	Poorly diff. adenoca.	4.3±0.2	T	H
H-154	Poorly diff. adenoca.	7.0±0.2	H	L
H-81	Squamous cell ca.	3.7±0.3	H	T
Breast Cancer				
H-31	Papillotubular ca.	8.7±0.3	L	L
H-71	Papillotubular ca.	11.0±0.8	L	L
H-62	Medullary tubular ca.	6.4±0.5	H	L
Colorectal Cancer				
H-26	Well diff. adenoca.	9.6±0.5	I	H
H-110	Well diff. adenoca.	9.7±0.9	I	H
H-143	Well diff. adenoca.	4.4±0.4	H	I
Pancreatic Cancer				
H-48	Well diff. adenoca.	9.5±0.6	L	H
H-171	Well diff. adenoca.	13	I	L

* Serum levels in host mice are classified as : H ; high, I ; intermediate, L ; low, T ; trace

All but one of them were established from primary or metastatic tumor of each patient without previous chemotherapy. The volume doubling time of each tumor line ranged from 4 to 13 days.

A piece of each tumor excised to 2-3mm cube was inoculated subcutaneously on the back of the mice at 5-8 weeks of age. The animals were divided into groups consisting of 7 mice each when estimated tumor volume reached a level of approximately 100 mm^3, and the size of each tumor was measured in 3 dimensions twice weekly during the experiment. They were kept in the vinyl isolator throughout the study period except for the temporary transfer to a clean bench for tumor transplantation and drug administration.

The drugs used were 3 fluoropyrimidine compounds; tegafur, UFT and 5'-DFUR. They were administered orally once a day except Sunday, 25-30 times in total, at a dose of 100, 17.5 and 123 mg/kg, respectively. Dosage of each drug adopted was maximal tolerated dose predetermined for the treatment schedule. After termination of each experiment the therapeutic effect of each drug was evaluated by the inhibition rate (I.R.) based on the following equation:

$$\text{Inhibition rate} = 100 - \frac{\text{Mean tumor weight of treated group}}{\text{Mean tumor weight of control group}} \times 100(\%)$$

When the inhibition rate was 58% or more, the drug was evaluated as effective. Histological changes of each tumor were also examined.

3. RESULTS

Fig. 1 shows an example of single-drug chemotherapy with
graded doses of 5'-DFUR on a breast cancer, H-62, xenografted in nude mice. The solid lines of the treated groups are situated lower as compared with the dotted line of
the untreated control. A dose response relationship was
clearly noted between graded doses of 5'-DFUR and their
antitumor effects.

Effect of 5´-DFUR on Growth of Human Breast Cancer Xenograft (H-62-26) in Nude Mice

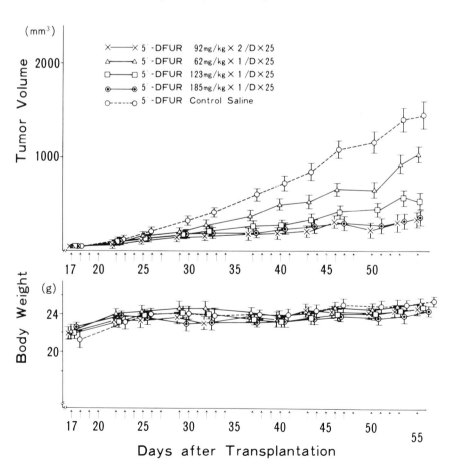

FIGURE 1   Effect of oral administration of 5'-DFUR at a graded dose levels on growth of a human breast cancer xenografts(H-62-26) in nude mice. On the abscissa the number of days following tumor transplantation is plotted and the short arrow shows the day of treatment. Each point and vertical bar represents the average and standard error of estimated tumor volume.

As indicated in the lower panel, the side effects of the drugs were monitored from changes in body weight.

Fig.2 shows an experiment in which animals bearing pancreatic cancer(H-171) were treated with each one of the 3 compounds. Daily treatment with 123 mg/kg of 5'-DFUR succeeded almost completely in inhibiting the tumor growth, whereas 100 mg/kg of tegafur and 17.5 mg/kg of UFT remained in the slight or moderate suppression of the growth. The inhibition rates of 5'-DFUR, tegafur and UFT were 81, 21 and 43%, respectively. The differences of response between 5'-DFUR versus tegafur and 5'-DFUR versus UFT were statistically significant at a level of $p < 0.001$ and 0.05, respectively.

Simultaneous comparison of the antitumor activity between the 2 or 3 drugs were made in some tumor lines. Table 2 indicates the effects of tegafur compared with those of UFT on 3 gastric, 2 colorectal and 3 breast cancers xenografted in nude mice.

Chemotherapy with Fluorinated Pyrimidine Drivatives on Human Pancreatic Cancer Xenografts (H-171-4) in Nude Mice

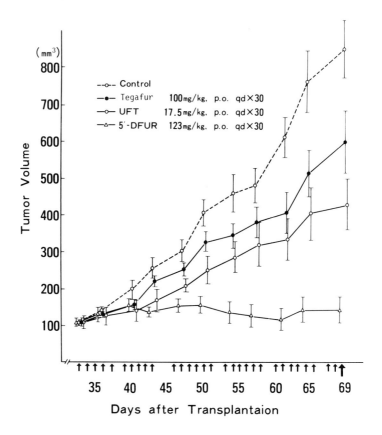

FIGURE 2   Chemotherapy with 3 fluorinated pyrimidine derivatives, tegafur, UFT and 5'-DFUR, on human pancreatic cancer xenografts(H-171-4).   Each curve represents changes of mean volume with standard error of 7 tumors in the control and treated groups.

TABLE 2

Inhibition Rate to Tegafur versus UFT against Human
Gastrointestinal and Breast Cancer Xenografts in Nude
Mice

Drug	Tegafur	UFT[a]	
Dosage (mg/kg/d×25~30)	100	17.5	20
Gastric Cancer			
H-55 (well)	64[b]		77
H-111 (well)	59	67	
H-154 (por)	43	63	
Colorectal Cancer			
H-110 (well)	61	66	
H-143 (well)	61	66	
Breast Cancer			
H-31 (pap-tub)	56		78
H-62 (med. tub)	10		24
H-71 (pap-tub)	0 **[c]	50	

a) Uracil plus tegafur in molar ratio 4 : 1
b) Each number shows inhibition rate (I.R.) : $(1 - T/C) \times 100 (\%)$
c) **: significantly defferent between the 2 drugs at p<0.01

The inhibition rates of UFT were superior to those of
tegafur in every tumor. But, the pattern of sensitivity
to UFT among these tumors was very similar to that to tegafur. This implicates that the mode of action will be similar between these two drugs. In a breast cancer line(H-
71), the difference of the response between the drugs was
stastically significant(p<0.01) by the student's t test.

Simultaneous comparisons of the inhibitory effects of
5'-DFUR versus tegafur or the 3 drugs were shown in Table
3. In all of 8 experiments, 123 or 100 mg/kg of 5'-DFUR
revealed higher inhibition rate than 100 mg/kg of tegafur.
Among them, the effect of 5'-DFUR was significantly supe-

rior to that of tegafur in each 2 gastric and breast cancers and each one rectal and pancreatic cancers. Direct comparison of UFT and 5'-DFUR was made in 4 experiments. In 2 gastric cancers(H-106 and H-81), UFT exibited higher inhibition rate, whereas the results were reversed in 2 other tumors; each one pancreatic and breast cancers.

TABLE 3

Comparative Studies of Effects of 5'-DFUR, Tegafur, and UFT on Human Cancer Xenografts in Nude Mice

Drug Dosage (mg/kg/d×25~30)	5'-DFUR 100	5'-DFUR 123	Tegafur 100	UFT 17.5
Gastric Cancer				
H-23 (mod)		68	25**	
H-55 (well)	98		70*	
H-1 1 1 (well)	61		45	
H-1 0 6 (por)		44*		67
H-8 1 (sq)		93		95
Colorectal Cancer				
H-26 (well)		91	38**	
Pancreatic Cancer				
H-1 7 1 (well)		81	21***	43*
Breast Cancer				
H-3 1 (pap-tub)		99	95*	
H-62 (med, tub)		4 1	1 5	
H-7 1 (med, tub.)		68	0***	50*

Each number shows inhibition rate (I.R.); $(1 - T/C) \times 100 (\%)$
* : p<0.05, ** : p<0.01, *** : p<0.001

Table 4 summarizes the results of the experimental chemotherapy with tegafur, UFT and 5'-DFUR against 15 lines of human cancer xenografts in nude mice. If a drug was judged as effective to a cancer when I.R. was 58% or more, tegafur was effective in 6 out of 15 human cancer lines(40%), i.e., 3 gastric, 2 colorectal and one breast cancers.

TABLE 4

Response Rate to Tegafur, UFT and 5'-DFUR against 15 Human Cancer Xenografts in Nude Mice

Drug	Grade of Response[a]						% Responder	
	−	±	+	⧺	⧺	⧻	≧ +	≧ ⧺
Tegafur	4[b]	5	3	2	0	1	40%	7%
UFT	3	1	8	1	2	0	73%	13%
5'-DFUR	3	1	4	1	3	3	73%	40%

a) Evaluated by inhibition rate (I.R.): $(1 - T/C) \times 100\%$; −, I.R. < 40; ±, I.R. from 40 to 57; +, I.R. from 58 to 69; ⧺, I.R. from 70 to 79; ⧺, I.R. ≧ 80; ⧻, tumor shrinkage to a volume smaller than the starting one.
b) Each number indicates number of cases in each grade of response

In UFT, 11 out of 15 lines(73%), i.e., 6 gastric, each 2 colorectal and breast and 1 pancreatic cancer lines, were counted as effective. 5'-DFUR was also effective in 11 lines(73%), i.e., 5 gastric, 3 breast, 2 colorectal and 1 pancreatic cancers. If inhibition rate of 80% or more was counted as responder, response rates of tegafur, UFT and 5'-DFUR were 7, 13 and 40%, respectively.

4. DISCUSSION

Since 1974, attempts have been made in our laboratory

to transplant malignant human tumors and 45 out of 175 specimens have been established as serially transplantable tumor xenografts(4). The results of 5 experimental chemotherapies with human cancers xenografted to nude mice were directly compared with the clinical responses to the same treatment observed in each donor patient, and close correlation of the results between the original and transplanted tumors was found(5). Recently, 15 lines of human gastrointestinal and breast cancers have been selected for the secondary screening panel, and 14 drugs in clinical use or under development were evaluated as a single agent chemotherapy(3).

In the present study, long term daily treatment with UFT at a maximal tolerated dose showed higher response rate than that of tegafur. As far as the 2 drugs were concerned, the experimental results coincided well with the clinical results. Equimolar dose of 5'-DFUR also exhibited higher response rate than that of tegafur. Although comparative studies of UFT versus and 5'-DFUR have been continued, UFT showed higher inhibition rate in 2 gastric cancers and 5'-DFUR in 2 other cancers so far. Among the 3 drugs, 5'-DFUR led the most frequently to the shrinkage of treated tumor. These experimental results will be expected to show the good coincidence with the clinical phase II results of the same type of cancer in the near future.

Thus, one of the superiority of the human tumor-nude

mouse panel in the study of cancer chemotherapy is to make
the accurate and quick comparison between the analoguous
drugs possible.   Giuliani et al(6) reported the effects
of new doxorubicin analogues, 5-FU and BCNU on 9 xenografts of human colorectal cancers with close relation to the
clinical activity.   Apart from the wide superficial screening panel of NCI(1,2), the methods adopted by this study this study and Giuliani et al. appear to be desirable
as a predictive secondary screening to be performed immediately before clinical trial with the aim to determine
the organotropic property of the test agents.

REFERENCES

1.   Houchens DP, Ovejera AA, Sheridan MA, et al. (1979)
     Therapy for mouse tumor and human tumor xenografts
     with the antitumor antibiotic AT-125. Cancer Treat
     Rep 63: 473-476.

2.   Ovejera AA, Houchens DP. (1981) Human tumor xenografts
     in athymic nude mice as a preclinical screen for anti-
     cancer agents. Seminars in Oncology 8: 386-393.

3.   Fujita M, Fujita F, Taguchi T. (1983) Chemosensitivity
     of human gastrointestinal and breast cancer xenografts
     in nude mice and predictability to clinical response
     of anticancer agents. In Proc 4th Intl Workshop on
     Immune-Deficient Animals in Exper Res (ed) B Sordat.
     Basel, Karger (in press).

4.   Taguchi T, Fujita M, Usugane M. (1977) Heterotrans-
     plantation of various human and canine tumors into
     nude mice. In Proc 2nd Intl Workshop on Nude Mice
     (eds) T Nomura, N Ohsawa, N Tamaoki and K Fujiwara.
     University of Tokyo Press, pp. 305-312.

5.   Fujita M, Hayata S, Taguchi T. (1980) Relationship of
     chemotherapy on human cancer xenografts in nude mice
     to clinical response in donor patient. J Surg Oncol
     15: 211-219.

6. Giuliani FC, Zirvi KA, Kaplan NO, et al. (1981) Chemotherapy of human colorectal tumor xenografts in athymic mice with clinically active drugs. Int J Cancer 27: 5-13.

Fluoropyrimidines in Cancer Therapy
K. Kimura, S. Fujii, M. Ogawa, G.P. Bodey, P. Alberto, eds.

DISCUSSION

Hoshi: Dr. Sadée, did you find any intermediates which are derivates of 5-FU?

Sadée: I have shown you the structures of those intermediates that we have identified, including the hydroxylated metabolites as well as the dehydrogenated metabolites.

Hoshi: Do the hydroxylated metabolites contain the 5-FU moiety in the molecule?

Sadée: Yes, and the tetrahydrofuranyl moiety with a double bond in it, produced by a dehydrogenating enzyme, which would be another circulating intermediate. Probably this drug would be active because it is fairly labile chemically. It might even undergo chemical conversion to 5-FU. However, the concentration of this potential intermediate is relatively low. So, if you would make the drug and inject it in lieu of tegafur, it probably would be rather toxic at equimolar doses.

Hoshi: Is 2' hydrolysis specifically localized in the gastrointestinal tract?

Sadée: No, the activities expressed per gram wet weight actually would only be about one in the liver and about 0.6 in the GI tract and about 0.3 in the brain. So, the liver still has the highest activity, but it is not like cytochrome P-450 where the liver has, maybe, tenfold more or a hundredfold more activity than in the brain or in a tumor.

Majima (Chiba Cancer Center, Chiba): I would like to ask Dr. Sadée a few questions. First, you said that tegafur is cleaved in the cell at the C-2' or C-5' positions. If I am not mistaken, you mentioned that metabolites produced by cleavage by P-450 are not redistributed. Is the 5-FU concentration that we see after tegafur administration in human beings solely due to cleavage at the C-2' position?

Sadée: No, that is not what I meant. The concentrations of 5-FU that are circulating are generated by several pathways. However, 5-FU plasma levels are so low that they do not contribute to the toxicity or to the effects. Therefore, it doesn't really matter which pathway it is. But

it appears to me that Dr. Fujii has now 'tricked' the
system into providing more 5-FU to the circulation by
blocking the catabolic pathway. If you add uracil, then
you will block the metabolism of 5-FU in the liver and
allow more of the drug to be activated and redistributed.
So that is an additional factor that has to be taken into
account.

Majima: Recently, we have found that when we give tegafur
to human beings over a long time, they develop serious
toxicity manifested as anosmia. We wonder if the metabolism
of tegafur in brain cells is different from other organs
of the body.

Sadée: The brain contains rather low levels of cytochrome
P-450, so that pathway may not be an important one, although some brain cells may contain enough of this enzyme.
The products are not only 5-FU but also the tetrahydrofuranyl moiety. Thus, we have to consider what happens to
the tetrahydrofuranyl moiety. In the brain, there is
activation to 4-hydroxybutanal; and we have found that
4-hydroxybutanal is not as efficiently oxydized to 4-
hydroxybutyric acid in the brain as it is in the liver.
So there are differences. In addition, I would like to
emphasize that 4-hydroxybutylic acid is also a neuroactive
compound, but I do not know whether it contributes to the
neurological effects of tegafur.

Majima: Also, some cat studies have indicated that 5-FU is
metabolized to fluroacetate and flurocitrate in the brain.
Does this contribute to toxicity in any chronic way?

Sadée: I don't know.

Spears: Regarding neurologic toxicity, Dr. Stephen Howell
used large doses of 5-FU administered by continuous infusion and attempted to protect against the side effects
with standard oral doses of allopurinol. He thought that
there was an increase in the neurologic toxicity due to
5-FU. However, he did not indicate any olfactory toxicity,
but mainly ataxia and cerebellar problems.

Loo: Quite some time ago, in 1978, my colleagues at M.D.
Anderson reported in *Cancer Research* the work we have done
in patients with tegafur. The results are at some variance
with what has been described today. I want to point out
that in our studies we gave a tremendous dose of tegafur
(5 g/m^2) to patients, and in five of the eight patients
the concentration of 5-FU derived from the tegafur was
extremely high, on the average of 1.7 µg/ml, and persisted
for at least 50 hours or longer. The second point I want
to make is that tegafur penetrates into the CSF quite
readily and the 5-FU level later measured in the CSF is
also very high.

Sadée: I just want to comment briefly that there has been
controversy about the blood levels of 5-FU after tegafur

administration. We have felt that a dehydrometabolite which is chemically very labile and very easily decomposes to 5-FU. So there are differences in the assays, and there are also differences in the dose study, as mentioned by Dr. Loo. Very high doses could, in effect, lead to higher 5-FU levels.

Hara: Dr. Sadée, I have been deeply impressed by your excellent presentation. I understand that there are two major metabolic pathways which involve P-450 and the soluble enzyme. You said that you did not use human tissue, but used rabbit liver tissue. Did you use any other tissues such as intestine, kidney or spleen of rabbit?

Sadée: We did use brain and intestines and found the same activity. I think similar activity is also found in rats, but we did not use human tissue. That is why I pointed out your work that shows an additional, or a different enzyme activity in human tumors. I think that the same principles, in terms of the philosophy behind my study, apply; but it must still be determined what the precise enzyme is that activates tegafur in human tumors as well as in normal human tissues.

Tsukagoshi (Cancer Chemotherapy Center, Tokyo): Dr. Spears, do you have any data on the differences in thymidylate synthetase activity among various human cancer tissues, or between normal and tumor tissues?

Spears: I presented some of the work that will be submitted for publication soon. This was largely done in gastro-intestinal malignancies, and most of these were colorectal carcinomas. The level of enzyme inhibition at an average of one to two hours after 5-FU bolus administration intravenously was approximately 80% in the tumors. This was somewhat greater in two breast cancers that we studied. In these two tumors there was a slightly greater percentage of inhibition but also a much lower absolute level of free enzyme. We were unable to correlate antitumor response with this effect in patients with colorectal cancers. However, one of the breast cancer patients achieved a complete response to single-agent 5-FU, and the other achieved disease stabilization. So, at least in those two cases, we had a correlation with enzyme inhibition, although it may be the tumor tissue type that correlated instead. I presented the results in normal liver and showed that in this case there was less enzyme inhibition. This correlated with lower FdUMP and higher dUMP levels in the liver. The liver is not a target organ for 5-FU toxicity. The closest that we have come to studying that is normal human mucosa which we studied in two patients at approximately one to two hours after 5-FU bolus administration. The results were very similar to those found in the liver. However, the GI tract is not a target organ for 5-FU toxicity following bolus administration. What we would really like to know is the results in normal bone marrow, and those

135

studies have yet to be done.

Tsukagoshi: Do you think the enzyme levels correlate with the side effects generally?

Spears: I think that is something that remains to be determined. A particularly important question is whether or not continuous infusion produces similar kinds of pharmacokinetic inhibition data or whether the mode of administration changes the mechanism of action against the tumor cells.

H. Fujita: I would like to ask Dr. Sadée a question. Where is the intermediate 3' or 4' hydroxy-tegafur or dehydro-tegafur produced? Is it in the liver microsomes?

Sadée: I think you should know that better than I do because you have done some of those studies. I do think that the liver microsomes are the major site. The hydroxylation is most likely mediated by microsomal enzymes. It is possible that during hydroxylation, at either C-5' or the other position, there is a secondary reaction that introduces a double bond rather than an OH group.

H. Fujita: How greatly do these intermediates contribute to antitumor activity?

Sadée: In my opinion, the hydroxylated metabolites are exceedingly low in plasma. Most of them are not activated to a significant extent to 5-FU, as has been discussed and published by Dr. Loo, for instance. We have only found one hydroxylated metabolite that is very efficiently cleaved to 5-FU, and that is the beta-D-4'-hydroxy-tegafur. This metabolite is actually very interesting because it is a very good substrate for thymidine phosphorylase. That is the only metabolite we know of that has a specific mechanism for activation to 5-FU.

H. Fujita: Dr. Spears, have you measured the 5-FU levels in sensitive tumors and in resistant tumors?

Spears: No, we did not measure the parent drug, unfortunately. We did do plasma pharmacokinetics in a handful of patients and found, in the one breast cancer patient who showed a complete response to 5-FU, a very large plasma 5-FU clearance level that perhaps correlated with a larger area under the curve of exposure of the tumor to 5-FU.

Kimura: Dr. Sadée, do you have any suggestions as to how to activate tegafur?

Sadée: Do you mean how to produce derivatives that would be more active or how to make tegafur more active per se? One approach, which I have already suggested, is to hydroxylate tegafur at the beta-D-4' position. This would result in a very active prodrug. You could introduce a double bond which would probably result in a faster release of 5-FU. You might want to try cytochrome P-450 induction, as proposed by Dr. Fujii, for instance. In this case,

136

however, you have to make sure that the 5-FU is redistributed. Thus, I think a combination of enzyme induction and tegafur administration plus uracil would probably be successful in releasing more drug. On the other hand, I do not think that this is really very desirable because we do not need more drug release, but we need more specific drug release; and those are two quite different issues.

Bertino: Dr. Spears, I missed how you did the assay exactly. Do you fortify your enzyme extracts when you measure thymidylate synthetase with methylene tetrahydrofolate or do you measure the level of the enzyme without the presence of methylene tetrahydrofolate? That might be a very important limiting factor in terms of enzyme activity: whether or not there is sufficient folate there to saturate the enzyme.

Spears: I think that is a critical question also, and we have looked at it both ways - with or without added 5, 10-methylene tetrahydrofolate. One of the problems in human studies is that we are dealing with a post-5-FU treated tumor that has some bound enzyme and some free enzyme. When we add the folate, we actually stabilize ternary complex that is there. If we do the assay without added folate, there may be a destabilization of the bound enzyme so that we get an artifactual increase in apparent free enzyme compared to using added tetrahydrofolate. These are kinetic complications that cannot be examined with single biopsies. I think that the Houghton suggestion that in the untreated tumor what is the FdUMP binding capacity in the absence of added folate, addresses the question regarding potential sensitivity of the tumor. I think that is an important thing to study. In all of the data that we have shown, we have added excess folate cofactor. In some animal tumors that we have studied, we have done the initial tumor processing in the presence of folate and have not found a great difference in the amount of enzyme inhibition. One think I have been impressed with in our animal tumors is the ability of the endogenous folates to bind FdUMP to the enzyme.

Fujii: Have you ever tried to purify the enzymes?

Sadée: No, we have not attempted to do that yet.

Fjuii: Do you think M-1 and M-2 are produced by tissues other than the liver?

Sadée: We have not done that. Dr. Spears, dUMP levels may have two functions, (1) inhibit the binding of FdUMP to thymidylate synthetase, but also (2) elevated levels of dUMP. These effects are most likely associated in all tissues with a very large excretion or production of deoxyuridine which inhibits thymidine uptake very effectively (in many cells to the order of 10 micromolar dUrd in the medium); therefore, you may have different effects on dUMP. Do you consider the thymidine bypass in your studies?

Spears: I think it would be very important to consider whether or not salvage pathway synthesis of DNA could occur. Dr. Bruce Chabner has stated that he feels the thymidine levels in blood are not sufficiently high for salvage pathways to be active enough for DNA synthesis in most tumors. However, of course, thymidine levels in tumors - especially those that are undergoing necrosis and perhaps even in response to 5-FU - could generate enough thymidine to rescue the tumors. We have not been able to look at that experimentally, but I think that is a future goal. There are those who feel that drugs such as dipyridamole can be used as thymidine kinase salvage pathway inhibitors, but I don't think that any inhibitors are yet known that would be strong enough to permit suitable experiments.

Sommadossi: Dr. Fujii, it is well known that uracil inhibits 5-FU catabolism, but I am surprised about the significant difference of the 5-FU/uracil ratios when we compare the in vitro and the in vivo data. You showed, if I understood, that there is about 30% inhibition of 5-FU catabolism in the presence of 100 times or sometimes 1,000 times more uracil than 5-FU, using liver slices. However, it can be seen, in the in vivo situation, that there is a greater inhibition with smaller ratios ranged from 1:4 to 1:10. How can you explain that? On the basis of the data that we generated with Dr. Diasio and that we presented last May to the AACR, it appears that to estimate the exact degree of the inhibition of 5-FU catabolism by different agents, such as uracil, we need to measure the intracellular $5\text{-}FUH_2$ levels, in an intact cell system. For instance, we found that with a ratio of 1:7 for 5-FU/uracil, inhibition of 5-FU catabolism represented about 90%. Could you give us an explanation why these ratios are so high in your experiments?

Fujii: Yes, that is a problem. In the case of the enzymes Km of degradation enzymes is almost same for two substrates, uracil and 5-FU, but we used slices or cells. Under these conditions, uracil inhibited degradation of 5-FU at 1,000 times 5-FU. We cannot explain this phenomenon, so we need to do more studies.

Tsukagoshi: Dr. Syrkin, we have had experience with the combination of psychotropic agents including chlorpromazine, in which adriamycin resistance is overcome to some extent and in which the antitumor effects of these compounds are enhanced. In your study, does the combination of phenazepam or aminazine with 5-FU overcome the 5-FU resistance to some extent, or does it enhance it, or does it remain at the usual level of antitumor effect?

Syrkin: Unfortunately, we have not yet used any 5-FU-resistant tumor strains.

Kimura: What about the efflux or influx of 5-FU in combination with the psychotropic agents? Anthracycline and vincristine incorporations are much affected by these psychotropic agents. So, in your case, membrane interaction probably has something to do with this enhancement of antitumor effect. What would you think?

Syrkin: In our laboratory we used only physiological methods, and until now we have not studied this at the biochemical level in order to discover the mechanism of this interaction. I think that future study will produce some very important results. It will be necessary to study the mechanism of biochemical interaction.

Kimura: Dr. Syrkin, you talked of tegafur in combination with aminazine or phenazepam increasing tumor growth inhibition. Is that a selective toxicity for tumor tissues? Do you have any results for normal tissue, pathologically or biochemically?

Syrkin: I do not think it is selective because we have seen an increase of toxicity in normal tissues. For example, we have seen an increase in LD_{50} with the combination of tegafur with chlorpromazine, and we have seen an increase in leukopenia. Therefore, unfortunately, I do not think that we have a selective increase in antitumor activity.

Majima: Dr. Loo, the combination of 5-FU, PALA and TdR is very interesting. As a clinician, I am wondering whether the pharmacokinetic and pharmacodynamic effects are the same for host cells and tumor cells. Otherwise the combination won't improve the therapeutic index.

Loo: I'm glad somebody is supporting what I have been preaching for years; namely, that whenever you attempt to modify the pharmacokinetics of an antitumor agent (antimetabolites, in particular), you seldom modify the therapeutic index. In fact, in my experience, I have never seen any improvement because you do not produce selectivity simply by modulating one of the biochemical pathways. This kind of attempt is, in my view, futile.

Fujii: Dr. Loo, you said that FUdR appears in the blood after the administration of the combination of 5-FU and thymidine. Have you examined the effect of thymidine on the antitumor effect of FUdR in vitro?

Loo: The reason we attribute the effect completely to thymidine itself and thymine derived from the thymidine is that we have also studied the pharmacokinetic interaction of 5-FU with PALA. This was not done clinically, but this was done in the dog. It is our experience, at least regarding the pharmacokinetics of 5-FU, that dogs and humans resemble each other very closely. Therefore, we speculated that PALA exerts a negligible effect on the pharmacokinetics and the metabolism of 5-FU. Since this interaction was not detectable in the dog, most likely there wouldn't be any in people either.

Fujii: I have done experiments in vitro, and thymidine did not influence the gross antitumor activity of 5-FU using cell culture, but did inhibit the antitumor effect of FUdR.

Loo: My only comment is that I always feel that in the in vitro situation you bypass most of the pharmacokinetic barriers, and the model most likely is not a very good one compared with in vivo studies. Thus, whenever we attempt to prove something, we always go to animals - rodents or the dog - rather than to a tissue culture or cell culture or an isolated enzyme system.

Spears: How did you get the clinical approval to do serial lung biopsies on patients with lung cancer over so many hours? This is a very difficult thing to justify from the clinical standpoint.

Loo: That question would best be addressed to my colleague, Dr. Bodey, but I believe there was some clinical justification.

Bodey: Serial biopsies were only performed on patients with subcutaneous metastases. The patients were fully informed of the nature of the experiments and agreed to participate.

Woolley: I would just like to comment on something that I think I understood Dr. Syrkin to say. In commenting on the neurotoxicity of 5-FU, he stated that at the therapeutic concentrations that he was using he saw very little if any neurotoxicity of 5-FU. We have been studying 5-FU in conjunction with allopurinol and have used doses of 1,500 to 2,000 mg/m^2 of 5-FU to protect against myelosuppression. At those doses, the neurotoxicity of 5-FU is quite substantial. I would agree that doses commonly used (in the range of 600 to 1,200 mg/m^2) cause minimal neurotoxicity, but at higher doses (above 1,500 mg/m^2), neurotoxicity may be substantial and frequently dose limiting. Is that your experience also?

Syrkin: Yes.

Sommadossi: I have a question for Dr. Hoshi about his very interesting talk. I believe that in terms of the intracellular pharmacokinetics of 5-FU and its metabolites the FU catabolites are produced in the systemic circulation, and not formed within the ascites?

Hoshi: If HCFU changes to 5-FU, the other pathways are similar to 5-FU. This is not specific to HCFU.

Fujii: Dr. Hoshi, where is the site of absorption of HCFU, the stomach or the intestines?

Hoshi: The intestines, of course. Don't you agree?

Fujii: At a lower pH HCFU is very stable, but at a higher pH it is unstable. You said that you found a high level of

HCFU in the blood. Also, you said that the level is achieved to the maximum very fast - within one hour. How do you explain that?

Hoshi: The pH of the intestinal content in the duodenum is approximately 5.6; therefore, HCFU is stable. HCFU is rapidly transported to the intestine, and rapid absorption occurs.

Woolley: I would just like to make a comment. Dr. Tattersall and I have experience with the combination of 5-FU and allopurinol. It is an excellent method of modifying the granulocytopenia produced by 5-FU. It is quite clear that you can attenuate the toxicity of 5-FU by using allopurinol. The dose of allopurinol is quite important, but if used appropriately, you can modify the toxicity of 5-FU either given as a continuous infusion or given as a bolus injection. It is very interesting that you are seeing antitumor activity, which of course is the important thing. If you rescue the tumor along with the bone marrow, then you really accomplish nothing, as Dr. Loo pointed out. There are at least two randomized trials that are beginning. One designed by the Southeast Cancer Study Group uses either 5-FU alone or 5-FU plus allopurinol in colon cancer. In that trial, the failures with 5-FU and allopurinol then receive 5-FU alone. Thus, we will see whether or not patients who failed to respond to 5-FU and allopurinol will subsequently respond to 5-FU alone. There is another study in Argentina that has a similar design.

Tattersall: In our study, I think we only had four patients with gastric cancer who were treated with 5-FU plus allopurinol, and two of them responded. Your responses seem to be predominantly in that tumor type with both of the schedules that you have used. I wonder if this should encourage the Americans to look at it in gastric cancer rather than colon cancer, where a much bigger series has in fact already been accumulated by Stephen Howell and others. I think the response rate in colorectal cancer is about 15%, whereas in gastric cancer, your series and ours together, suggest that there may be a better response rate.

Ogawa: Dr. Syrkin, you listed only 'responses' and I wonder what kind of responses you obtained - complete or partial? I also wonder if you have any data about the duration of remission.

Syrkin: The duration of remission is approximately four months. We consider an objective response as a decrease in the size of tumor by more than fifty percent.

Sadée: Dr. Hara, I just have a brief question about how you interpret the generation of 5-FU with your in vitro studies using the isolated enzyme thymidine phosphorylase. Can you really make the statement that the increased levels of 5-FU in the tumors correlate with the levels of thymidine phosphorylase activity in those same tumors? If you have a high formation of 5-FU in the tumor when compared with other tissues and if you compare the amount of thymidine phosphorylase in those tissues with the amount of 5-FU produced, then you have an argument for saying that this is really the enzyme which activates tegafur.

Hara: In malignant tumors the activity is much higher than it is in normal tissues.

Fujii: Did you identify 5'-deoxyribose-1-phosphate or phosphorylated tetrahydrofuran?

Hara: No, I didn't.

Fujii: What was the rate of enzyme activity of thymidine phosphorylase for tegafur compared with natural substrates such as thymidine?

Hara: We just tried to purify thymidine phosphorylase, and we partially succeeded. We only used this partially purified thymidine phosphorylase.

Woolley: Dr. Fujita, you mentioned an organic germanium compound you were working with. Could you say any more about that?

H. Fujita: Germanium-132 is a low-molecular immunomodulator which is an interferon and NK-cell inducer. It is now in phase I or phase II studies in Japan. Tegafur or HCFU in combination with G-132 is undergoing clinical study.

Sadée: I think what we should consider during this discussion is what we should actually measure for the selection of a prodrug. What biochemical parameters are important? Furthermore, what biochemical reactions correlate with the response in any individual – from one patient to the next? Finally, what models are important in terms of predicting antitumor effects in humans? Maybe this could be a major theme for the discussion.

Niitani (Nihon Medical School, Tokyo): Dr. Fujita, the doses of each drug that you used in the experiment seem to be so different. How did you determine the dose of each drug?

M. Fujita: It is the maximum tolerated dose (MTD) and the same treatment schedule: 123 mg/kg of 5'-DFUR is equimolar to 100 mg/kg of tegafur.

Majima: How about the dose of UFT?

M. Fujita: The dose of UFT is also an MTD. In some experiments it was shown to be slightly toxic, so we reduced the dose.

Majima: Dr. Fujita, you mentioned G-132 and fluorinated pyrimidine combinations. What is the rationale for the pharmacokinetic and pharmacodynamic point of view? Also, why did you choose G-132? This one is not well studied yet.

H. Fujita: In Japan, immunochemotherapy is widely tried in clinical situations, e.g., in stomach cancer very long-term chemotherapy with tegafur, and some immunomodulators such as OK-432, which is a hemolytic streptococci product, and PS-K, which is a basidiomycetes product, are very widely used with tegafur. Recently, germanium-132 has been developed and this drug has very low toxicity. It can be used both orally and intravenously, daily, for a very long time with tegafur. Many bacterial immunoadjuvants have inhibitory action on P-450, and therefore the activation of tegafur is greatly reduced. I have experimented with these three immunoadjuvants used in Japan for P-450 activity and 5-FU production of tegafur. OK-432 and anaerobic corynebacterium, or BCG, inhibit the activation of tegafur. These combinations interfere with the activation of tegafur, but G-132 and PS-K do not inhibit its activation. Thus, I think that this combination is suitable.

Fujii: Dr. Sommadossi, you said that in the case of the 5'-DFUR you find a high level of 5-FUH_2 in the blood. Is this true for 5-FU infusions?

Sommadossi: We get approximately the same amount of 5-FUH_2 after administration of about one gram of 5-FU by IV bolus. However, we did not compare, in the same patient, the amounts of 5-FUH_2 formed after administration of 5-FU or 5'-DFUR. In addition, saturation of the conversion of 5-FU to 5-FUH_2 induces maximum levels of 3 or 4×10^{-5}M. Furthermore, the very slow decline for 5-FUH_2 is similarly found after administration of 5'-DFUR or 5-FU.

Hara: Dr. Sommadossi, you determined the level of 5-FU and 5'-DFUR after administration of 5'-DFUR; but this is not important because it is clear that 5'-DFUR is activated in the tissue. Thus, the tissue level is the most important thing. Did you check the levels in tumor tissues and in normal tissues?

Sommadossi: No, we didn't check. It is true that the activation in tissues is very important, but from the results that we presented, it appears that the clearance equals the hepatic blood flow for 5'-DFUR and in consequence, the production of 5-FU might result essentially from the liver. Therefore, it is important to know the amount of 5-FU in the systemic circulation. About the CNS toxicity observed after administration of 5'-DFUR, I would like to mention that we did some determinations of 5'-DFUR and 5-FU in CSF during CNS toxicity. However, we couldn't find any direct correlation between the observed toxicity and the amounts of these compounds.

Tattersall: I would like to ask all the speakers if there is any evidence to suggest that the rate of administration of 5-FU makes any difference on the relative effect on RNA metabolism versus DNA metabolism. Is there any evidence to suggest, for example, that high peaks are more important than continuous levels?

Sadée: I think that this is a particularly difficult question, but also a very important question to address. We have looked in tissue cultures at DNA- and RNA-related actions of 5-FU, and it appeared that the RNA-directed effects of 5-FU in mouse lymphoma S-49 tissue culture were more pronounced relative to DNA-related effects with continuous exposure. Thus, there may be a difference that favors RNA effects over the long run, but that is only in tissue culture, and in vivo it may be entirely different.

Woolley: The available data on infusion of drugs, particularly into the hepatic arterial circulation, suggest that continuous infusion would be more effective than a pulse type of administration of either 5-FU or FUDR. Clinical responses have occurred in patients who received continuous infusion of these drugs, after they failed to respond to ether bolus or loading dose administration of the same drugs given peripherally.

Sadée: It should also be considered that a sublethal dose of thymidylate inhibition will slow down the cell progression through the cell cycle and will prevent the cells from getting into G_1, where some of the RNA-directed effects occur. I think that very clearly a time effect is important here. Even FUDR in vivo in patients appears to be acting primarily through the conversion to 5-FU. So we do have, always, both actions likely to be present, and both actions will affect each other to a significant extent.

CLINICAL ASPECTS: NEW DRUGS

Fluoropyrimidines in Cancer Therapy
K. Kimura, S. Fujii, M. Ogawa, G.P. Bodey, P. Alberto, eds.

UFT, A NEW ANTICANCER DRUG

Kiyoji Kimura and Shoji Suga

1. INTRODUCTION

UFT is not a newly synthesized drug, but a newly combined drug of uracil(U) and tegafur(FT), with a U/FT molar ratio of 4, developed based on experimental rationale defined by Fujii et al(1,2). Details of experimental studies are fully discussed by Fujii et al in this volume(3).

Prior to introducing clinical results of UFT, fundamentals of oral use of FT should be elucidated. Firstly, it is based on experimental results of studies on cell-killing kinetics and pharmacokinetics of 5-fluorouracil (5-FU) and FT. Secondly, it is also based on our previous experiences of oral administration of various anti-cancer drugs in the treatment of leukemia and lymphoma.

2. CELL-KILLING KINETICS

The cell-killing kinetics of anticancer drugs have been extensively studied with an attempt at enhancing the chemotherapeutic efficacy from viewpoints of schedule and route of drug administration(4,5). In order to measure the survival rate of proliferative tumor cells, soft agar

cloning assays as single cell culture techniques have
been utilized.   Colony-forming cells serve as a measure
of the number of tumor cells with extensively proliferative capacity.   In these in vitro experiments four cultured cell lines including Yoshida sarcoma, L-1210 leukemia, P3HRI and OAT derived from oat cell carcinoma of the
lung were used.   In cultured L-1210 cells colony-forming
efficiency was 99.5%.   The survival tumor cells following exposure to varied concentrations of anticancer drugs
at a given period of time were determined by soft agar
cloning assay using the four cell lines.

   Figure 1 illustrates cell-killing curves of 5-FU.

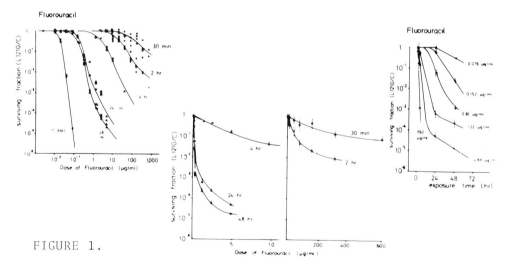

FIGURE 1.

Dose response curves plotted on logarithmic scale of
L-1210 cell-killing patterns against 5-FU at various
exposure time are shown in the upper left of the figure.
When the exposure time was 30 minutes, no more than 2 log
cells in 10^6 cell population could be killed, despite of
high concentrations of 5-FU.   The result thus indicates

that the action of 5-FU is cytostatic at shorter exposure time.

On the contrary, cells were effectively killed with longer exposure time, in spite of lower concentration of 5-FU; for example, at 11th day of exposure with a concentration of less than 10^{-2} μg/ml. The semi-log plotted dose response curves shown in the lower left of Figure 1 confirmed the above tendency. The surviving fraction curves initially declined exponentially with exposure times of more than 24 hours, and finally reached to the point where an increase of concentration resulted in no further cell kill. The dose response curves became plateau at this point. The maximum reduction in the surviving fraction of L-1210 cells was dependent on the duration of exposure time of 5-FU, but independent on the concentration of 5-FU. The semi-log plotted curves of exposure shown in the right portion of the figure indicate that the action of 5-FU is time-dependent. The cell-killing effect becomes more profound with prolonged exposure time, despite of low concentrations of 5-FU.

The cell-killing curves of FT are shown in Figure 2, which suggest that FT possess a greater tendency of time-dependency compared with 5-FU. Thus, cell-killing patterns of 5-FU and FT could be summarized as; 1) cytostatic, 2) concentration-independent, and 3) time-dependent. The experimental results strongly suggest that a low dose of FT be administered for a longer period of time in order to provide total killing of L-1210 cells;

that is, a long-term administration of low dose FT is more effective than a short-term administration of high dose of FT.

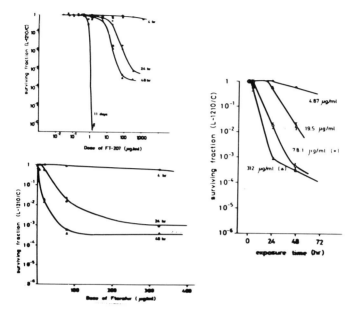

FIGURE 2. Cell-killing curves of FT

The minimum inhibitory concentrations (MIC) of 5-FU and FT at 11th day of exposure were approximately 0.05 μg/ml and 6 μg/ml. The reduction of 1 log cell in 10^6 cells implies a more than 90% tumor regression in a clinical setting, which is highly attractive for cancer chemotherapists.

Our experimental studies have demonstrated that alkylating agents and anticancer antibiotics such as adriamycin and mitomycin C exhibit characteristics of concentration-dependency, in contrast to time-dependent agents such as antimetabolites, vinca alkaloids and L-asparaginase(4,5,6,7).

150

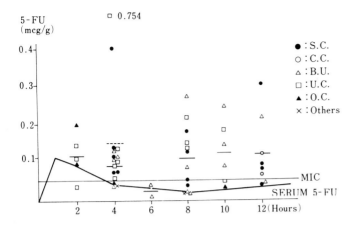

S.C. : Stomach cancer, C.C. : Colon cancer, B.C. : Breast cancer,
U.C. : Uterus cancer, O.C. : Ovarian cancer.

FIGURE 3. 5-FU levels in tumor tissues after
administration of 300 mg of UFT

3. PHARMACOKINETICS

Pharmacokinetic studies on 5-FU and FT in animals
revealed that FT was absorbed rapidly from gastrointestinal tract, and in blood the concentration of 5-FU, an
active substance of FT, remained higher and longer in
comparison with that of intravenous administration of FT
(8,9). This finding led to an oral use of FT.

The aim of UFT therapy is to enhance chemotherapeutic effects of FT by high 5-FU concentration and long-lasting
5-FU levels in tumor tissues, with less toxicity to the
host. With a purpose of confirming 5-FU concentration
in tumor tissues after UFT administration, UFT at a dose
of 200 mg/m^2 was given to patients with various types of
cancer at 2, 4, 6, 8 and 12 hours prior to operation.
Both 5-FU and FT levels in tumor and normal tissues of
48 operated cases were measured. 5-FU levels in blood

151

and tumor tissues after administration of 200 mg/m^2 of UFT are depicted in Figure 3.

In spite of a decrease in blood level of 5-FU at 4 hours after UFT administration, 5-FU levels in tumor tissues remained high; exceeding of 0.05 μg which is determined as MIC. 5-FU levels in serum, normal and tumor tissues at 4, 8, and 12 hours after 200 mg/m^2 UFT administration to patients with stomach cancer are shown in Figure 4

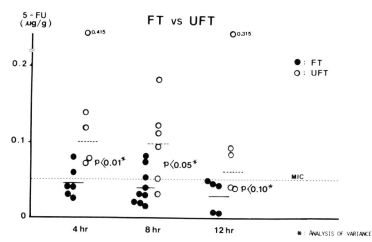

FIGURE 4. 5-FU levels in serum, normal and tumor tissues after administration of 200 mg/m^2 of UFT

5-FU levels in tumor tissues were 1.5 to 3 times higher than those in normal or serum, suggesting selective toxicity of UFT for stomach cancer. 5-FU levels in tumor tissues at 4, 8, and 12 hours after administration of 200 mg/m^2 of either FT alone or UFT in patients with stomach cancer are shown in Figure 5. 5-FU levels after UFT administration were significantly higher compared to FT alone. Consequently, clinical efficacy of UFT was expected.

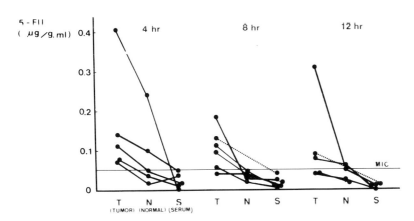

FIGURE 5.   5-FU levels in tumor tissues after administration of 200 mg/m^2 of UFT versus 200 mg/m^2 of FT alone

4.   CLINICAL STUDY

A Phase I study of UFT on 170 patients with various solid tumors was performed in 21 institutions(10).
At single doses of 2-20 mg/kg of UFT, nausea was associated in a few patients.   Subsequently, UFT was administered on a daily chronic schedule with escalating doses from 100 mg/day up to 900 mg/day.   The dose-limiting toxicity was gastrointestinal disturbance such as nausea, vomiting and diarrhea, which occurred in most patients receiving a daily dose of more than 750 mg.   An optimal dose on a daily chronic schedule was determined to be 200 mg/m^2/day.

In our current study UFT was given at a dose of 200 mg/m^2 b.i.d. to a total of 16 patients with advanced gastric cancer: one complete and 6 partial responses (43.7%) were obtained and the remaining 9 patients showed stable disease.   Later on 5 patients were included in this study and all patients were subsequently administered a

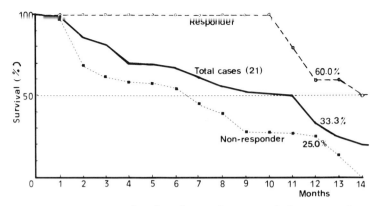

FIGURE 6. Survival of patients with gastric cancer after onset of UFT therapy

combination of UFT and mitomycin C (UFTM). The median duration of survival was 14 months for responders, while that for non-responders was 6.3 months, with an overall survival of 11 months as shown in Figure 6.

Major toxicity encountered during UFT treatment included mild diarrhea and skin pigmentation which occurred in approximately 10% of the patients; however, neither hematologic nor hepatic toxicity was observed.

5. CASE REPORT

Figures 7, 8 and 9 show the cases effectively treated with UFT of 200 mg/m^2 b.i.d. orally.
Case 1 (M.N.): A 77-year old female was referred to National Nagoya Hospital due to abdominal pain and an abdominal mass having a diagnosis of advanced gastric cancer, with a palpable tumor of 5x5 cm in size at epigastric region. Borrmann type 2 cancer was developed at gastric angle area and the biopsy of the lesion revealed a well-differentiated adenocarcinoma (Figure 7-a). UFT at a dose of 200 mg/m^2 orally b.i.d. was initiated and the

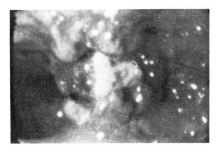 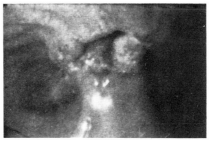

a) before UFT therapy   b) 3 wks after therapy

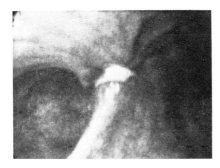 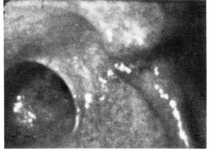

c) 7 wks after therapy   d) 3 mos after therapy

FIGURE 7.   Gastroendoscopic changes after UFT therapy
            (Case 1:M.N.)

shrinkages of tumor size and carcinomatous ulcer were
observed at 3 weeks after onset of UFT treatment (Figure
7-b).   Further improvement of the lesion was evident at
7 weeks from initiation of UFT by endoscoy (Figure 7-c).
At 3 months ulcer was disappeared (Figure 7-d).   She
received UFT in out-patient clinic and survived for 3.5
years.   This case suggests that a long-term administration of UFT is essential in order to achieve complete
response.

Case 2 (K.S.): A 75-year old male visited our Hospital
due to dysphagia and emaciation.   Radiographic examination revealed a remarkable narrowness of the gastric cavity due to invasion of gastric cancer (Figure 8-a).   One

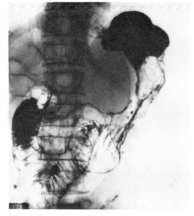 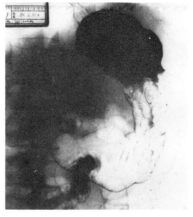

a) before UFT therapy   b) 8 wks after therapy

FIGURE 8. Changes on X-ray film after UFT therapy
(Case 2:K.S.) A defect shadow on X-ray
film was remarkably improved after UFT
therapy.

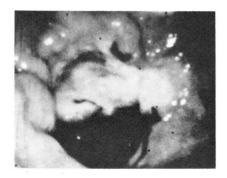 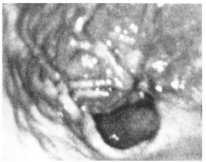

a) before UFT therapy   b) after UFT therapy

FIGURE 9. Gastroendoscopic changes after UFT therapy
(Case 3:T.M.) Gastric cancer of Borrmann
type 2, 6 cm in diameter fluoroscopically,
at the anterior wall of the corpus(a) was
improved, showing a p.m. type-like appearance of gastric cancer after 5 wks of
UFT therapy.

month after onset of UFT treatment the narrowness of gastric wall was reduced in association with subjective improvement of dysphagia (Figure 8-b).   However, UFT treatment was discontinued since thrombocytopenia was developed.   The patient survived for 5 months.

156

Case 3 (I.M.). A 81 year-old female admitted due to a sudden episode of massive hematemesis was diagnosed as gastric cancer of Borrmann type 2 adenocarcinoma (Figure 9-a). Endoscopic findings at 5 weeks after onset of UFT therapy showed flatness and disappearance of malignant regions surrounding cancerous ulcer (Figure 9-b).

6.   DISCUSSION

UFT has demonstrated its selectively higher concentration and longer retention of 5-FU in tumor tissues of gastrointestinal and other tumors compared to those in normal tissues of humans.   Similar results eliciting the difference of 5-FU concentration in normal and tumor tissues are reported by Taguchi et al(11) and Fukui et al (12).

A 43.7% response rate with a median survival of more than one year in responders was obtained in our current study on UFT, which is superior to a 22% in 41 evaluable patients treated with FT alone, achieving the median survivals of 10.5 months for responders and 4.8 months for non-responders(13).   Summarizing published data of UFT a 27.5% response rate was accumulated in 49 responders of 178 patients(14). Furue et al, on the contrary, reviewed published literature concerning oral FT and reported an overall response rate of 20.2% for advanced gastric cancer(15).

A comparative retrospective analysis of clinical efficacy of UFT versus FT elucidates benefits of UFT therapy: UFT achieved 10 partial responses (28%) of 30 evaluable patients with advanced gastric cancer, whereas FT alone yielded 8 partial responses (24.4%) of 33 patients (16). In addition, gastrointestinal toxicity associated with UFT was nearly identical to that associated with FT. Pigmentation was observed in the minority of patients.

Fujii et al have indicated that the enhancement of antitumor effect of UFT depends on inhibition of degradation of 5-FU and increase of phosphorylation activity from 5-FU to F-dUMP. In order to confirm this hypothesis we explored our study on thymidine phosphorylase activity using normal and tumor tissues of human stomach cancer. The result demonstrated that thymidine phosphorylase activity in tumor tissues was significantly greater than that in normal tissues, suggesting that FT be transformed to 5-FU in tumor tissues.

In conclusion, a combination of uracil and FT(UFT) has enhanced antitumor activity of FT against gastric cancer, without increasing toxicity of FT.

Recently, a clinical study of UFT has been extended to a Phase III study of UFT in combination with mitomycin C (UFTM therapy) for the treatment of gastric cancer. Details of UFTM trials are presented by Suga et al in this volume (17).

REFERENCES

1. Fujii S, Ikenaka K, Fukushima M et al. (1978) Effect
   of uracil and its derivatives on antitumor activity
   of 5-fluorouracil and its derivatives on antitumor
   activity of 5-fluorouracil and 1-(2-tetrahydrofuryl)-
   5-fluorouracil. Gann 69: 763-777.

2. Fujii S, Kitano K, Ikenaka T et al. (1979) Effect
   of co-administration of uracil or cytosine on the
   antitumor activity of clinical doses of 1-(2-tetra-
   hydrofuryl)-5-fluorouracil and levels of 5-fluoroura-
   cil in rodents. Gann 70: 209-214.

3. Fujii S, Ikenaka K, Shirasaka T (1984) Attempts on
   enhancement of antitumor activity of masked fluoropyrimidines. In: Fluoropyrimidines in Cancer Therapy.
   (eds) K Kimura, S Fujii, M Ogawa, GP Bodey and P
   Alberto, Excerpta Medica, Amsterdam (this volume).

4. Shimoyama M (1975) Cytocidal action of anticancer
   agents: Evaluation of the sensitivity of cultured
   animal and human cancer cells. In: Comparative Leukemia Research 1973, Leukemogenesis. (eds) Y Ito and
   RM Dutcher, University of Tokyo Press, Tokyo, pp.
   711-722.

5. Shimoyama M (1976) Implication of cell-kill-kinetics
   of anticancer agents in the design of optimal therapeutic schedules. Jpn J Cancer Chemother 3: 1103-1110.

6. Kimura K, Kumaoka S, Kanagami H et al. (1972) Chemotherapy of cancer (16). Theory and practice of oral
   administration of anticancer drugs. 69th Annual
   Meetings of Japanese Society of Internal Medicine,
   p. 981 (Abstract).

7. Kimura K (1975) Studies on a device of administration
   methods of anticancer drugs and its clinical effects.
   Jpn Geriat Med 13: 97-101

8. Fujita J, Kimura K (1971) Characteristic patterns
   of in vivo distribution of various anti-cancer agents.
   In: Advances in Antimicrobial and Antineoplastic
   Chemotherapy. (eds) M Hejzla, M Semonsky and S Masák,
   Urban & Schwarzenberg,München-Berlin-Wien, pp. 313-
   316.

9. Fujita H (1971) Comparative studies on the blood level,
   tissue distribution, excretion and inactivation of
   anticancer drugs. Jpn J Clin Oncol 12: 151-162

10. Taguchi T, Furue H, Koyama Y et al. (1980) Phase I study of UTF (uracil plus futraful preparation). Jpn J Cancer Chemother 7: 966-972.

11. Taguchi T, Nakano Y, Fujii S et al. (1978) Determination of 5-fluorouracil levels in tumors, blood, and other tissues. Jpn J Cancer Chemother 5: 1167-1172.

12. Fukui Y, Imabayashi N, Nishi M et al. (1980) Clinical study on the enhancement of drug delivery into tumor tissue by using UFT. Jpn J Cancer Chemother 7: 2124-2129.

13. Konda C (1975) The effect of oral and rectal administration of N-(2-tetrahydrofuryl)-5-fluorouracil in the treatment of advanced cancer. Jpn J Cancer Clin 21: 1044-1050.

14. Suga S, Kimura K, Yokoyama Y et al. (1982) Studies on the designing of chemotherapy for gastric cancer in man, based on the tumor tissue concentration of anticancer agents. Gastroenterologia Japonica 17: 295-300.

15. Furue H, Nakao I, Kaneko T et al. (1975) Chemotherapy for gastric cancer. Jpn J Cancer Chemother 2: 351-359.

16. Watanabe H, Yamamoto S, Naito T (1980) Clinical results of oral UFT therapy under cooperative study. Jpn J Cancer Chemother 71: 1588-1596.

17. Suga S, Kimura K, Yoshida Y et al. (1984) UFTM chemotherapy for gastric cancer: Effectiveness and survival between UFTM and surgical treatment in patients with Borrmann type 4 gastric cancer. In: Fluoropyrimidines in Cancer Therapy. (eds) K Kimura, S Fujii, M Ogawa, GP Bodey and P Alberto, Excerpta Medica, Amsterdam (this volume).

Fluoropyrimidines in Cancer Therapy
K. Kimura, S. Fujii, M. Ogawa, G.P. Bodey, P. Alberto, eds.

CLINICAL STUDIES OF A NEW FLUORINATED PYRIMIDINE, 1-HEXYLCARBAMOYL-5-FLUOROURACIL (HCFU)

Yoshiyuki Koyama and The Cooperative Study
Group of HCFU

1-Hexylcarbamoyl-5-fluorouracil (HCFU) was developed by Hoshi, Kuretani and others of the National Cancer Center Research Institute, as one of a number of masked compounds of 5-FU in 1976 (1).

The compound has marked antitumor activity against L-1210 and C-1498, ascites sarcoma 180, Nakahara-Fukuoka sarcoma, adenocarcinoma 755 and Ehrlich's ascites carcinoma (2). It has also antitumor activity by oral administration against Lewis lung carcinoma (3, 4), B16 melanoma (3) and spontaneous mammary carcinoma in mice (5). The drug orally administered has a wider antitumor spectrum and a greater antitumor activity against mouse leukemia than 5-FU and tegafur (3).

The chemical structure of HCFU is given in Figure 1. Coversion to 5-FU is considered either directly (without being subjected to enzymatic changes) or through intermediate metabolites such as 1-ω-carboxypentylcarbamoyl-5-FU (CPEFU) and 1-ω-carboxypropylcarbamoyl-5-FU (CPRFU) by hepatic enzymes (6, 7) (FIGURE 2).

FIGURE 1   Structure of 1-hexylcarbamoyl-5-fluorouracil (HCFU) (M. Wt. 257.26).

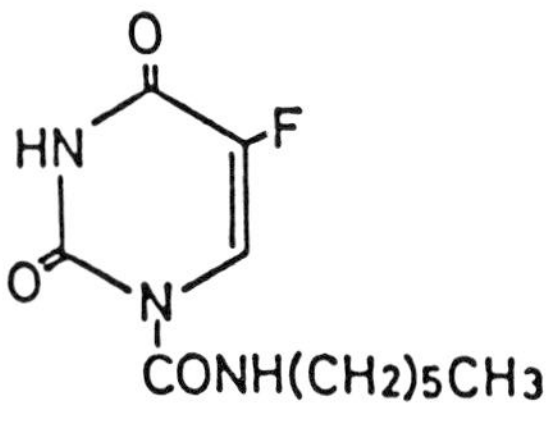

FIGURE 2   Possible metabolic pathways of HCFU.

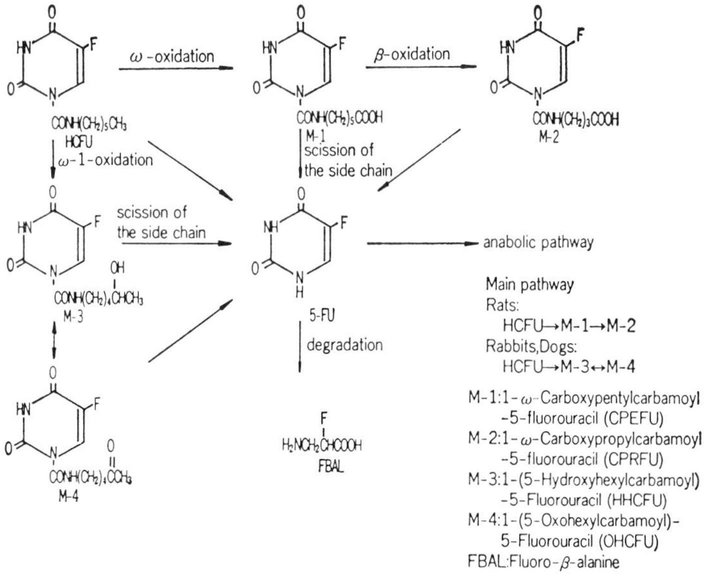

Pharmacokinetic study : Fujita (8) studied pharmacokinetics of HCFU in rabbits and mice bearing Sarcoma 180. HCFU orally adminis- tered was gradually absorbed from gastrointestinal tracts, and HCFU and its metabolites (CPEFU, CPRFU etc.) persisted for several hours in the tissues and they were successively converted to 5-FU. HCFU, its metabolites and 5-FU distributed highly in the stomach, kidney and urinary bladder and slightly in the brain and spleen. A relati- vely high concentration of 5-FU was detected in tumor tissues and the lung, lip, rectum, skin etc.

The production of 5-FU from HCFU was not influenced by pre- treatment of phenobarbital and glutathione or CCl_4. This indicates that conversion of HCFU to 5-FU is not mainly depend on the liver.

The serum levels of HCFU fraction (HCFU and its metabolites) and 5-FU by a single dose of HCFU administered orally in cancer patients, are shown in FIGURE 3 (10). Their maximum serum levels were found

162

two to four hours after administration and gradually decreased there-after. Their serum levels were dependent on doses given.

FIGURE 3   Serum concentrations of 5-FU and HCFU fraction.

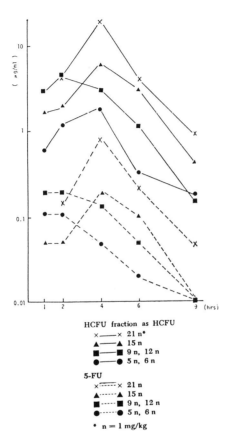

HCFU fraction as HCFU
×————× 21 n*
▲————▲ 15 n
■————■ 9 n, 12 n
●————● 5 n, 6 n

5-FU
×┄┄┄× 21 n
▲┄┄┄▲ 15 n
■┄┄┄■ 9 n, 12 n
●┄┄┄● 5 n, 6 n

* n = 1 mg/kg

Phase I Study : A phase I study of HCFU was done in 11 institutions of the Co-operative Study Group of HCFU (11). The characteristic toxic effects were a transient hot sensation and pollakiuria, which occurred 15 - 120 minutes after oral administration and continued for 30 minutes to four hours and then subsided spontaneously. Gastrointestinal disturbances such as nausea, vomiting, anorexia and diarrhea, which are common with 5-FU administration, also occurred but did less frequently. Hematopoietic and hepatic toxicities were slight and no renal or other cumulative toxicity was observed.

The maximum tolerated dose for a single oral administration was estimated to be between 400 and 500 mg/m^2 and the optimal daily dose for continuous administration was considered to be between 300 and 600 mg/m^2, with divided daily administration. From results of serum levels studies, the favorable clinical dose was 200 mg every six hours (800 mg/day), maintaining the serum level of 5-FU more than 0.1 μg/ml for 24 hours (12).

To clarify the cause of these characteristic toxicity, Horikomi and others (13) investigated the effects of HCFU and its main metabolite CPEFU on the single neuron activity of the preoptic area in the rat and found that electrophoretic application of HCFU or CPEFU increased the discharge rate of warm-sensitive neurons and decreased the rate of cold-sensitive neurons. They found, moreover, that sulpiride, a neuroleptic agent, inhibits spontaneous discharge of warm-sensitive neurons and facilitates that of cold-sensitive neurons. These findings suggest that the heat sensation caused by HCFU might be explained by its effect on the thermosensitive neurons in the pre-optic area and may be relieved with sulpiride.

Horikomi and others (14) also found that CPEFU markedly accelerates bladder movement in the cat, rabbit and rat. This phenomenon disappeared in the spinal cord cat and postcollicular-midpontine decerebrated cat, but still remained in the intercollicular-prepontine decerebrated cat. This suggests that pollakiuria caused by HCFU is due to CPEFU stimulation on the micturition reflex center in the brain stem. Chlorpromazine and sulpiride inhibit the acceleration of bladder movement and relieved pollakiuria caused by HCFU.

164

Phase II Study : A phase II study (15, 16, 17, 18) was performed in thirty-six institutions (TABLE 1), on nationwide scale, beginning September 1978. Patients, histologically diagnosed as having a carcinoma and who had progressive disease, performance status of 0 to 3 and no intense disturbances in renal, hepatic and/or bone marrow functions, were selected. Pretreated cases had to have a two-weeks therapy-free interval after their last treatment and had to show no evidence of effectiveness of treatment.

TABLE 1 Co-operative study group of HCFU

Yoichi Kasai, M.D.	[1] Hokkaido University, Faculty of Medicine
Takeo Wada, M.D.	[2] Sapporo Medical College
Akira Wakui, M.D.	[3] The Research Institute for Tuberculosis and Cancer, Tohoku University
Sei-ichi Yoshida, M.D.	[4] Saitama Cancer Center Hospital
Osamu Takatani, M.D.	[5] National Defense Medical College Hospital
Hisashi Majima, M.D.	[6] Chiba Cancer Center Hospital
Hiroshi Sato, M.D.	[7] University of Chiba, School of Medicine
Yoshiyuki Koyama, M.D. (Chairman)	[8] National Medical Center Hospital
Yasuo Koyama, M.D.	[9] National Cancer Center Hospital
Tatsuo Saito, M.D., and	[10] Cancer Institute and Cancer Chemotherapy Center,
Makoto Ogawa, M.D.	Japanese Foundation for Cancer Research
Ichiji Ito, M.D.	[11] Tokyo Metropolitan Komagome Hospital
Yoshio Hara, M.D.	[12] Tokyo Metropolitan Ebara Hospital
Hisashi Furue, M.D.	[13] Teikyo University, School of Medicine
Satoru Kasama, M.D., and	[14] University of Tokyo, Faculty of Medicine
Tadao Niijima, M.D.	
Hikoo Shirakabe, M.D.	[15] Juntendo University, School of Medicine
Kazuei Ogoshi, M.D.	[16] Niigata Cancer Center Hospital
Terukazu Muto, M.D.	[17] Niigata University, School of Medicine
Nobu Hattori, M.D.	[18] Kanazawa University, Faculty of Medicine
Kiyoji Kimura, M.D.	[19] National Nagoya Hospital
Kazuo Ohta, M.D.	[20] Aichi Cancer Center Hospital
Tatsuhei Kondo, M.D.	[21] Nagoya University, School of Medicine
Toru Yasutomi, M.D.	[22] National Kyoto Hospital
Haruto Uchino, M.D., and	[23] Kyoto University, Faculty of Medicine
Yorinori Hikasa, M.D.	
Susumu Majima, M.D.	[24] Kyoto Prefectural University of Medicine
Toshio Terasawa, M.D.	[25] Center for Adult Diseases
Goro Kozaki, M.D.	[26] Osaka University, Medical School
Tetsuo Taguchi, M.D.	[27] Research Institute for Microbial Disease, Osaka University
Katsuji Sakai, M.D.	[28] Osaka City University, Medical School
Takashi Shimoyama, M.D.	[29] Hyogo College of Medicine
Shigemasa Koga, M.D.	[30] Tottori University, School of Medicine
Ikuroh Kimura, M.D., and	[31] Okayama University, Medical School
Kunzo Orita, M.D.	
Takao Hattori, M.D.	[32] Research Institute for Nuclear Medicine and Biology, Hiroshima University
Motonosuke Furusawa, M.D.	[33] National Kyushu Cancer Center Hospital
Kiyoshi Inokuchi, M.D.	[34] Kyushu University, Faculty of Medicine
Mansei Nishi, M.D.	[35] Kagoshima University, School of Medicine
Kazuo Yunoki, M.D.	[36] Institute for Cancer Research, Faculty of Medicine, Kagoshima University

HCFU (300   600 mg/m^2) was orally administered in two to four divided doses in form of tablets or fine granules every day for more than four weeks, until side effects appeared. The number of patients entered in the study was three hundred and sixty; 172 males and 188 females. Age of patients ranged from five to 86 years and the median age was 59.7.

Results of the HCFU treatment were evaluated by the committee on evaluation of clinical effects of HCFU (Chairman : Dr. Saito, Co-operative Study Group of HCFU) according to the Criteria of Japan Society for Cancer Therapy for "Evaluation of Clinical Effects of Cancer Chemotherapy on Solid Tumors" (19, 20) (TABLES 2 and 3), which are almost the same as those of WHO (21). In cases of malignant pleural or peritoneal effusion, complete response (CR) is assumed when disappearance of tumor cell in the fluid and complete disappearance of effusion are obtained, by two observations not less than four weeks apart (TABLE 4).

TABLE 2   Objective response in measurable disease

1. *Complete response (CR)*.	The disappearance of all known disease, determined by 2 observations not less than 4 weeks apart.
2. *Partial response (PR)*.	(1) 50% or more decrease in total tumor size of the bidimensionally measurable lesions which have been measured to determine the effect of therapy by 2 observations not less than 4 weeks apart. (2) 30% or more decrease in total tumor size of the single dimension which have been measured to determine the effect of therapy by 2 observations not less than 4 weeks apart. In addition, there can be no appearance of new lesions or progression of any lesion.
3. *No change (NC)*.	A 50% decrease (or a 30% decrease in single dimension) in total tumor size cannot be established nor has a 25% increase in the size of one or more measurable lesions been demonstrated.
4. *Progressive disease (PD)*.	A 25% or more increase in the size of one or more measurable lesions, or the appearance of new lesions.

TABLE 3   Objective response in unmeasurable disease

1. *Complete response (CR)*.	Complete disappearance of all known disease for at least 4 weeks.
2. *Partial response (PR)*.	Estimated decrease in tumour size of 50% or more for at least 4 weeks.
3. *No change (NC)*.	No significant change for at least 4 weeks. This includes stable disease, estimated decrease of less than 50%, and lesions with estimated increase of less than 25%.
4. *Progressive disease (PD)*.	Appearance of any new lesion not previously identified or estimated increase of 25% or more in existent lesions.

TABLE 4   Tentative criteria for the evaluation of malignant pleural or peritoneal effusion

A. *Complete response (CR)*
Disappearance of tumor cells in pleural or peritoneal effusion and the complete disappearance of pleural or peritoneal effusion by 2 observations not less than 4 weeks apart.
B. *Partial response (PR)*
Disappearance of tumor cells in pleural or peritoneal effusion and the distinct reduction of pleural or peritoneal effusion by 2 observations not less than 4 weeks apart.
C. *No response*
Failure in A and B.

274 out of 360 cases were evaluable and there were 252 cases of solid tumors (108 gastric carcinoma, 53 breast cancer, 41 colorectal carcinoma and others) and 22 cases of malignant effusion (TABLE 5). There were 11 cases excluded in which radio- or chemotherapy of other drugs was combined during HCFU treatment, 67 cases dropped out in which HCFU treatment was less than four weeks and 8 unevaluable cases. There were 5 CRs (4 breast and one colorectum) and 55 PRs (21 stomach, 16 colorectum, 15 breast, each one of pancreas, lung and other) and the response rate (RR) was 23.8% in solid tumors. In gastric carcinoma, there were 21 PRs and the rate was 19.4%, whereas in colorectal carcinoma, there were one CR and 16 PRs and the RR was 41.5%. In mammary carcinoma, there were 4CRs and 15 PRs and the RR was 35.8%. In cases of malignant effusions, there were 7CRs (4 stomach, 2 ovary and one unknown) with 31.8% response rate. There were 4CRs out of 9

cases in gastric carcinoma and the RR was 44.4%, and 2 CRs out of 2
cases in ovarian carcinoma (TABLE 6).

TABLE 5   Evaluation of HCFU in solid tumor

Primary sites	No. of entered cases	No. of evaluated cases	No. of cases				Response rate %	
			CR	PR	NC	PD		
Esophagus	4	3	–	–	–	3	0	(0/3)
Stomach	140	108	–	21	56	31	19.4	(21/108)
Pancreas	6	3	–	1	2	–	33	(1/3)
Liver	29	18	–	–	14	4	0	(0/18)
Colorectum	55	41	1	16	14	10	41.5	(17/41)
Lung	14	10	–	1	5	4	10	(1/10)
Breast	65	53	4	15	24	10	35.8	(19/53)
Kidney	2	2	–	–	2	–	0	(0/2)
Uterus	1	1	–	–	1	–	0	(0/1)
Ovary	3	2	–	–	2	–	0	(0/2)
Others	9	7	–	–	6	1	0	(0/7)
Unknown	5	4	–	1	1	2	25	(1/4)
Total	333	252	5	55	127	65	23.8	(60/252)

Excluded cases   10   (During HCFU treatment combined other therapy)
Dropped cases   63   (HCFU treatment less than 4 weeks)
Unevaluated cases 8
                                      (HCFU Co-operative Study Group)

TABLE 6   Evaluation of HCFU in malignant pleural or peritoneal
           effusion

Primary sites	No. of entered cases	No. of evaluated cases	Response CR	No response	Response rate %	
Esophagus	1	1	–	1	0	
Stomach	11	9	4	5	44.4	(4/9)
Pancreas	2	2	–	2	0	
Colorectum	4	3	–	3	0	
Lung	1	1	–	1	0	
Breast	2	1	–	1	0	
Uterus	1	1	–	1	0	
Ovary	2	2	2	–	100	(2/2)
Others	2	1	–	1	0	
Unknown	1	1	1	–	100	(1/1)
	27	22	7	15	31.8	(7/22)

(HCFU Co-operative Study Group)

The average period of overall partial response was 13.4 weeks and that of complete response was 31.1 weeks. A significant difference $(p < 0.05)$ was observed between the response rate obtained with a daily dose of 400 mg/m^2 or more and that seen when lower doses were used (TABLE 7).

TABLE 7   Relation between daily dose and response rate of HCFU

| Daily dose (mg/m²) | No. of cases | | | | Response rate % |
	Response*	No change†	Progressive‡ disease	Total	
< 300	5	16	6	27	18.5
300 ≤	11	28	22	61	18.0
400 ≤	18	27	16	61	29.5§
500 ≤	11	9	5	25	44.0§
600 ≤	1	2	1	4	25.0§
Total	46	82	50	178	25.8

* CR + PR + response in effusion.
† NC.
‡ PD + no response in effusion.
§ Significant difference $(P < 0.05)$.

Toxicity of HCFU was studied in the 360 cases entered. 152 cases (42.2%) showed some side effects, with most experiencing a hot sensation (16.4%), then pollakiuria (15.3%), anorexia (16.9%), nausea and vomiting (13.1%), general fatigue (11.7%), urgency to defecate (6.4%), and diarrhea (5.8%) (TABLE 8). Among the side effects, those which were peculiar to HCFU were transient hot sensation, pollakiuria and urgency to defecate. These kinds of side effects were mainly observed early in the treatment (FIGURE 4) and they were controlled by sulpiride and chlorpromazine.

TABLE 8   Toxicity of HCFU

	No. of cases		Incidence %
Entered cases	360		
Cases without toxicity	208		57.8
Cases with toxicity	152		42.2
Anorexia	61	(9)	16.9
Hot sensation	59	(7)	16.4
Pollakiuria	55	(8)	15.3
Nausea or vomiting	47	(11)	13.1
General fatique	42	(3)	11.7
Urgency to defecate	23	(3)	6.4
Diarrhea	21	(1)	5.8
Sweat	10		2.7
Fever	8		2.2
Dizziness	6		1.7
Skin rash	5	(2)	1.4
Oral ulcer	4	(1)	1.1
Epilation	4		1.1
Pigmentation	3		0.8
Tendency to bleeding	2		0.6
Others	13	(2)	3.6

( ) : Cases in which treatment was discontinued
due to toxicity

The incidence of hematological toxicity of grade 2 or more by the WHO grading was observed to be 5.9% for hemoglobin, 2.8% for white blood cells, 1.8% for the platelet count. Incidence of hepatic and renal toxicity of grade 1 or more was 2.6% for total bilirubin, 2.3% for SGOT, 1.7% for SGPT, 3.8% for BUN and 2.8% for creatinine (TABLE 9).

A phase III study is going on comparing HCFU to tegafur or 5-FU combined with mitomycin C or adriamycin in gastric and colorectal carcinoma on a nationwide scale. Combined treatment of HCFU with radiotherapy is performed in head and neck tumors.

FIGURE 4   Time of appearance of (a) hot sensation (43 cases), (b) pollakiuria (41 cases) and (c) urgency to defecate (17 cases) after the first day of treatment

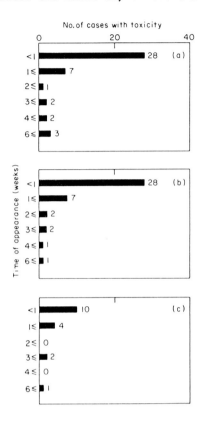

TABLE 9   Hematological, hepatic and renal toxic effects of HCFU by WHO grading

Item	Hematology (Grade 2 by WHO)			Biochemistry (Grade 1 by WHO)				
	WBC	Hb	Pl	T.Bil	GOT	GPT	BUN	Creat
Patients tested	251	185	224	156	177	177	157	108
Abnormal cases	7	11	4	4	4	3	6	3
Incidence (%)	2.8	5.9	1.8	2.6	2.3	1.7	3.8	2.8

SUMMARY AND CONCLUSION :

1-Hexylcarbamoyl-5-fluorouracil (HCFU), a masked compound of
5-FU, has a wider antitumor spectrum than 5-FU and tegafur.

Co-operative phase I and II studies have been carried out in 36
institutions. Optimal daily doses for clinical use ranged from 300
to 600 mg/m^2 and a higher response rate was obtained with doses of
400 mg/m^2 or more. The drug is available in case whose liver function is disturbed.

360 cases were entered in the study and 274 cases were evaluable.
Partial responses (PR) were obtained 21 out of 108 evaluable cases
with gastric carcinoma and the response rate (RR) was 19.4%. In 41
colorectal carcinoma the rate was 41.5%, including one complete response (CR) and 16 PRs. The RR in breast cancer was 35.8%, with 4CRs
and 15 PRs. Overall response rate of solid tumors were 23.8%,
including 5 CRs and 55 PRs. The average period of partial response
was 13.4 weeks and that of CR was 31.1 weeks.

The incidence of gastrointestinal toxicities, such as anorexia,
nausea, vomiting, was similar to those of 5-FU and tegafur. However,
unusual central nervous toxicities such as hot sensation, pollakiuria
and urgency to defecate were observed in approximately 16% of the
cases, early in the treatment and these side effects could be controlled by sulpiride.

REFERENCES :

1. Hoshi A, Iigo M, Nakamura A, Yoshida M, Kuretani K.
   (1976) Antitumor activity of 1-hexylcarbamoyl-5-fluorouracil in
   a variety of experimental tumors. Gann 67 : 725-731.

2. Hoshi A, Yoshida M, Inomata M, Iigo M, Ando N, Kuretani
   K. (1980) Antitumor activity of metabolites of 1-hexylcarbamoyl-

5-fluorouracil and related compounds against L1210 leukemia in vivo and L5178Y lymphoma cell in vitro. J Pharm Dyn 3 : 478-481.

3. Iigo M, Hoshi A, Nakamura A, Kuretani A. (1978) Antitumor activity of 1-hexylcarbamoyl-5-fluorouracil in Lewis lung carcinoma and B16 melanoma. J Pharm Dyn 1 : 49-54.

4. Tsuruo T, Iida H, Naganuma K, Tsukagoshi S, Sakurai Y. (1980) Inhibition of murine colon adenocarcinomas and Lewis lung carcinoma by 1-hexylcarbamoyl-5-fluorouracil. Cancer Chemother Pharmacol 4 : 83-87.

5. Tokuzen R, Iigo M, Hoshi A, Kuretani K. (1980) Effects of 1-hexylcarbamoyl-5-fluorouracil on spontaneous mammary adenocarcinoma in mice. Gann 71 : 724-728.

6. Kobari T, Iguro Y, Ujiie A, Namekawa H. (1980) Metabolism of 1-hexylcarbamoyl-5-fluorouracil, a new antitumor agent, in rats, rabbits and dogs. Current Chemotherapy and Infectious Disease, Amer Society of Microbiology : 1584-1586.

7. Kono A, Tanaka M, Eguchi S, Hara Y. (1979) Determination of 1-hexylcarbamoyl-5-fluorouracil and its metabolites in biomedical specimens by high-performance liquid chromatography. J Chromatography 163: 109-113.

8. Fujita H, Ogawa K. (1981) In vivo distribution and activation of 1-hexylcarbamoyl-5-fluorouracil (HCFU). Jpn J Clin Pharmacol Ther 12 : 233-243.

9. Okabayashi K, Koyama Y, Maruyama K, Okazaki N, Sakano T, Ise T. (1979) Clinical trials of a new antitumor drug, 1-hexylcarbamoyl-5-fluorouracil. Jpn J Clin Oncol 9 : 35-39.

10. Koyama Y. & HCFU Clinical Study Group (1980) Absorption and excretion of a new oral antitumor drug, 1-hexylcarbamoyl-5-fluorouracil (HCFU) in cancer patients. Jpn J Clin Oncol 10 : 83-92

11. Koyama Y, Koyama Y. (1980) Phase I study of a new antitumor drug, 1-hexylcarbamoyl-5-fluorouracil (HCFU) administered orally : An HCFU Clinical Study Group Report. Cancer Treat Rep 64 : 861-867.

12. Hara Y, Kono A, Tanaka M. (1982) Clinical study of 5-fluorouracil (5-FU) serum concentration by oral administration of a new fluorinated pyrimidine, 1-hexylcarbamoyl-5-fluorouracil (HCFU). Jpn J Cancer Chemother 9: 293-300.

13. Horikomi K, Muramoto K, Araki K, Henmi Z, Sakai K. (1980) Effects of 1-hexylcarbamoyl-5-fluorouracil (HCFU) and 1-ω-carboxypentylcarbamoyl-5-fluorouracil (CPEFU) on hypothalamic neurons

in the rat.   Jpn J Clin Pharmacol Ther 11: 17-25.

14. Horikomi K, Ozeki K, Mitsushima T, Henmi Z, Maruyama K,
    Majima H, Sakai Y. (1980) Effects of 1-hexylcarbamoyl-5-
    fluorouracil (HCFU) and its metabolites on bladder movement (in
    Japanese) Jpn J Clin Pharmacol Ther 11 : 27-36.

15. Koyama Y. (1980) Phase II study of a new fluorinated pyrimidine,
    1-hexylcarbamoyl-5-fluorouracil (HCFU), Co-operative Study Group
    of HCFU. Jpn J Cancer Chemother   7 : 1181-1190.

16. Taguchi T.& Osaka Cancer Chemotherapy Co-operative Study Group
    (1980) Clinical trial of 1-hexylcarbamoyl-5-fluorouracil (HCFU)
    by co-operative study group.   Jpn J   Cancer Chemother
    7 : 1191-1197.

17. Koyama Y. (1981) 1-Hexylcarbamoyl-5-fluorouracil (HCFU) - a
    masked 5-fluorinated pyrimidine. Cancer Treat Rev 8 : 147-156.

18. Koyama Y. (1982) Phase II study of Carmofur (HCFU) fine gra-
    nules (Co-operative study group of HCFU). Jpn J Cancer Chemother
    9: 906-914.

19. Koyama Y. (1979) Standard for clinical evaluation of cancer
    chemotherapy. J Jpn Soc Cancer Ther 14: 52-53.

20. Koyama Y. (1981) Criteria for evaluation of clinical effects of
    cancer chemotherapy on solid tumors. (eds) T. Saito
    et al, Criteria for Evaluation of Clinical Effects of Cancer
    Chemotherapy and Immunotherapy and Development of Antitumor Drugs,
    Science Forum Ltd. (Tokyo) pp. 28-39.

21. WHO Handbook for Reporting Results of Cancer Treatment (1979) WHO
    Offset Publication No. 48, pp. 22-25, World Health Organization,
    Geneva.

© 1984 Elsevier Science Publishers B.V.
Fluoropyrimidines in Cancer Therapy
K. Kimura, S. Fujii, M. Ogawa, G.P. Bodey, P. Alberto, eds.

PHASE I, II & III TRIALS OF INTRAVENOUS 5'-DEOXY-5-FLUOROURIDINE

Pierre Alberto, Reto Abele, Bernadette Mermillod
Walter Weber and Francesco Cavalli

5-Fluorouracil (5-FU) is an antitumor agent of limited activity producing objective tumor regressions in approximately 20 % of patients with cancer of the breast, the stomach, the pancreas, the large bowel, the oropharyngeal tract and the prostate (1,2,3,4). In spite of this poor responses, 5-FU remains a major component of frequently used chemotherapy regimens. Two reasons for this are the absence of cross resistance with other active agents and the lack of a better treatment for digestive tract tumors. 5-FU is used with many different dose schedules, by intravenous or oral routes. In all of them, the maximum tolerated dose is limited by myelosuppression and digestive toxicity. It may be speculated that a higher rate of tumor response could be achieved with an active analog of 5-FU producing a lesser degree of hematologic and digestive toxicity.

5'-Deoxy-5-fluorouridine (5'-DFUR) is a new fluoropyrimidine (5) with improved hematologic tolerance. Its chemical structure consists in a 5-FU molecule attached to a pseudopentose. This compound cannot be directly phosphorylated and incorporated into nucleic acids (6). 5'-DFUR is intra-cellularly transformed into 5-FU by a nucleoside phosphorylase and, therefore, acts as an intracellular prodrug (6,7). Experimental observations have demonstrated a higher level of activity of this enzyme in tumors than in normal tissues (7,8). In mice, tho LD50 of 5'-DFUR is 10 times higher than that of 5-FU, and an equivalent level of antitumor activity produces less myelosuppression (9). The disposition of 5'-DFUR in humans follows a non linear process, with an apparent elimination halftime increasing from 10 minutes for a single dose of 1 g/sq.m. to 30 minutes for 15 g/sq.m. Two metabolites are detected in the plasma, 5FU and 5,6 di-hydrofluorouracil, the initial compound on the catabolic pathway (10).

PHASE I STUDIES

In order to determine the maximum tolerable dose of 5'-DFUR in such a manner that a direct comparison with 5-FU could be possible, we selected a treatment schedule with 5 consecutive rapid I.V. injections repeated every 3 weeks (11). This schedule is identical to the one most extensively studied for 5-FU. Starting from an initial dose of 300 mg/sq.m. daily, a dose of 5000 mg/sq.m. daily was reached in 6 steps. The patients had advanced malignancies not amenable to any other form of treatment. They had initial values superior to 3500 and 120'000/mm3 for leukocytes and platelets and inferior to 120 and 20 micro-moles/liter for serum creatinine and bilirubin. Their performance index was superior to 40 on the Karnofsky scale. No intra-patient escalation was allowed. Blood counts were repeated twice weekly and serum chemistries once weekly. Electrocardiogram and audiogram were performed immediately before and after completion of the trial. Tumor responses were determined according to standard criteria whenever possible.

The characteristics of the 30 patients treated are shown in table 1. Only 4 had prior chemotherapy, including 2 with 5-FU. A total of 66 courses of 5'-DFUR were administered. No patient received more than 4 courses.

TABLE 1   Patient characteristics

	N. of patients
Patients in study	30
Female/male	15/15
Primary tumor	
Lung, non-small cell types	6
GI tract adenocarcinoma	20
Other	4
No prior treatment	25
Radiotherapy alone	1
Chemotherapy alone	4
Median age in years (range):	63 (38-82)
Median performance index (range):	70 (50-80)

Four to 8 patients were entered at each dose level.
Tables 2 and 3 indicate the hematologic toxicity. Leukopenia, particularly granulocytopenia, was more pronounced
than thrombopenia. A moderate degree of leukopenia appeared with 2000 mg/sm.m. daily. The 2 patients treated at
5000 mg/sq.m. daily experienced a reversible agranulo-
cytosis. The dose related myelosuppression was not increased when the treatement was repeated. Non hematologic
toxic reactions are shown in table 4. The most frequent
was gastro-intestinal and consisted of nausea, vomiting
and mucositis. The 2 patients with 5000 mg/sq.m. developed a severe stomatitis. Cardiac toxicity was observed in
2 patients with 1000 mg/sq.m., consisting in precordial
pain appearing during the treatment, displacement of ST
segments in the ECG and elevation of serum creatine-
kinase. Neurologic symptoms were observed in 3 patients,
expressed by somnolence, fatigue and ataxia. Four patients

TABLE 2   5' DFUR   induced leukocyte toxicity

Dose (mg/sq.m./day)	median lowest counts / mm3 (1st course / subsequent courses)	
	leukocytes	granulocytes
300	9700/11900	8300/not available
1000	7300/5400	4500/3500
2000	6200/6100	3500/3100
3000	4100/5100	2200/3800
4000	2300/4500	800/1500
5000	1500/----	200/----

TABLE 3   5'-DFUR - induced platelet toxicity

Dose (mg/sq.m./day)	median lowest counts / mm3 (1st course / subsequent courses)
	platelets
300	389000/133000
1000	234000/195000
2000	217000/196000
3000	185000/162000
4000	120000/134000
5000	108000/------

complained of a sensation of "hot-skin", particularly in the face and pelvis. This symptom seems to be indentical with that recently reported by japanese investigators with alkylcarbamoyl-derivatives of fluorouracil (12). One patient had a partial alopecia after 5000 mg/sq.m. daily.

TABLE 4   5'-DFUR   induced non-hematologic toxicity

| Toxic reaction | N. toxic reactions at each dose (mg/sq.m./day) | | | | | |
	300	1000	2000	3000	4000	5000
nausea-vomiting	1	1	3	2	3	1
stomatitis	0	2	1	0	1	2
ECG changes	0	2	0	0	0	0
CNS symptoms	2	0	0	1	0	0
alopecia	0	0	0	0	0	1
N. of patients	5	8	4	4	7	2

Antitumor activity was recorded in one patient with gastric adenocarcinoma and in one patient with adenocarcinoma of the lung. It was concluded from these observations that disease oriented Phase II studies were warranted, and that the dose for Phase II trials should be 4000 mg/sq.m. in patients without previous dose related myelosuppression, and 3000 mg/sq.m. for the other patients.

In another Phase I study (13), 5'-DFUR was given in weekly short term I.V. infusions. Granulopenia was observed with 10 g/sq.m. weekly and the maximum tolerated dose was 15 g/sq.m. weekly. Stomatitis, "hot-skin" in the pelvis, alopecia and neurologic toxicity were also observed.

PHASE II STUDIES

A Phase II study in advanced colorectal adenocarcinoma was recently completed by the Swiss Cancer Group SAKK (14). Fourty-two patients were treated with five successive daily rapid I.V. injections of 5'-DFUR, 4000 mg/sq./m. in patients without prior chemotherapy, and 3000 mg/sq.m.

in other patients. The therapeutic result was assessed
after 2 treatments, 3 weeks apart. Patients had histologically proven adenocarcinoma of the colon or rectum and
measurable lesions in the liver and lung. Initial values
for leukocytes, platelets, serum creatinine and bilirubin
were the same as in Phase I. Blood counts, serum chemis-
try, clinical examination, evaluation of toxicity and
tumor measurements were repeated weekly. Patients characteristics are shown in table 5. Thirty-one patients received two full courses. Three of them had unfortunately
incomplete study documentation, and one was treated with
wrong doses. Twenty-seven were fully evaluable for tumor
response and toxicity. Seven responses were observed, one
complete response in the liver, and 6 partial responses in
liver and lung. The toxicity is summarized in table 6 and
7. Only 5 treatment courses produced a leucopenia of less
than 2000/mm3 and no one was inferior to 1000/mm3. Thrombopenia was observed in one patient only. As in the Phase
I trial, nausea vomiting and mucositis were the most frequently occuring non-hematologic toxic reactions. Neurologic complications were seen in 33 % of the patients, consisting in fatigue, dizziness, ataxia and in a few cases
mental confusion. These symptoms never occurred during the
first course, and seem to be related to the duration of
treatment. They represent a major problem and may lead to
the discontinuation of therapy despite of tumor response.
This toxicity is rapidly reversible upon cessation of
5'-DFUR application. Cardiac toxicity was observed in
5 cases. In 3 patients transient arrhythmia and minor ECG
changes were the only pathologic findings. One patient
complained of ischemic chest pain with ECG lesions suggesting coronary ischemia. One patient treated through a
central catheter located in the right atrium had a reversible cardiac arrest during the fourth course of treat-

ment. Skin reactions were registred in 6 patients, consisting in "hot-skin", erythema and cutaneous desquamation. Four patients complained of hair loss.

TABLE 5   Eligible patient characteristics

Total number	42		
Female/male	15/27		
Median age (range)	62 years (35-74)		
Median performance status	1 (0-2)		
Prior treatment			
surgery	29		
surgery + radiotherapy	6		
surgery + chemotherapy	1		
surgery + radiotherapy + chemotherapy 1			
none	5		
Prior tumor :	colon	sigmoid+rectum	total
number of patients	14	28	42
N. of patients with			
intraabdominal relapses	11	17	28
liver metastases	7	18	25
lung metastases	4	12	16
soft tissues metastases	4	8	12
other	2*	0	2

*1 in bone and 1 in brain

In another Phase II series 20 patients with oropharyngeal squamous cell carcinoma received the same treatment
schedule (15). The tumor response after 2 treatment courses could be evaluated in 12 patients, with 1 complete and
2 partial responses, 7 stable diseases and 2 tumor progressions. The toxicity was more severe than in patients

TABLE 6   Hematologic toxicity (colo-rectal carcinoma)

| | N. of evaluable patients | | | |
| | first course | | second course | |
Lowest count/mm3 for leukocytes and platelets	leukocytes	platelets	leukocytes	platelets
≥4000 and ≥100000	19	35	17	26
3000-3900 and 75000-99000	8	2	6	2
2000-2900 and 50000-74000	9	0	4	0
1000-1900 and 25000-49000	4	0	1	0
<1000 and <25000	0	1	0	0
Total	40	38	28	28

TABLE 7   Non-hematologic toxicity (colo-rectal carcinoma)

| | N. of patients with WHO grade | | | | % toxic |
Type	1	2	3	4	patients
Nausea+vomiting	9	5	2	0	38
Mucosal	5	7	3	1	38
Neurologic	2	6	5	1	33
Cutaneous	3	3	0	0	14
Cardiac	2	1	0	2	12
Hair loss	3	0	1	0	10

with other tumor types. Four patients had a leukopenia of less than 1000/mm3. Two of them developed infectious complications and one died of meningeal infection. Gastrointestinal toxicity was frequently observed. Neurological toxicity was present in 5 patients, with one transient coma. Skin erythema and desquamation were seen in 3 patients. Laryngeal edema was observed in 3 haevily preirradiated patients. One patient died in cardiogenic shock, possibly related to the treatment. As for other antitumor agents, patients with advanced head and neck cancer seem to be more exposed to the toxic manifestations of 5'-DFUR. Other Phase II trials are in progress with the same schedule in patients with breast carcinoma and malignant melanoma. Other EORTC study groups have Phase II studies in progress using the same schedule or a weekly intravenous dose of 12 g/sq.m. in short perfusion.

PHASE III STUDIES

Japanese studies with oral 5'-DFUR are in progress or have already been completed. In Europ, a Phase III study is presently in activity, conducted by the Swiss Cancer Group SAKK. In this study, patients with colo-rectal cancer are randomized to receive in five consecutive days every 3 weeks by rapid I.V. injection either 5-FU, 450 mg/sq.m. or 5'-DFUR, 4000 mg/sq.m. Patients with prior chemotherapy are not eligible. No interim report is available. However, early observations suggest that the level of toxicity of both regimens is equivalent and that neurologic symptoms are more frequent with 5'-DFUR.

CONCLUSION

Many important informations are still lacking concerning the activity of 5'-DFUR in human tumors and concerning the long term tolerance of this compound in cancer patients. In particular, the therapeutic activity of this new drug in tumor types generally resistant to 5-FU is largely unknown. Also, the influence of the duration of intravenous perfusions upon antitumor activity and patient tolerance, particularly for what concerns the neurological side effects, remains to be cleared. The tolerance of 5'-DFUR in drug combinations should also be investigated, as well as the interaction with compounds known for their modification of the cytotoxicity of 5-FU. The mechanism responsible for the neurotoxicity should be investigated.

The activity of 5'-DFUR in tumors such as colorectal cancer, head and neck cancer and breast cancer indicates that this new fluoropyrimidine deserves a place in modern tumor chemotherapy, and that an intensive effort of clinical and pharmacological investigations with this compound is warranted.

REFERENCES

1. Ansfield FJ, Ramirez G, Mackman S, et al. (1969) A ten-year study of 5-fluorouracil in disseminated breast cancer with clinical results and survival times. Cancer Res 29: 1062-1066.

2. Moertel CG. (1978) Chemotherapy of gastrointestinal cancer. N Engl J Med 299: 1049-1051.

3. Amer MH, Al-Sarraf M, and Vaitkevicius VK. (1979) Factors that affect response to chemotherapy and survival of patients with advanced head and neck cancer. Cancer 43: 2202-2206.

4. Scott WW, Gibbons RP, Johnson DE, et al. (1975) Comparison of 5-fluorouracil (NSC-19893) and cyclophosphamide (NSC-26271) in patients with advanced carcinoma of the prostate. Cancer Chemother Rep 59: 195-201.

5. Cook AF, Holman MJ, Kramer MJ, et al. (1979) Fluorinated pyrimidine nucleosides. 3. synthesis and antitumor activity of a series of 5'-deoxy-5-fluoropyrimidine nucleosides. J Med Chem 22: 1330-1335.

6. Armstrong RD and Diasio RB. (1980) Metabolism and biological activity of 5'-deoxy-5-fluorouridine, a novel fluoropyrimidine. Cancer Res 40: 3333-3338.

7. Ishitsuka H, Miwa M, Takemoto K, et al. (1980) Role of uridine phosphorylase for antitumor activity of 5'-deoxy-5-fluorouridine. GANN 71: 112-123.

8. Fujita H, Nakagawa H, and Ogawa K. (1982) Pharmaco-kinetics of 5'-deoxy-5-fluorouridine (5'-DFUR) by oral administration. 13th International Cancer Congress, Seattle, USA.

9. Bollag W, and Hartmann HR. (1980) Tumor inhibitory effects of a new fluorouracil derivative: 5'-deoxy-5-fluorouridine. Europ J Cancer 16: 427-432.

10. Sommadossi JP, Aubert C, Cano JP, et al. (1983) Kinetics and metabolism of a new fluoropyrimidine, 5'-deoxy-5-fluorouridine, in humans. Cancer Res 43: 930-933.

11. Abele R, Alberto P, Seematter RJ, et al. (1982) Phase I clinical study with 5'-deoxy-5-fluorouridine, a new fluoropyrimidine derivative. Cancer Treat Rep 66: 1307-1313.

12. Koyama A, and Koyama Y. (1980) Phase I study of a new antitumor drug, 1-hexylcarbomoyl-5-fluorouracil (HCFU), administered orally: an HCFU clinical study group report. Cancer Treat Rep 64: 861-867.

13. Gouveia J, Ribaud P, Schwarzenberg L, et al. (1981) Phase I study of 5'-deoxy-5-fluorouridine (DFUR). Abstract N° 683, 12th International Congress of Chemotherapy, Florence.

14. Abele R, Alberto P, Kaplan S, et al. (in press). Phase II study of doxifluridine in advanced colo-rectal adenocarcinoma. J Clin Oncol.

15. Abele R, Kaplan E, Grossenbacher R, et al. (in press) Phase II study of doxifluridine in advanced squamous cell carcinoma of the head and neck. Europ J Cancer Clin Oncol.

© 1984 Elsevier Science Publishers B.V.
Fluoropyrimidines in Cancer Therapy
K. Kimura, S. Fujii, M. Ogawa, G.P. Bodey, P. Alberto, eds.

A PHASE II STUDY OF ORAL 5'-DEOXY-5-FLUOROURIDINE: 5'-DFUR COOPERATIVE GROUP STUDY

Kazuo Ota and Kiyoji Kimura

1. INTRODUCTION

5'-Deoxy-5-fluorouridine (5'-DFUR) is a new derivative of 5-fluorouracil (5-FU) synthesized by Cook et al. (1) (Figure 1). Experimental studies have shown its superiority to 5-FU in various animal tumor models in terms of the chemotherapeutic index (2, 3). It was found to be converted to 5-FU by uridine phosphorylase in mice (3) and by thymidine phosphorylase in humans (4, 5). In addition, uridine phosphorylase was found to be abundant in sarcoma-180 solid tumor, leading to a significantly higher conversion to 5-FU and 5-FU concentrations in the tumor than in normal tissues (3). The concentration of the active form of 5-FU therefore reaches higher levels in tumor tissues than in normal tissues or in peripheral blood of animals (6, 7) and humans(8). Accordingly, the side effects are diminished while antitumor activity is increased.

Clinical trials of 5'-DFUR by i.v. administration have been performed in Europe. In Japan, however, the drug was firstly administered by oral administration. Preliminary results of the phase II study of oral 5'-DFUR conducted by the Cooperative Study Group involving 94 institutions in Japan are overviewed.

5′-Deoxy-5-fluorouridine
(m. w. 246.19)

5-Fluorouracil
(m. w. 130.08)

FIGURE 1   Structures of 5'-DFUR and 5-FU.

2.   EARLY PHASE II STUDY

2.1. Response

In an early phase II study the optimal dose of 800 mg/m^2/day was considered to be tolerable. Response rates in 104 cases are described in Table 1. Five complete and 4 partial responses were observed in 30 cases with breast cancer, and efficacy was recognized also in some cases of head and neck, stomach, colorectum and pancreas cancer.

2.2. Side effect

The side effects reported in the early phase II study are summarized in Table 2. Gastrointestinal toxicities, especially diarrhea, were observed most frequently. In 46% of patients side effects were observed and the administration was stopped in 20% of patients due to the side effects, indicated by the numbers in parentheses.

TABLE 1 Response of 5'-DFUR by primary site in early phase II study

Primary site	CR	PR	MR	NC	PD	Total
Head and neck		1		2		3
Salivary gland				1		1
Thyroid				5		5
Esophagus				2		2
Stomach		1	3	13	10	27
Colorectum	1		1	5	3	10
Liver				3	1	4
Cholangioma				1		1
Pancreas		1		2	1	4
Lung				8	2	10
Breast	5	4	1	16	4	30
Renal cell				1	1	2
Others				5		5
Total	6	7	5	64	22	104

CR: complete response, PR: partial response, MR: minor response, NC: no change, PD: progressive disease

2.3. Determination of optimal dose

Response and side effects of 5'-DFUR in relation to daily dosage is described in Table 3. Responses were obtained at a level of 800 mg/m^2/day or above. Comparing the two groups; that is, the group receiving 800 mg/m^2/day and the group receiving more than 800 mg/m^2/day, no significant difference was seen in efficacy. However, a lower incidence of side effects was observed at the daily dose of 800 mg/m^2. The optimal dose was therefore determined to be 800 mg/m^2/day, and further phase II study using this dose was performed.

TABLE 2   Side effects of 5'-DFUR in early phase II study

Symptoms	No. of cases where side effects appeared	Incidence rate (%)
Digestive system		
Diarrhea	32 (18)	19.3
Nausea	21 (10)	12.7
Vomiting	7 (7)	4.2
Anorexia	18 (7)	10.8
Epigastric pain	8 (4)	4.8
Stomatitis	3	1.8
Others	3 (1)	1.8
Others		
Fatigue	2 (1)	1.2
Pigmentation	4 (1)	2.4
Fever	2 (2)	1.2
Others	14 (8)	8.4
Hematology		
Leukopenia ($<4000/mm^3$)	11 (3)	6.6
Thrombocytopenia ($<100,000/mm^3$)	3 (2)	1.8
Anemia RBC $<3 \times 10^6/mm^3$ Hb $<11g/dl$	5 (2)	3.0
Liver function		
SGOT increased	4	2.4
SGPT increased	2	1.2

Total number of patients: 166
Number of cases where side effects appeared: 77 (46.4%)
Number of cases where administration was stopped due to side effects: 34 (20%)

3.   PHASE II STUDY

3.1. Patients

Patients characteristics entered into the study are shown in Table 4.   Early and late phase II studies were carried in 415 cases: 306 cases were evaluable for

TABLE 3 Response and side effects of 5'-DFUR in relation to daily dosage

Dosage (mg/m^2/day)		400	600	800	1000	1200	1400	1600	1800	2400
Response	CR	0	0	5	0	1	0	0	0	
	PR	0	0	6	0	0	1	0	0	
	Response rate (%)	0/5	0/18	11/67	0/5	1/6 (16.7)	1/1 (100.0)	0/1	0/1	
		0/23		(16.4)	2/14 (14.3)					
		NS								
Overall side effects	Incidence rate (%)	3/6 (50.0)	9/30 (30.0)	46/107 (42.9)	5/9 (55.6)	7/9 (77.8)	1/1 (100.0)	1/2 (50.0)	1/1 (100.0)	1/1 (100.0)
		12/36 (33.3)			16/23 (69.6)					
		NS			P< 0.1					
Diarrhea	Incidence rate (%)	0/6	3/30 (10.0)	20/107 (18.7)	3/9 (33.3)	3/9 (33.3)	1/1 (100.0)	1/1 (100.0)	1/1 (100.0)	0/1
		3/36 (8.3)			9/23 (39.1)					
		P< 0.1			P< 0.05					

response including 230 cases with measurable lesions. There were 91 male and 139 female patients with a mean age of 59 years (range: 18 to 86). The median performance status was 1.

3.2. Response

Clinical efficacy of 5'-DFUR in 230 measurable cases is summarized in Table 5. In breast cancer, 9 complete and 10 partial responses were achieved out of 71 cases, with a response rate of 27%. In colorectal cancer, complete and partial responses were achieved each in 2 cases out of 40, with a response rate of 10%. In stomach cancer, partial response was achieved in 9 of 55 cases, with a response rate of 16%. Although the number

TABLE 4 Background of patients treated with 5'-DFUR

Overall treated cases	:	415
Non-evaluable cases	:	109
Evaluable cases	:	306
Non-measurable cases	:	76
Measurable cases	:	230
Sex	:	91 Males, 139 Females
Age	:	59 (18 - 86)
Performance status	:	1 (Median)

of cases was small in head and neck cancer, the response rate was 40%, and in pancreas cancer the response rate was 33%; however, no response was obtained in lung cancer. The overall response rate was 16%. Similar response rate was observed in either group with or without prior chemotherapy including 5-FU and/or tegafur.

Response parameters are described in Table 6. Among 19 breast cancer patients who responded, the decrease in lesion size was observed within 35 days on the average. This corresponded to a total mean dosage of 5'-DFUR administered of 40g. The mean durations of response in patients achieving complete and partial responses were over 165 or 145 days, respectively. Time to response appeared longer in colorectal cancer compared to breast cancer.

3.3. Side effects

The side effects of 5'-DFUR are detailed in Table 7. The side effects were noted in 46% of 415 cases. Diarrhea was highest in frequency and occurred in 22%.

TABLE 5　Response of 5'-DFUR by primary site in phae II study

(Measurable cases)

Primary site	CR	PR	MR	NC	PD	Total	CR + PR (%)
Head and neck		2		3		5	40.0
Salivary gland				1		1	
Thyroid			1	5	1	7	
Esophagus					1	1	
Stomach		9	6	27	13	55	16.4
Colorectum	2	2	2	23	11	40	10.0
Liver				5	5	10	
Cholangioma				1		1	
Pancreas		2	1	1	2	6	33.3
Lung				15	9	24	
Breast	9	10	7	29	16	71	26.8
Renal cell				1		1	
Others				7	1	8	
Total	11	25	17	118	59	230	15.7
Prior chemotherapy (−)	2	11	7	40	13	73	17.8
(+)	9	14	10	78	46	57	14.6

TABLE 6　　　　Parameters of response

Mean
(Min. ~ Max.)

Primary site	by the Onset of response		Duration of response	
	Time required (days)	Total dosage (g)	Response	Days
Breast	35 (9 — 98)	40 (11— 118)	CR	165 < (28 ~ 475<)
			PR	145 < (84 ~ 217<)
Stomach	25 (5 — 85)	29 (6— 102)	PR	103 < (53 ~ 178<)
Colorectum	77 (13 — 164)	92 (16— 197)	CR	228 < (76 ~ 380<)
			PR	151 (99 ~ 191<)
Others	38 (15— 66)	39 (18— 52)	PR	160 < (29 ~ 262<)

TABLE 7   Side effects of 5'-DFUR in phase II study

Symptoms	No. of cases where side effects appeared	Incidence rate (%)
Digestive system		
Diarrhea	93 (41)	22.4
Nausea	48 (20)	11.6
Vomiting	15 (11)	3.6
Anorexia	54 (25)	13.0
Epigastric pain	3 (1)	0.7
Stomatitis	5 (1)	1.2
Others	21 (8)	5.1
Others		
Fatigue	7 (1)	1.7
Pigmentation	5 (5)	1.2
Fever	2 (2)	0.1
Others	27 (14)	6.5
Hematology		
Leukopenia ($<4000/mm^3$)	18 (6)	4.3
Thrombocytopenia ($<100,000/mm^3$)	8 (3)	1.9
Anemia RBC $<3 \times 10^6/mm^3$ Hb $<11g/dl$	2	0.5
Liver function		
SGOT increased	3 (1)	0.7
SGPT increased	4 (1)	1.0

Total number of patients: 415
Number of cases where side effects appeared: 190 (45.8%)
Number of cases where administration was stopped due to side effects: 60 (14.5%)

Gastrointestinal toxicities such as diarrhea, anorexia, nausea and vomiting, were factors in stopping administration. Leukopenia less than $4,000/mm^3$ was however seen in only 4%. The number of cases who interrupted the drug due to the side effect was 60 (15%), as indicated by the numbers in parentheses.

The first case is a 56-year old female with recurrent breast cancer. The previous chemotherapy consisted of cyclophosphamide, adriamycin and 5-FU (CAF), and hormonal therapy with tamoxifen. Both regimens were ineffective. Metastasis to the brain and multiple bones, and disturbance of consciousness were observed. Radiotherapy was given for brain metastasis. She was also given 1,200 mg of 5'-DFUR daily. The metastasized lesion at the 2nd lumbar and 7th cervical vertebrae became ossified after the therapy (Figure 2) and a locally recurrent lesion of 5 x 5 cm breast cancer

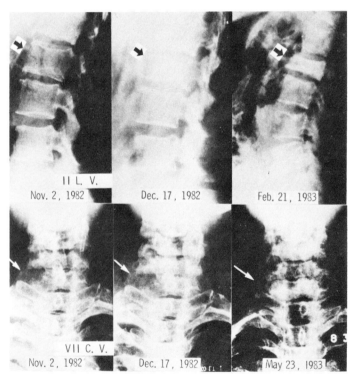

FIGURE 2 Breast cancer with bone metastasis: 56-year-old
female treated with 5'-DFUR from Nov. 20, 1983.

completely disappeared.

The second case is a 59-year old female of previously untreated colon cancer with lung metastasis. She was given 1,200 mg of 5'-DFUR daily, requiring frequent interruptions of administration due to

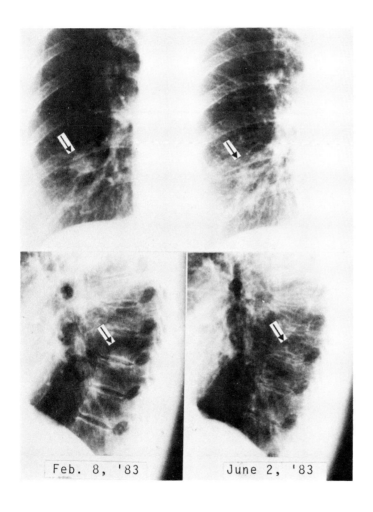

FIGURE 3 Colon cancer with lung metastasis: 59-year-old female treated with 5'-DFUR from Feb. 15, 1983.

diarrhea. Metastatic lesions in the lung decreased in
size remarkably after 6 weeks of therapy as shown in
Figure 3, and the response continued for 6 months.

The third case is a 74-year old female also with
previously untreated rectal cancer and lung metastasis.
She was given 1,200 mg 5'-DFUR daily for over 6 months.
Metastatic lesions in the lung decreased in size
markedly as shown in Figure 4. Duration of response was
more than 3 months, and no any side effects were
observed.

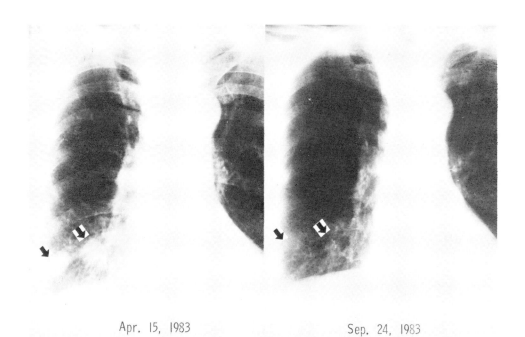

Apr. 15, 1983   Sep. 24, 1983

FIGURE 4 Rectal cancer with lung metastasis: 74-year-old
         female treated with 5'-DFUR from Apr. 21, 1983.

4. DISCUSSION AND CONCLUSION

Phase II study of oral 5'-DFUR in various cancer patients was carried out at multiple institutions. The optimal dose was determined to be 800 $mg/m^2/day$. Good responses were observed in breast, stomach, colorectum, pancreas and head and neck cancers, but not in lung cancer. It is noteworthy that in cases receiving prior chemotherapy including fluoropyrimidines, good responses were seen, suggesting that 5'-DFUR is much highly activated to the active form of 5-FU in tumor tissues. As to side effects, gastrointestinal toxicities such as diarrhea, nausea and vomiting were found to be dose-limiting factors. Leukopenia was also observed in some cases, but the bone marrow suppression was mild. In conclusion, oral 5'-DFUR seems to be effective for breast, stomach and colorectal cancers without producing severe side effects. To evaluate the clinical usefulness of this compound further randomized trials in comparison with other fluoropyrimidines should be conducted.

REFERENCES

1. Cook AF, Holman MJ, Kramer MJ, et al. (1979) Fluorinated pyrimidine nucleotides.3. Synthesis and antitumor activity of a series of 5'-deoxy-5-fluoropyrimidine nucleotides. J Med Chem 22: 1330-1335.

2. Bullag W, Hartmann HR. (1980) Tumor inhibitory effects of a new fluorouracil derivative: 5'-deoxy-5-fluorouridine. Eur J Cancer 16: 427-432.

3. Ishitsuka H, Miwa M, Takemoto K, et al. (1980) Role of uridine phosphorylase for antitumor activity of 5'-deoxy-5-fluorouridine. Gann 71: 112-123.

4. Shirasaka T, Nagayama S, Kitano S, et al. (1980) Pyrimidine nucleoside phosphorylase in rodents and human. Jpn J Cancer Chemother 8: 262-269.

5. Kono A, Hara Y, Sugata S, et al. (1982) Activation of 5'-deoxy-5-fluorouridine by thymidine phosphorylase in human tumors. Chem Pharm Bull 31: 175-178.

6. Fujita H, Ogawa K, Nakagawa H. (1983) Pharmacokinetics of 5'-deoxy-5-fluorouridine (5'-DFUR) by oral administration. J Jpn Soc Cancer Ther 18: 916-926.

7. Suzuki S, Hongu Y, Fukazawa H, et al. (1980) Tissue distribution of 5'-deoxy-5-fluorouridine and derived 5-fluorouracil in tumor-bearing mice and rats. Gann 71: 238-245.

8. Hara Y. (1983) Enzymatic conversion of 5'-deoxy-5-fluorouridine and tegafur to 5-fluorouracil in human tumor tissue. Proceedings of the International Symposium on Fluoropyrimidines 1983, Nagoya (this volume).

Fluoropyrimidines in Cancer Therapy
K. Kimura, S. Fujii, M. Ogawa, G.P. Bodey, P. Alberto, eds.

TEGAFUR AND 5-FLUOROURACIL + PALA REGIMENS IN METASTATIC CANCER

Gerald P. Bodey, Agop Y. Bedikian, Gabriel N. Hortobagyi
and Manuel Valdivieso

1. INTRODUCTION

Although substantial progress has been made in the treatment of metastatic cancer, effective therapy remains to be discovered for several common malignancies. Consequently, the search for new agents remains an important endeavor in cancer research. 5-Fluorouracil (5FU) remains an important agent for the treatment of many adenocarcinomas. Attempts have been made to build upon this experience by synthesizing new analogues, and by enhancing the effect of 5-fluorouracil by biochemical modulation. This paper will report the experience at M. D. Anderson Hospital with the analogue, tegafur, and with 5FU combinations aimed at biochemical modulation.

2. TEGAFUR REVISITED

Tegafur, a furanidylpyrimidine analogue of 5FU was synthesized in the Soviet Union. The spectrum of activity of tegafur was similar to 5FU in animal tumor systems but it was much less toxic. In their initial clinical trials, a dose of 15-20 mg/Kg intravenously q 12 hr was selected. Therapy was continued to a total dose of 30-40 g. Only minimal side-effects, consisting of nausea and vomiting and diarrhea were reported. They found response rates (complete + partial + minor) of 26% in gastric carcinoma, 31% in rectal carcinoma and 40% in breast carcinoma (1). Studies conducted by several Japanese investigators confirmed the activity of tegafur in adenocarcinomas.

We initiated clinical trials with tegafur, administering the drug intravenously in single daily doses for 5 days at 2 to 3 week intervals (2). The maximum tolerated dose with this schedule was 2 $gm/M^2/d$. Hematological toxicity occurred in only 7% of patients. Dose-limiting toxicities were severe vomiting, ataxia and dizziness.

Pharmacological studies were conducted in 8 patients who received single doses of 5 gm/M^2 tegafur (3). The plasma disappearance of tegafur was exponential with a terminal half-life of 8.8 hr. The drug was converted to 5FU and plasma concentrations of this compound were maintained above 1.7 µg/ml for at least 48 hr. The concentrations of 5FU derived from tegafur were substantially greater than those achieved by continuous infusion of 5FU at the maximum tolerated dose ($1.1g/M^2$). Hence, tegafur appeared to act as a sustained release preparation of 5FU. However, some investigators have not been able to detect similar concentrations of 5FU after tegafur administration.

Numerous studies were conducted with tegafur in combination regimens, using short intensive courses of

therapy. For example, tegafur was combined with adriamycin and cyclophosphamide (ACFTOR) for the treatment of
breast carcinoma, and compared to previous experience
with the FAC regimen (4). All of these patients also
received BCG immunotherapy. It was anticipated that since
tegafur caused less myelosuppression than 5FU, that it
would be possible to administer higher doses of the
ACFTOR regimen. The complete remission rate for the 91
evaluable patients treated with AFTOR was 20% compared to
19% for the 105 evaluable patients treated with FAC. The
overall response rates were 66% and 76% respectively. The
hematological toxicities of the 2 regimens were similar.
For example, during the first course of therapy, the
median lowest neutrophil count was $800/mm^3$ (range, 300-
$2600/mm^3$) in patients receiving FAC compared to $1100/mm^3$
(range, $0-4400/mm^3$) in patients receiving ACFTOR. Important non-hematological toxicities are shown in Table 1.
Several significant toxicities were observed more often
with the ACFTOR regimen. While nausea and vomiting were
common with both regimens, severe vomiting occurred much
more frequently in patients receiving ACFTOR. This led
to substantial weight loss and necessitated hospitalization of some patients for fluid and electrolyte
replacement. Lethargy, dizziness, fever, chest pain,
hypotension, and visual and personality changes were
observed only in patients who received ACFTOR. Hence,
the substitution of tegafur for 5FU in the FAC regimen

TABLE 1   Toxicities of FAC and ACFTOR regimens

	FAC	ACFTOR
Vomiting	86	84
Severe Vomiting	7	34
Weight Loss >5 lbs	2	76
Stomatitis	22	12
Weakness	4	22
Lethargy, Dizziness	0	9
Chest Pain	0	7
Visual and Personality Changes	0	3

Expressed as percent of patients

did not permit the administration of higher doses of chemotherapy, did not improve response rates, and resulted in unpleasant side-effects.

Subsequently, pharmacology studies were conducted which demonstrated that tegafur was reliably absorbed from the gastrointestinal tract and that low-dose, long-term administration could avoid the acute unpleasant side-effects of tegafur. These observations rekindled an interest in the use of tegafur. We conducted a phase I trial of oral tegafur, beginning with a dose of 0.5 $g/M^2/d$ for 21 days, repeated at 3 week intervals (5). The drug was administered in 2 or 3 divided doses. The maximum tolerated dose was 1.25 g/M^2 and the dose-limiting toxicity was diarrhea. Neurological toxicity, consisting of speech difficulties, confusion and dizziness did occur at doses $\geq$ 1g/M^2/day but they were infrequent. Myelosuppressive toxicity was also minimal. Toxicity occurred more frequently in patients with pre-existent liver impairment.

Subsequently, we participated in a multicenter prospective randomized trial of oral tegafur vs intravenous 5FU at a dose of 1 g/M^2/day for 21 days q 28 days. The dose was reduced in patients with liver impairment. 5FU was given at a dose of 500 mg/M^2/day x 4 days, then 250 mg/M^2/day q 2 days x 4 at 4 week intervals. The 2 regimens were equally effective in this disease. No complete remissions were obtained; 6 (19%) patients treated with 5FU and 7 (20%) patients treated with tegafur achieved a partial response. The median duration of partial responses was 4 mos with both drugs. The important toxicities of the 2 regimens are presented in Table 2. Hematologic toxicity of tegafur was negligible while that of 5FU was moderate. Diarrhea and mucositis were more common with 5FU whereas malaise and skin rash were more common with tegafur. The multicenter results were similar to those obtained at our institution. These results have rekindled an interest in tegafur, suggesting that it could be used in preferance to 5FU in combination regimens because of its minimal myelosuppression.

TABLE 2   Toxicities of oral tegafur vs intravenous 5FU in
           colorectal carcinoma

	5 FU	TEGAFUR
Evaluable Courses	121	170
Myelosuppression	32	2
Vomiting	22	22
Diarrhea	41	27
Mucositis	34	26
Malaise	42	57
Dizziness	3	6
Skin rash	10	31

Expressed as percent of courses

3. BIOCHEMICAL MODULATION OF 5FU

Attempts have been made to enhance the antitumor
effect of 5FU through biochemical modulation.   Although
several agents have been used, this discussion will focus
on thymidine and N-(phosphonoacetyl)-L-aspartate (PALA).
The combination of 5FU plus thymidine acts synergistically against several animal tumor systems, including mouse
AKR, L1210 and P388 leukemias, CD8F1 breast carcinoma and
colon carcinoma 26.   However, there is some controversy
about the enhanced effect of the combination over 5FU
against the latter tumor.   Several mechanisms have been
proposed to account for this synergistic effect.   Thymidine competes with those enzymes which metabolize 5FU,

thus reducing the rate of catabolism of 5FU and prolonging the plasma half-life. Thymidine may act as a source of deoxyribose-enhancing conversion of 5FU to 5-fluoro-2' deoxyuridine. Also, thymidine could protect cells from the DNA blockade of 5FU and shunt 5FU into fraudulent RNA which causes greater lethality (7).

An early phase II study in humans demonstrated that thymidine enhanced the cytotoxicity of 5FU to bone marrow cells (8). Partial remissions were obtained in patients with adenocarcinomas and lymphomas, including patients who had received 5FU previously. The administration of thymidine with 5FU to patients with colorectal carcinoma decreased the plasma clearance of 5FU, increased the plasma concentration, reduced renal clearance of 5FU, and enhanced its conversion to 5'fluorodeoxyuridine (9). Concomitant 5FU plus continuous infusion of thymidine enhanced the toxicity of 5FU, including mucositis, myelosuppression and gastrointestinal toxicity (10). Neurological toxicity was also caused by the combination, consisting of lethargy, confusion, disorientation and nystagmus (8). Whether or not thymidine enhanced the therapeutic efficacy of 5FU could not be determined from these studies.

PALA is a transition state inhibitor of asparatate transcarbamylase, an early enzyme in the pathway of de novo pyrimidine nucleotide biosynthesis. 5FU is a late inhibitor of the pyrimidine biosynthetic pathway; hence, these agents might be expected to act synergistically in combination. In tumor cell lines, PALA enhanced the incorporation of 5FU into fraudulent RNA. The combination caused greater inhibition of thymidylate synthetase than 5FU alone, whereas PALA alone had no effect. The combination was more active than either agent alone against experimental colon and Lewis lung carcinomas. They also acted synergistically to inhibit the growth of human mammary carcinoma cell lines in vitro.

We evaluated two schedules of 5FU plus PALA in patients with colorectal carcinoma (11). Fifteen evaluable patients were randomized to receive either PALA 1-2.5 g/M^2 and 5FU 240-600 mg/M^2 once weekly or PALA 400-1000/M^2/d and 5 FU 200-500/M^2/d for 5 days at 4 week intervals. Partial responses were observed in 4 of the 24 patients receiving the weekly schedule and 3 of the 26 patients receiving the 5 day schedule. The responses lasted a median of 3 months. Myelosuppression was mild with both regimens. Major toxicity included skin rash, stomatitis and diarrhea which were more frequent and severe with the weekly schedule. In this study, the addition of PALA to 5FU enhanced the toxicity but did not enhance the therapeutic efficacy, and neither schedule studied was found to be superior.

The combination of PALA + 5FU has also been evaluated in patients with advanced breast carcinoma, refractory to other antitumor agents (12). Most of these patients had received lower doses of 5FU in previous combination regimens. Patients were randomly assigned to one of the following regimens: PALA 800 mg/M^2/d x 5 d q 2 wks; or PALA 400 mg/M^2/d x 5d + 5FU 300 mg/M^2/d x5d q4 wks; or 5FU 400 mg/M^2/d x 5d q 3 wks. The results of this study are presented in Table 3.

TABLE 3 Results of PALA and 5FU regimens in refractory breast carcinoma

	PALA	5FU	PALA + 5FU
Evaluable Patients	19	11	35
Complete Remission	0	0	1 (3%)
Partial Remission	1 (5%)	2 (18%)	10 (29%)
Stable Disease	5 (26%)	3 (27%)	16 (46%)
Progression	13	6	8

All of the responders in each arm of the study had received prior 5FU therapy and their disease was no longer responding to this therapy. If stable disease is considered a response, then the differences in response rates between the combination and the single agents is statistically significant (p < 0.01). The patient who achieved a complete remission with PALA + 5FU remains in remission for > 9 mos. The median duration of partial remission was 5 months and of stable disease was 3 mos. Myelosuppression was mild with each regimen. Skin rash, mucositis and gastrointestinal toxicities were the major toxicities and occurred more often in patients receiving PALA.

Casper et al. have conducted a phase I trial of 5FU + PALA, using a different schedule (13). Initially they administered 2 gm/M^2 PALA, followed 3 hrs later by 5FU 200-500 mg/M^2. Doses were repeated weekly x 3 followed by a 2 wk observation period. They determined that much lower doses of PALA inhibited pyrimidine synthesis. Consequently, they devised a second schedule whereby PALA 250 mg/M^2 was given 24 hrs before 5FU 750 mg/M^2. With the former schedule, dose-limiting toxicities were skin rash, diarrhea and mucositis. The dose-limiting toxicity with the second schedule was leukopenia. Only minor responses were seen in this phase I study. They concluded that the optimum approach to this combination was to use a dose of PALA of 250 mg/M^2 which would cause adequate enzymatic blockade and permit the administration of maximum doses of 5FU for its antitumor effect.

The combination of PALA + 5FU + thymidine has been shown to be substantially more active than 5FU + thymidine against colon carcinoma 26. This combination caused a large increase in 5FU incorporation into tumor RNA. Consequently, we conducted a phase I trial of this combination in patients with adenocarcinomas (14). PALA 1 gm/M^2 was given on day 1, and thymidine 30 g and 5FU 150-300 mg/M^2 on day 2. Courses were repeated at 4 wk intervals. The majority of patients had received a fluoropyrimidine previously. The results of this study are shown in Table 4.

TABLE 4 PALA + Thymidine + 5FU in adenocarcinoma

Patients	28
Complete Remission	1
Minor Response	1
Stable Disease	8
Progression	18

There were only one complete remission and one minor response among the evaluable patients. Both responses occurred in patients with colorectal carcinoma. Dose-limiting toxicities were gastrointestinal (vomiting, mucositis, diarrhea) and neurological (ataxia, headache, weakness). Significant myelosuppression was observed when the dose of 5FU was escalated to 250-300 mg/M^2. This drug combination resulted in a significant prolongation of the plasma half-life of 5FU. Although the anticipated biochemical effects of thymidine and PALA on 5FU were observed, the clinical results were disappointing. Hopefully, other schedules and combinations will prove to be more effective.

REFERENCES

1. Blokhina NG, Vozny EK, Garin AM. (1972) Results of treatment of malignant tumors with ftorafur. Cancer 30: 390-392.

2. Valdivieso M, Bodey GP, Gottlieb JA, et al. (1976) Clinical evaluation of ftorafur. Cancer Res 36: 1821-1824.

3. Lu K, Loo TL, Benvenuto JA, Benjamin RS, et al. (1975) Pharmacologic disposition and metabolism of ftorafur (abstract). Pharmacologist 17: 202.

4. Hortobagyi GN, Blumenschein GR, Tashima CK, et al. (1979). Ftorafur, adriamycin, cyclophosphamide and BCG in the treatment of metastatic breast cancer. Cancer 42: 398-405.

5. Bedikian AY, Bodey GP, Valdivieso M, et al. (1983) Phase I evaluation of oral tegafur. Cancer Treat Rep 67: 81-84.

6. Bedikian AY, Stroehlein J, Korinek J, et al. (1983) A comparative study of oral tegafur and intravenous 5-fluorouracil in patients with metastatic colorectal cancer. Cancer Clin Trials (in press).

7. Martin DS, Stolfi RL, Sawyer RC, et al. (1980) An overview of thymidine. Cancer 45: 1117-1128.

8. Woodcock TM, Martin DS, Damin LEM, et al. (1980) Combinaton clinical trials with thymidine and fluorouracil: a phase I and clinical pharmacologic evaluation. Cancer 45: 1135-1143.

9. Au JLS, Rustum YM, Ledesma EJ, et al. (1982) Clinical pharmacological studies of concurrent infusion of 5-fluorouracil and thymidine in treatment of colorectal carcinomas. Cancer Res 42: 2930-2937.

10. Kirkwood JM, Ensminger W, Rosowsky A, et al. (1980) Comparison of pharmacokinetics of 5-fluorouracil and 5-fluorouracil with concurrent thymidine infusions in a phase I trial. Cancer Res 40: 107-113.

11. Bedikian AY, Stroehlein JR, Karlin DA, et al. (1981) Chemotherapy for colorectal cancer with a combination of PALA and 5-FU. Cancer Treat Rep 65: 747-753.

12. Mann G, Hortobagyi G, Buzdar A, et al. A comparative study of PALA, PALA/5-FU and 5-FU in advanced breast cancer. To be published.

13. Casper ES, Vale K, Williams LJ, et al. (1983) Phase I and clinical pharmacological evaluation of biochemical modulation of 5-fluorouracil with N-(phosphonacetyl)-L-aspartic acid. Cancer Res 43:2324-2329.

14. Chiuten DF, Valdivieso M, Benvenuto JA, et al. A phase I-II clinical and pharmacologic study of thymidine, 5-fluorouracil and PALA given in combinations. To be published.

© 1984 Elsevier Science Publishers B.V.
Fluoropyrimidines in Cancer Therapy
K. Kimura, S. Fujii, M. Ogawa, G.P. Bodey, P. Alberto, eds.

DISCUSSION

Blokhina: I have two questions for Dr. Kimura. First, how long did the conventional course of treatment by UFT last in cases of cancer of the stomach? Second, did you use maintenance therapy after the conventional course?

Kimura: We used UFT therapy as long as possible. Now we are trying UFTM for induction therapy. For induction therapy of stomach cancer, UFTM is better than UFT alone. UFTM is a combination of UFT and mitomycin C. After that, long-term administration of UFT alone can be given for maintenance. Sometimes consolidation therapy is performed with UFTM, whereas UFT is used for maintenance.

Syrkin: I have a question for Dr. Koyama. One of the side effects of HCFU was hot sensation. I am interested as to whether it is possible to predict this side effect from the experimental data on preclinical toxicity.

Y. Koyama: There is no way of predicting this peculiar toxicity from the preclinical results. We found this from the phase I studies.

O'Connell: I wanted to comment on one of Dr. Bodey's clinical trials in that we are in the process of conducting a phase II trial of the PALA-5-FU-thymidine combination in patients with advanced untreated colorectal carcinoma. Our schedule is a bit different from the schedule used by Dr. Bodey. We elected to give the full single-agent dose of PALA (4 g/m^2) on day 1. Twenty-four hours later, thymidine (15 g) is given over a 30-minute period followed by a single intravenous bolus of 5-FU (200 mg/m^2). This regimen was based on the elegant pharmacokinetic and biochemical studies that Dr. Loo presented at the previous session as well as the in vivo animal model data of Dr. Schabel. To date, we have observed eight of 31 patients with objective tumor responses, including some with rather remarkable reductions in hepatomegaly and abdominal masses and subcutaneous metastases. Interestingly, this has been seen primarily in patients with anaplastic (grade 3 or 4) type of colorectal carcinomas or rapidly progressing tumors. Thus, we have a continued interest in this type of approach, particularly for patients with rapidly progressive tumors.

Yan Sun (Cancer Institute and Hospital, CAMS, Peking): I am very interested in the CNS toxicity associated with 5'-DFUR. Is any further data available, such as the 5-FU level in the CSF, EEG examination data, or autopsy findings? 5'-DFUR does not have any CNS toxicity, but it is well known for 5-FU. One of the remote toxicities of 5-FU is cerebral or cerebellar degeneration. Does this occur with 5'-DFUR?

Alberto: Concerning CNS toxicity and related laboratory exploration, unfortunately I have no answer. We did not regularly check either the EEG or the cerebrospinal fluid.

Ota: In our study of oral administration of 5'-DFUR, we have had no such CNS toxicity. Only diarrhea is a dose-limiting toxicity.

Bodey: I think that the results that Dr. O'Connell mentioned are of considerable interest. We had given a dose of PALA of only 1 g/m^2 on day 1, and then the thymidine dose was 30 g on day 2, and the 5-FU dose was 150-300 mg/m^2 on day 2. It is of particular interest to me, Dr. O'Connell, that your dose of PALA is considerably higher than the dose that we gave, and yet Dr. Martin and his colleagues have suggested that the most appropriate approach is to use a lower dose of PALA because you achieve the same biochemical modulation at a lower dose. This would then allow you to give higher doses of 5-FU.

O'Connell: As it turns out, we were actually able to give essentially the same 5-FU dose in combination with the full single-agent dose of PALA. Although I don't think we can draw any comparative conclusions because your population of patients was predominantly a group previously treated with the fluorinated pyrimidines (and that may have accounted for your low response rate), the responses that we have observed may challenge the appropriateness of the urinary tests in determining what the proper dose of a biochemical modulating compound should be.

Kimura: I would like to add some comments to what Dr. Alberto said. In Japan, we use 5'-DFUR orally. You use the same drug intravenously. You heard the opinion given in Dr. Ota's report. In your opinion, which is better - intravenous or oral use?

Alberto: I must say that when we started with the phase I studies with this drug, it was from the beginning an agreement between the Japanese investigators and us that they should use it orally and we should use it intravenously. It was based on this agreement that we worked with this drug intravenously. Personally, I prefer to avoid oral administration for the first step when the toxic dose is not known. Probably, people in Japan are more disciplined than patients in Europe, and you probably do not have this difficulty of never being sure that the patient has taken exactly what he was told to take.

Sadée: Several speakers proposed the notion that HCFU is, in fact, useful in cases with liver impairment. I think that this implies that other 5-FU prodrugs are ineffective. While I believe I understand the biochemical rationale, I do not know what the evidence is. The only piece of information was actually provided by Dr. Bodey, who said that in a patient with liver impairment tegafur was more toxic (implying that it certainly is still active). Since Dr. Koyama was the last speaker to mention that HCFU ought to be used preferably in cases with liver impairment, maybe I should ask him. What is the evidence that the other agents are not active?

Y. Koyama: I think it is based on Dr. Fujita's results. Could you comment?

H. Fujita: In our animal experiments using mice bearing sarcoma 180, pretreatment with carbon tetrachloride resulted in very low 5-FU tissue levels after tegafur administration. When tegafur was given to patients at the Saitama Cancer Center, patients with very high SGOT, jaundice, or high alkaline phosphatase had very low 5-FU levels when compared to patients with normal liver function. However, 5-FU levels after HCFU administration to mice were not reduced by pretreatment with carbon tetrachloride. The activation of HCFU is not influenced with liver impairment.

Bodey: Dr. Sadée, in terms of the liver toxicity in the patients who had impairment of liver function (generally as a consequence of tumor metastases), we saw more myelo-suppression with tegafur and also more nausea and vomiting. I am not aware that there was any difference in the response rate between those patients and patients who did not have such liver impairment. It was primarily a difference in the toxicities.

CLINICAL ASPECTS:
METHODS OF ADMINISTRATION

Fluoropyrimidines in Cancer Therapy
K. Kimura, S. Fujii, M. Ogawa, G.P. Bodey, P. Alberto, eds.

CLINICAL STUDIES OF RECTAL ADMINISTRATION OF TEGAFUR

Chihiro Konda

1. INTRODUCTION

Currently tegafur is one of the most broadly used anticancer agents in cancer chemotherapy in Japan. This agent is administered by a variety of routes for systemic chemotherapy, including intravenous, oral and rectal administration. Rectal administration of tegafur has been firstly proposed in our hospital in 1973 and thereafter extensively studied in Japan. It is notable that tegafur is the first and only one anticancer agent safely applied to rectal administration for clinical use. This compound was proved a unique quality that it was well absorbed from the rectum without any local damages. Thereafter it appeared in blood and produced a peak of blood concentration in the early period of time after rectal administration (1,2). This finding was very similar to those of intravenous or oral administration of tegafur. The acute toxicity indicated as value of LD_{50} in rats by rectal administration of tegafur demonstrated no significant difference among intravenous, intraperitoneal, intramuscular and oral administration of the drug. This fact also suggested that tegafur was well absorbed from the rectum.

After absorption from the rectum the larger amount of tegafur appeared in the caval vein blood rather than in the portal vein blood (3). Accordingly, rectally absorbed tegafur might be not only diminished the first pass through liver and less decomposed to 5-fluorouracil and others primarily by liver, but also more readily distributed to all tissues compared to orally administered tegafur. Furthermore, rectally administered tegafur appeared in lymph with high concentration (3). It was well known that tegafur slowly cleft to 5-fluorouracil in vivo. It was proved that tegafur and its metabolites revealed in blood, lymph or tissues with the sustained high concentration for long period of time after rectal administration (3). Such a feature of pharmacokinetics by rectal administration was favorable for the cytotoxicity of tegafur or 5-fluorouracil to be enhanced by longer exposure to tumor cells in vitro (4). From these facts as mentioned above, chemotherapy with rectal administration of tegafur seems to be rational.

This study is concerned with the clinical results of rectal administration for cancer chemotherapy in our hospital.

2. PATIENTS AND METHODS

Patients with a variety of cancer treated in our hospital were subjected to this study. For the convenient application of tegafur, a suppository was prepared, cont-

aining tegafur of 0.75 or 1.0g in the aliphatic base,
Witepsol W-35. This suppository melts at 36 to 37^0C and
liquifies within three to four minutes. Tegafur is releas-
ed from the suppository within 25 minutes at all.

Rectal administration of tegafur with the suppository
was designed in two protocols as shown in Table 1.

TABLE 1   Protocols of rectal administration of tegafur

Protocol	Dosage of tegafur	Interval of administration
I	0.75 or 1.0g	q 12 hours
II	0.75 or 1.0g	q 24 hours

In protocol I the suppository contained tegafur was
administered twice a day and in protocol II it was given
once a day in the consecutive days. They terminated
the administration by progression of disease or by severe
toxicity.

Evaluation of the response was based on the criteria
designed by the Japanese Society of Cancer Therapy.
Complete response was defined as the complete disappearance
of all detectable disease. Partial response was defined as
50% or more reduction of measurable tumors without simultaneous progression of other tumors or without development
of new metastasis. Others were defined as minor response,

stable disease or progressive disease.

3. RESULTS

A total of 273 patients were entered in this study.
One hundred and forty patients were evaluable for response, 117 patients were evaluable only for the toxicity,
and 10 patients were inadequate for any evaluation. The
response rates by primary site of cancer are illustrated
in Table 2. Overall response rate was observed in 10%, 14
patients out of 146 with a variety of cancers. All were
evaluated as a patial response. Protocol I produced a 22%
response rate, 12 of 54 patients, while protocol II produced a 2% response rate, 2 of 92 patients. In protocol I
8 responders were observed in 20 patients with cancer of
the stomach, 1 in 12 with the lung and all of 2 with the
breast, respectively. While in protocol II each one responder was observed in 15 patients with cancer of the
lung and in 12 with the breast, respectively.

The response rates related to prior chemotherapy with
fluoropyrimidines are shown in Table 3. In protocol I a
22% response rate, 6 of 27 patients previously untreated,
was observed and a 32% response rate, 6 of 19 patients
previously treated with fluoropyrimidines, respectively.
In protocol II each one responder was observed in 41
patients previously untreated and in 44 previously treated with fluoropyrimidines.

The response rates related to a variety of metastases

are illustrated in Table 4.

TABLE 2   Response rates related to primary sites of
           cancer

Primary sites	protocol I		protocol II		total	
Esophagus	0/2		0/1		0/3	
Stomach	8/20	40%	0/38		8/58	14%
Colorectum	1/8	13%	0/9		1/17	6%
Liver	0/1		0/1		0/2	
Pancreas	0/1		0/1		0/2	
Biliary tracts	0/2		0/1		0/3	
Lung	1/12	8%	1/15	7%	2/27	7%
Breast	2/2		1/12	8%	3/14	21%
Head and neck	–		0/3		0/3	
Cervix	0/2		0/2		0/4	
Ovary	0/1		0/1		0/2	
Kidney	–		0/3		0/3	
Urinary tracts	0/1		–		0/1	
Primary unknown	0/1		0/3		0/4	
Others	0/1		0/2		0/3	
Total	12/54	22%	2/92	2%	14/146	10%

Both in protocol I and in protocol II different response
rate was observed in a variety of metastatic sites of
cancers.

TABLE 3   Response rates related to prior chemotherapy

Prior chemotherapy	protocol I		protocol II	
None	6/27	22%	1/41	2%
Fluoropyrimidines	6/19	32%	1/44	2%

TABLE 4   Response rates related to a variety of
metastatic sites of cancers

Metastatic sites	protocol I		protocol II	
Lymph node	9/15	60%	3/11	27%
Liver	3/8	38%	0/18	0%
Lung	0/11	0%	0/20	0%
Soft tissue	0/3	0%	1/4	24%
Intraabdominal mass	6/18	33%	0/20	0%
Primary sites	1/18	6%	0/24	0%

Lymph node metastasis responded in 60%, 9 of 15 patients received protocol I, while it responded in 27%, 3 of 11 patients received protocol II. Liver metastasis responded in 38%, 3 of 8 patients received protocol I, while none of 18 received protocol II. Lung metastasis responded neither protocol I nor protocol II. Soft tissue metastasis responded in only one of 4 patients receiving

protocol II. Intraabdominal metastatic mass responded in
33%, 6 or 18 patients received protocol I, while
not in any of the 20 patients receiving protocol II.
Additionally, primary sites of cancer responded only in
6%, one of 18 patients receiving protocol I, and
not in any of the 24 patients receiving protocol II.

TABLE 5   Patient distribution by dose for the initiation
           of response

Dose for the initiation of response : g	protocol I			protocol II		
	A	B	C	A	B	C
-10	3	1	-	-	-	-
10-	2	3	-	2	-	-
20-	3	-	1	1	-	-
30-	-	1	1	-	-	-
40-	1	1	-	-	-	-
50-	-	2	2	-	-	-
60-	-	-	-	-	-	-
80-	-	-	-	-	-	-
100-	-	1	-	-	-	-

A: lymph node metastasis, B: intraabdominal metastatic
mass, C: liver metastasis

    Patient distribution by dose for the initiation of
the response in a variety of metastasis is listed in
Table 5. Initiation of response on lymph node metastasis
by protocol I was obtained at a total dose of tegafur

less than 30g in 0 of 9 responders. However, initiation of
response on intraabdominal metastatic mass by protocol I
was obtained at a same total dose in 4 of 9 responders.
A total dose of tegafur more than 30g was necessary for
obtaining initiation of response on liver metastasis in
all of patients. Response on intraabdominal metastatic
mass was obtained at a total dose of 30g or more in 5 of
9 responders. Exceptionally, one patient obtained
initiation of response at a total dose of 100g or more.

TABLE 6   Patient distribution by duration of response
           related to primary sites of cancer

Duration of response: months	stomach	breast	lung	colorectum	total
-3	3	2	2	1	8
3-	3	-	-	-	3
6-	1	1	-	-	2
9-	-	-	-	-	-
12-	1	-	-	-	1

Patient distribution by duration of response related
to primary sites of cancer is illustrated in Table 6.
Duration of response lasted 3 months or less was observed
in 8 of 14 responders, while the duration lasted more
than 3 months was in 6, including 5 with cancer of the

stomach and one with the breast. Furthermore, the duration more than 6 months was in 3, and more than 12 months only in one, respectively.

TABLE 7   Incidence of hematological toxicity

	protocol I		protocol II		total	
No. of evaluable patients	46		92		138	
Leukopenia ($-$ 4,000)	4	9%	8	9%	12	9%
Anemia ($-$ 350 x 10^4)	10	22%	18	20%	28	20%
Thrombocytopenia ($-$ 7 x 10^4)	4	9%	8	9%	12	9%

Incidence of hematological toxicity is shown in Table 7.

Incidence of leukopenia was observed each in 9% out of evaluable 46 patients received protocol I and of 92 received protocol II. Incidence of anemia was found in 22% of the patients received protocol I and in 20% of the patients received protocol II. Incidence of thrombocyto-penia was found each in 9% of the patients received protocol I or protocol II. Furthermore, none of hematolog-ical toxicity were observed in 67% of the patients with protocol I and in 74% of the patients with protocol II.

TABLE 8   Incidence of clinical manifestations of
           toxicity

	protocol I		protocol II		total	
No. of evaluable patients	67		196		243	
Anorexia	16	24%	23	12%	39	15%
Nausea	11	16	8	4	19	7
Vomiting	8	12	8	4	16	6
Diarrhea	7	10	8	4	15	6
Stomatitis	6	9	5	3	11	4
Bleeding(anal)	6(6)	9(9)	4(1)	2(1)	10(7)	4(3)
Dizziness	2	3	5	3	7	3
Skin reaction	4	6	7	4	11	4
Pigmentation	6	9	8	4	14	5
Local pain	4	6	4	2	8	3
Others	2	3	8	4	10	4

    Incidence of clinical manifestations of toxicity is
listed in Table 8.
Clinical manifestations of toxicity occurred in 55% by
protocol I and in 33% by protocol II. In protocol I
anorexia occurred in 24%, nausea in 16%, vomiting in 12%,
diarrhea in 10%, stomatitis in 9%, anal bleeding in 9%,
pigmentation in 9%, and skin reaction and local pain each
in 6%. While in protocol II anorexia occurred in 12%, and

226

other manifestations including nausea, vomiting, diarrhea
in 5% or less. A variety of clinical manifestations of
toxicity was observed less frequently in protocol II than
in protocol I.

4. DISCUSSION

This study evaluated clinical efficacy of rectal
administration of tegafur designed in two protocols. The
higher response rates were obtained by protocol I in
patients with stomach and breast cancer.

Protocol I was notably effective on lymph node metastasis
and moderately on liver metastasis or intraabdominal
metastatic mass, while it was less effective on lung
metastasis or primary sites of cancers. The response of
protocol II was disappointingly low in a variety of
metastatic sites of cancers. Longer duration of the response was not obtained in this study. The duration of 6
months or more was found only in 3 of 14 responders including 2 of 8 responders with cancer of the stomach and 1
of 3 with the breast, respectively.

Hematological toxicity of the therapy was observed
less frequently. Difference in incidence of the toxicity
was found to be not significant between the two protocols.
The severity of leukopenia or thrombocytopenia was very
low as observed in oral administration of tegafur.

Incidence of clinical manifestations of toxicity was
not so high. The gastrointestinal disturbances were main

clinical manifestations of toxicity. Incidence of the
toxicity by protocol I was observed higher than that of
protocol II. No severe toxicity of CNS was not seen in
this study. As most of the manifestations were not
severe, the administration of tegafur could be continued
for obtaining the response, only occasionally modified the
dose or administration interval.

Protocol I of rectal administration of tegafur provided the notable prolongation of survival period in
patients with cancer of the stomach. Namely, median
survival time was 11.5 months in 19 patients received
protocol I, while it was 6.6 months in 38 patients
received protocol II. The results were superior to
median survival time of 5.5 months in 30 patients received oral administration of tegafur.

Rectal administration of tegafur is an effective
chemotherapy for cancer of the stomach.

REFERENCES

1. Akazawa A, Watanabe N, Yasuda Y, et al. (1974)
    Effects of suppository bases on rat rectal absorption
    of 1-(2-tetrahydrofuryl)-5-fluorouracil. Yakugaku
    34: 47-53.

2. Fujita H, Sugiyama M and Kimura K. (1976) Pharma-
    cokinetics of futraful (FT-207) for clinical appli-
    cation. Chemotherapy 8: 51-57.

3. Fujii S, Okuda H, Akazawa A, et al. (1975) Studies
    on the fate of 1-(2-tetrahydrofuryl)-5-fluorouracil
    (FT-207), a carcinostatic agent. III. Absorption,
    distribution, excretion and metabolism after rectal
    administration of FT-207. Yakugaku 95: 732-740.

4. Shimoyama M and Kimura K. (1973) Quantitative study
    on cytocidal action of anticancer agents. Saishin
    Igaku 28: 1024-1040.

© 1984 Elsevier Science Publishers B.V.
Fluoropyrimidines in Cancer Therapy
K. Kimura, S. Fujii, M. Ogawa, G.P. Bodey, P. Alberto, eds.

ORAL ADMINISTRATION OF 5-FLUOROURACIL AND TEGAFUR

Minoru Kurihara, Keiichi Miyasaka, Tsuguhiko Izumi
Yozo Sasaki and Toshiki Kamano

After some pioneer studies of oral administration of 5-FU in foreign and our countries[1-5], clinical application has been positively made by development of 5-FU dry syrup (d. s.) in Japan. Table 1 shows the clinical effects of 5-FU d.s. which were collected from Japanese Journal in the field of cancer treatment. The common dose schedule of 5-FU d.s. is daily 300 mg per body. Effective rates (>I-A, by Karnofsky's criteria) were 20.5% in overall 273 evaluable cases and 18.7% in 150 stomach cancers, 11.4% in 35 colon and rectum cancers and 34.7% in 49 breast cancers, respectively. Side effects which were collected from Japanese Journals were summarized in Table 2. Gastrointestinal side effects, such as anorexia, nausea, vomiting and diarrhea were recognized in less than 20% of cases, but causes the first reason to discontinue the administration. On the contrary, hematological toxicities were few and mild. Therefore, it is very often used even in out-patient clinic in Japan. Some marked effective cases of gastric cancers in radiological and endoscopic findings which have been seldom experienced in other chemotherapeutic drugs were reported by 5-FU d.s. administration.[6,7]

In order to confirm on the experimental basis that oral administration of 5-FU has effects on gastric cancer, ^{14}C-5-FU was administered orally and intravenously to dogs with gastric cancer induced by our method using ENNG[8] and normal beagles.

Method of administration of 2-^{14}C-5-FU

In case of oral administration 2-^{14}C-5-FU (Produced by CEA-IRF-SORIN, Specific activity: 45 to 55 mCi/mM) was diluted with 5-FU d.s., and 5.7 mg/kg (17/μCi/kg) to Dog No. 1 and 5.0 mg/kg (130 μCi/kg) to Dog No. 2 was infused under endoscopy into the stomach of each dog under anesthesia.

In case of intravenous administration, 2-^{14}C-5-FU was diluted with 5-FU injectabel solution, and 5.0 mg/kg (104 μCi/kg) to Dog No. 3 was intravenously administered under anesthesia.

The all 3 animals were sacrificed after 60 minutes.

Separation and quantitative analysis of 5-FU metabolites

The metabolites in the tumors and oragans were divided according to the method described by Schmidt - Thanhauser, and were separated according to the method described by Anada et al[9] who modified the method described by Chaudhuri.

Determination of 5-FU activating substances

100 mg of the tissue and 0.2 ml of plasma were treated by an automatic combustion system AROCA ASC-112.

TABLE 1   CLINICAL EFFECTS OF 5-FU (P.O.)

Tumor Site	5-FU dry syrup (d.s.)					5-FU tablet				
	evaluable cases	~0-C	I-A	I-B	response rate (>I-A,%)	evaluable cases	~0-C	I-A	I-B	response rate (>I-A,%)
Stomach	150	122	19	9	18.7	139	111	26	2	20.1
Colon, Rectum	35	31	4	0	11.4	31	22	6	3	29.0
Liver	9	5	4	0	44.4	13	11	1	1	15.4
Pancreas	5	5	0	0	0	5	4	1	0	20.0
Gallblader Bile duct	4	3	1	0	25.0	9	7	2	0	22.2
Breast	49	32	11	6	34.7	38	27	10	1	28.9
Miscellaneous	21	19	1	1	9.5	17	15	0	2	11.8
Total	273	211	40	16	20.5	252	197	46	9	21.8

TABLE 2   SIDES   EFFECTS OF 5-FU d.s. & 5-FU TABLET

	5-FU d.s.	5-FU tablet
Anorexia	19.4 (%)	14.3 (%)
Nausea	12.5	8.4
Vomiting	10.4	3.9
Diarrhea	11.6	3.4
Abdominal pain	2.4	0.7
Abdominal fullness	1.2	0.2
General fatigue	3.6	0.1
Stomatitis	2.7	2.9
Epilation	1.2	0.2
Pigmentation	0.9	0.1
Eruption	0.6	0.2
Fever	0.6	0.1
Glycosuria	0.6	0.6
Proteinuria	1.2	0.3
Leucocytopenia	10.1	7.1
Erythrocytopenia	2.4	0.2
Thrombocytopenia	4.2	2.9
None	46.6	58.1

The recovery rate of ^{14}C was more than 97%. The radioactivity was monitored by AROCA LSC-653, and dpm from the data were calculated by a computer. The determined values of radioactivity were converted into 5-FU values for convenience. The values in each tissue were shown as the mean level of 2 or 3 pieces.

RESULTS

5-FU concentration was measured in the tumorous tissues of the stomach, the intact tissues of the same stomach, lymphnodes and urine after 60 minutes of oral and intravenous administration. 5-FU values were shown in Table 3. In this study, 5-FU values were higher in cancer tissues than in normal tissues of stomach, not only in the superficial layer of the cancerous tissues, but also in the profound layer of the cancer tissues. Furthermore, 5-FU values in the oral administration were higher than those in the intravenous administration. On the contray, 5-FU values of lymphnodes and urine in the intravenous administration were higher than in the oral administration.

Constituents of 5-FU metabolites in Stomach

Table 4 shows the constituents of 5-FU metabolites observed in the tumorous tissues and the normal tissues of the stomach after oral administration to Dog No. 2 and after intravenous administration to Dog No. 3. The activating substances (5-FU, FUR and F-Nucleotide) were observed 75.6% in the cancerous tissues and 60.4% in the nomal tissues when administered by oral route and 22.7% in

TABLE 3 DISTRIBUTION OF RADIOACTIVITY IN THE STOMACH, LYMPHNODES AND URINE OF DOGS BEARING GASTRIC CANCER AFTER ADMINISTRATION OF $2-{}^{14}C-5-FU$

Dog No.	Weight (kg)	Dose 5-FU (mg/kg)	Dose ${}^{14}C$ (μCi/kg)	Route	Concentration of 5-FU				
					Stomach μg/g			Lymphnodes μg/g	Urine μg/ml
					Cancerous tissue		Normal tissue		
1	3.6	5.7	171	P.O.	2.62		1.64	.	.
2	5.0	5.0	130	P.O.	surface 5.28		surface 2.70	Pancreatic 0.23	
								Mesenteric 0.26	
								Submaxillary 0.30	0.04
								Axillary 0.21	
					deep 2.41		deep 0.53	Knee 0.21	
3	5.0	5.0	104	i.v.	surface 1.12		surface 0.68	Pyloric 0.58	
								Pancreatic 0.88	28.16
					deep 0.45		deep 0.44	Mesenterial 0.59	

TABLE 4 5-FU METABOLITES IN THE NORMAL AND CANCEROUS TISSUES OF
STOMACH IN DOGS BEARING GASTRIC CANCER

Dog. No.	Route	Stomach	Fraction				
			5-FU, FUR	F-Nucleotide	Urea	FUPA, FGPA	
2	P.O.	Cancerous tissue	75.0	0.6	2.1	22.7	
		Normal tissue	59.8	0.6	2.7	37.0	
3	i.v.	Cancerous tissue	21.7	1.0	22.7	73.9	
		Normal tissue	23.6	1.1	37.0	66.8	

(%)

the cancerous tissue and 24.7% in the normal tissue when administered by intravenous route. From these facts, oral administration is probably a route of administration to expect the direct effect against gastric cancer.

Five years ago, 5-FU tablet, which was aimed to reduce the side effect of lower G.I., such as diarrhea and abdominal pain, was developed. It is considered that tablet form is much longer sustained with diet in the stomach than d.s. form as shown in Fig. 1.

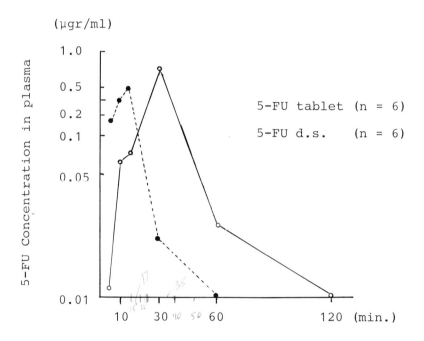

FIGURE 1   Absorption of 5-FU dry syrup and 5-FU tablet in Gastric Cancer Patients.
- Cross over administration of each form (200 mg as 5-FU) -

As the results of cooperative clinical study on 5-FU tablet by Tokyo Cancer Chemotherapy Cooperative Study Groups, 41 cases were evaluated as shown in Table 5. Dose schedule of 5-FU tablet was daily 300 mg per body, except for 3 cases which were administered 400 mg per body.

TABLE 5   CLINICAL EFFECTS OF 5-FU TABLET
(COOPERATIVE STUDY OF TOKYO CANCER CHEMO-
THERAPY CO-OPERATAIVE STUDY GROUP)

Tumor Site	Case No.	PR	NC + PD	Effective rate (%)
Stomach	27	5	22	18.5
Breast	6	2	4	33.3
Colon, Rectum	5	0	5	0
Duodenum	1	1	0	(100)
Lung	1	0	1	0
Esophagus	1	0	1	0
Total	41	8	33	19.5

Administration periods of 5-FU tablet were one to five months. Five PR cases were found in 27 gastric cancers (effective rate : 18.5%). In other cancers, two PR breast, and one PR duodenal cancer were found. Side effects of 5-FU tablet were shown in Table 6. It was rare to discontinue the administration of the drug in this trial.

TABLE 6. SIDE EFFECTS OF 5-FU TABLET

(COOPERATIVE STUDY OF TOKYO CANCER CHEMOTHERAPY COOPERATIVE STUDY GROUP)

		Weak		Strong		1	2	3	4	5	6	7	10	16 (W)
		↓	→	↓	→									
Anorexia	19.2%	3	3	1	3									
Nausea, Vomiting	11.5	2	2	0	2									
Diarrhea	7.7	0	2	1	1									
Stomatitis	9.6	1	3	0	1									
Itching	1.9	0	0	0	1									
Leukopenia	9.6	2	2	1	0									

↓ Weak and transient, → Weak and continuous
⬇ Strong and transient, ➡ Strong and continuous

Effective rate of cooperative study by Osaka Chemotherapy Cooperative Study Group was 23.3%[10]. Table 1 shows the clinical effects of 5-FU tablet which were collected from Japanese Journals. The common dose schedule is daily 300 mg per body. Effective rates (>I-A, by Karnofsky's Criteria) were 21.8% in overall 252 evaluable cases and 20.1% in 139 stomach cancers, 29% in 31 colon and rectum cancers and 29% in 38 breast cancers, respectively. Sides effects which were collected from Japanese Journals are shown in Table 2. Gastrointestinal side effects, such as anorexia, diarrhea, abdominal pain and hematological toxicities are less than that of 5-FU d.s. administration, respectively.

Thus, 5-FU tablet is considered as a useful chemotherapeutic drug, single or multi-combination with MMC and or ADR.

TABLE 7   THERAPEUTIC METHODS FOR G.I. CANCER
BY ANTICANCER AGENTS OF OUR GROUP

Single therapy	5-FU d.s. or tablet	300 mg/day P.O.
	tegafur cap. or granule	800 mg/day P.O.
Combined therapy	FMa	tegafur 800 mg/day + MMC i.a., 20 mg one shot
	tegafur or 5-FU	tegafur 800 mg/day or 5-FU 300 mg/day
	+ MMC	+ MMC i.v., 10 mg/ week
	(+ ADR)	(+ADR i.v., 30 mg/ week)

Effective cases of G.I. cancer have been also experienced by oral administration of tegafur in our group. Of the clinical cases treated with oral 5-FU (d.s., tablet), tegafur (capsule, granules) or multi-combination by

5-FU or tegafur + MMC, and or + ADR (Table 7.)

TABLE 8   TUMOR REGRESSION EFFECTS ON GASTRIC CANCER
          EVALUATED BY THE CRITERIA OF CANCER
          CHEMOTHERAPY FOR SOLID TUMORS

	Cases No.	CR	PR	NC	PD	Effective rate (%)
tegafur (P.O.)	23	1	1	17	4	8.7
5-FU (P.O.)	25	0	1	21	3	4.0
Subtotal	48	1	2	38	7	6.3
FMa	13	0	2	6	5	15.4
tegafur or 5-FU + MMC (+ ADR)	23	0	6	11	6	26.1
Subtotal	36	0	8	17	11	22.2
Total	84	1	10	55	18	13.1

84 were classified as evaluable according to the Criteria
of Cancer Chemotherapy for Solid Tumors and effective rate
resulted in 13.1% (Table 8.).   The effective rate in 48
cases treated with a single agent proved to be 6.3% and
that in 36 cases treated with multi-drug combination
22.2%.

REFERENCES

1. Chaudhuri NK, Mukherjee KL, Heidelberger C.
    (1958) Studies on Fluorinated Pyrimidines VII - The
    Degradative Pathway. Biochem Pharmacol I: 328-341.

2. Curreri AR, Ansfield FJ, McIver FA, et al. (1958)
    Clinical Studies with Fluorouracil. Cancer Rec 18:
    478-484.

3. Gold GL, Hall TC, Shinden BI, et al. (1959)
    A Clinical Study of 5-Fluorouracil. Cancer Res 19:
    935-939.

4. Khung CL, Hall TC, Piro AJ, et al. (1966)
    A Clinical Trial of Oral 5-Fluorouracil. Clin
    Pharmacol Therap 7: 527-533.

5. Kubo K, Tamura Z, Usami H. (1973) Distribution
    in tissues of 5-Fluorouracil and 5-Fluorouridylic
    acid after oral and intravenous administrations.
    Medicine and Biology 86: 69-72.

6. Naito T, Sato K, Harada M, et al.(1974) Clinical
    Report: Treatment of Advanced Stomach Cancer with
    Oral Administration of 5-Fluorouracil in Solution.
    Jpn J Cancer Chemother 1: 419-431.

7. Kurihara M, Shirakabe H, Izumi T, et al. (1981)
    X-ray and endoscopy in the evaluation of gastric
    cancer chemotherapy. In: Diagnosis and Treatment of
    Upper Gastrointestinal Tumors (eds) M Friedman, M
    Ogawa and D Kisner. Amsterdam-Oxford-Princeton.
    Excerpta Medica pp. 428-449

8. Kurihara M, Shirakabe H, Izumi T, et al. (1977)
    Adenocarcinomas of the Stomach Induced in Beagle Dogs
    by Oral Administration of N-Ethyl-N'-Nitro-N-Nitro-
    soguanidine. Zsch Krebsforsh u Klin Onkol 90:
    241-252.

9. Anada H, Nakamura N, Marumo H. (1974) Studies on
    the Metabolic Fate of 5-Fluorouracil in the Oral ad-
    ministration. Yakugaku Zashi 94: 1131-1138.

10. Taguchi T. (Osaka Cancer Chemotherapy Cooperative
    Study Group): Clinical Results of Co-operative Study
    on 5-Fluorouracil Tablets. Jpn J Cancer Chemother 6:
    737-741, 1979.

GROUP STUDY OF FLUORINATED PYRIMIDINES

Tokyo Cancer Chemotherapy Cooperative Study Group

The Tokyo Cancer Chemotherapy Cooperative Study Group is composed of 33 hospitals and universities in the Tokyo district. For ten years, our group has performed phase II and III studies on various anticancer agents. Fluorinated pyrimidines, tegafur (oral administration), tegafur (rectal administration), 5-FU dry syrup, and UFT have also been studied by our group.

ELIGIBILITY OF PATIENTS:

inoperable or recurrent cancer

histologically proven

measurable or evaluable

performance status of 0-3

age under 80 years

no double cancers

no serious hepatic dysfunctions

no serious renal dysfunctions

no serious bone marrow suppression

absence of previous treatment effects

CRITERIA OF RESPONSE:

Criteria of the Tokyo Cancer Chemotherapy Cooperative Study Group

markedly effective tumor regression of more than 90%

effective   50 - 90%

slightly effective   25 - 50%

no change

progressive

A decrease in ascites was excluded from evaluation of response.

METHOD OF ADMINISTRATION

Daily administration was carried out in all cases. The daily dose was as follows:

tegafur capsules (oral)   800 - 1200 mg for more than 6 weeks

tegafur suppositories (rectal) 750 mg twice a week for more than 3 weeks

5-FU dry syrup (oral)   300 - 400 mg for more than 4 weeks

UFT (oral)   600 mg for more than 4 weeks

TUMOR EFFECTS

Over all response rates of tegafur (oral), tegafur (rectal) and 5-FU dry syrup were 21.0%, 13.0% and 18.9%, respectively. Thus, there was no significant difference in response rates, but the rate was somewhat lower for tegafur suppositories. The response rates for gastric cancer were 23.7%, 9.1% and 22.9%, respectively. Therefore, there was also no significant difference in response rates for gastric cancer cases, but it was also somewhat low for tegafur suppositories. On the other hand, tegafur suppositories demonstrated a high response rate in colon cancer cases. No significant difference was noted in other tumor types. The response rate of lung cancer cases was extremely low for all dosage forms.

The tumor effect was correlated with the total dose, to some degree, for all agents. In responders, more than 50 g of tegafur, or more than 12 g of 5-FU was administered to determine tumor response. Tumor regression began within 4 weeks of initiating the administration. The tumor response appeared earlier in breast cancer than in gastrointestinal cancer.

Remission duration continued for more than 6 months in more than half of the cases (55.6%) treated by oral administration of tegafur, and more than one year in 14.8%; 10 weeks on the average for gastric cancer cases and 10 weeks even for colon cancer cases treated with tegafur suppositories; and for more than 6 months in half of the cases treated with 5-FU dry syrup.

TABLE 1 Response rate in patients treated with fluorinated pyrimidines

Pyrimidines	Entered	Evaluable	Markedly effective	Effective	Slightly effective	Responders	%
Tegafur capsules	116	100	6	15	6	27	27.0
Tegafur suppo.	96	69	5	4	12	21	30.4
5-FU dry syrup	85	74	11	3	6	20	27.0
5-FU capsules	32	29	3	3	0	3	10.3

TABLE 2 Response rate in stomach cancer patietns treated with fluorinated pyrimidines

Pyrimidines	Evaluable (cases)	Markedly effective	Effective	Slightly effective	No effect	Responders	%
Tegafur capsules	38	3	6	3	26	12	31.6
Tegafur suppo.	33	3	0	8	22	11	33.3
5-FU dry syrup	48	9	2	6	31	17	35.6
5-FU capsules	29	0	3	0	26	3	10.3

TABLE 3 Response rate in breast cancer patients treated with fluorinated pyrimidines

Pyrimidines	Evaluable (cases)	Markedly effective	Effective	Slightly effective	No effect	Responders	%
Tegafur capsules	17	1	5	1	10	7	41.2
Tegafur suppo.	6	0	2	1	3	3	50.0
5-FU dry syrup	5	1	0	0	4	1	20.0
5-FU capsules	2	0	0	0	2	0	0

TABLE 4 Response rate in lung cancer patients treated with fluorinated pyrimidines

Pyrimidines	Evaluable (cases)	Markedly effective	Effective	Slightly effective	No effect	Responders	%
Tegafur capsules	14	0	0	1	13	1	7.1
Tegafur suppo.	12	0	0	1	11	1	8.3
5-FU dry syrup	7	0	0	0	7	0	0
5-FU capsules	1	0	0	0	1	0	0

COMPARISON BETWEEN TEGAFUR CAPSULES AND UFT

Recently, a comparison between tegafur capsule and UFT was made by our group according to the criteria of the Ministry of Health and Welfare by this criteria, tumor regression of more than 50% was established as a partial response (PR). According to this stricter criteria, there were 13 responders, 16.3%, out of 80 evaluable cases treated with tegafur capsules. On the other hand there were 25 responders, 36.9%, out of 93 evaluable cases treated with UFT. Thus, a higher response was seen in cases treated with UFT. However, there were eight responders, or 24.2%, out of 33 evaluable cases with gastric cancer treated with tegafur capsules. On the other hand, there were 10 responders, or 27.8%, out of 36 evaluable cases with gastric cancer treated with UFT. UFT was found to be the most effective in colon cancer (66.7%), followed by breast cancer (33.3%), liver cancer (28.1%), and gastric cancer (27.8%). However, tumor response was not obtained in 16 lung cancer cases. The treatment duration until the appearance of response was 20.4 days on the average: 11.8 g was the average total dosage. Side effects were milder and less common with UFT than with tegafur capsules, as are mentioned later.

SIDE EFFECTS

The spectrum of side effects was similar among tegafur capsules, tegafur suppositories, 5-FU dry

TABLE 5 Comparison of UFT AND tegafur capsules

	Entered	Evaluable	CR	PR	MR	NC	PD	Responders	%
UFT									
Stomach cancer	53	36	0	10	2	16	8	10	27.8
Colon cancer	12	9	0	6	0	3	0	6	66.7
Liver cancer	7	7	0	2	0	3	2	2	28.6
Lung cancer	16	15	0	0	0	8	7	0	0
Breast cancer	14	12	0	4	0	6	2	0	33.3
Miscellaneous	18	14	0	3	0	6	5	3	21.4
Total	120	93	0	25	2	42	24	25	26.9
Tegafur									
Stomach cancer	43	33	0	8	2	16	7	8	24.2
Colon cancer	16	12	0	1	0	7	4	1	8.3
Liver cancer	2	1	0	1	0	0	0	1	100.0
Lung cancer	16	11	0	0	1	4	6	0	0
Breast cancer	15	12	1	1	1	8	1	2	16.7
Miscellaneous	12	11	0	1	3	4	3	1	9.1
Total	104	80	1	12	7	39	21	13	16.3

TABLE 6 Effects of fluorinated pyrimidines

	Tegafur (p.o.)		Tegafur (sup.)		5-FU dry syrup		5-FU capsules		UFT	
No. of cases	116 cases		88 cases		85 cases		32 cases		123 cases	
Fever	6	5.2%	1	1.1%	0	0	1	3.1%	0	0
Fatigue	20	17.2	5	5.6	1	1.1	8	25.0	7	5.7%
Anorexia	37	31.9	16	18.2	24	28.2	14	43.8	36	29.3
Nausea, vomiting	27	23.3	13	14.7	11	12.9	10	31.3	19	15.4
Diarrhea	19	16.4	10	11.3	9	10.5	3	9.4	7	5.7
Stomatitis	5	4.3	10	11.3	1	1.1	0	0	3	2.5
CNS toxicity	7	6.0	1	1.1	0		1	3.1	0	
Anal pain	0	0	2	2.2	0		0		0	
Skin rash	2	1.7	1	1.1	0		0		4	3.3
Alopecia	6	5.2	1	1.1	3	3.5	0		0	
Pigmentation	7	6.0	4	4.6	1	1.1	0		4	3.3
Leukopenia	7	6.0	6	6.8	0		1	3.1	6	4.9
Thrombocytopenia	5	4.3	6	6.8	0		1	3.1	4	3.3
SGOT elevation	12	10.3	18	20.5	0		3	9.4	0	
Glucosuria	0	0	1	1.1	0		0	0	0	
No side effects	22	19.0	53	60.2	46	54.1	14	43.8	68	55.3

syrup, and UFT. Major side effects were related to the digestive system, i.e. anorexia, nausea, vomiting, diarrhea, and stomatitis. Fatigue, CNS toxicity, skin rash, alopecia, and pigmentation were also occasionally seen. Bone marrow suppression such as leukopenia and thrombocytopenia, and liver dysfunction (elevation of SGOT) were seen in very few cases with any of the agents. The frequency of side effects was, however, somewhat higher with futraful capsules.

CONCLUSION

A sequential comparison was performed using four agents, tegafur capsules, tegafur suppositories, 5-FU dry syrup, and UFT by the Tokyo Cancer Chemotherapy Cooperative Study Group. The results of our study disclosed that there were no great differences in response rates, although they were somewhat lower for tegafur suppositories and definitely higher for UFT.

The frequency and spectrum of the side effects of all four drugs did not differ greatly, but they were somewhat milder with tegafur suppositories. Therefore, no definite difference was noted according to our dose schedule. However, UFT was thought to be one step advanced.

* Requests for reprints should be addressed to Hisashi Furue, M.D. Department of Internal Medicine, Teikyo University School of Medicine, 74 Mizonokuchi, Takatsu-ku, Kawasaki 213 Japan

REFERENCES

1. Watanabe H, Naito T, Uchiyama T, et al. (1974) Cooperative study on oral administration of Futraful. Tokyo Cancer Chemotherapy Cooperative Study Group. Jpn J Cancer Chemother 1: 111-121.

2. Nakatsu T, Uematsu Y, Suzuki Y. (1975) Oral administration of powder form of 5-fluorouracil to various carcinomas. Tokyo Cancer Chemotherapy Cooperative Study Group. Jpn J Cancer Chemother 2: 131-135.

3. Furukawa K, Kato R, and Hanaoka M. (1976) Clinical studies of futraful suppository by cooperative study group. Tokyo Cancer Chemotherapy Cooperative Study Group. Jpn J Cancer Chemother 3: 983-990.

4. Watanabe H, Yamamoto S, and Naito T. (1980) Clinical results of oral UFT therapy under cooperative study. Tokyo Cancer Chemotherapy Cooperative Study Group. Jpn J Cancer Chemother 7: 1588-1596.

Fluoropyrimidines in Cancer Therapy
K. Kimura, S. Fujii, M. Ogawa, G.P. Body, P. Alberto, eds.

SEQUENTIAL METHOTREXATE AND 5-FLUOROURACIL IN THE TREATMENT OF SOLID TUMORS

Joseph R. Bertino, Enrico Mini and Alberto Sobrero

1. INTRODUCTION

There is now a substantial body of evidence, produced in several experimental systems, both in vitro and in vivo, that indicates greater than additive cell kill may be obtained only when methotrexate (MTX) is administered before 5-fluorouracil (5 FU). Less than additive effects were observed with the reverse sequence (reviewed in 1,2)). Both of these drugs are widely used in combination for the treatment of solid tumors (e.g., CMF for breast cancer), without regard to sequence of administration; improved tumor response may result, if these drugs are scheduled optimally.

In this manuscript the biochemical and experimental tumor data obtained with the use of these two drugs in combination are reviewed, as well as clinical studies.

2. BIOCHEMICAL RATIONALE

5-FU may exert its lethal effects by inhibition of RNA synthesis or DNA synthesis (3) (Fig. 1). In both circumstances, conversion of 5-FU to 5-fluorouracil monophosphate (5-FUMP) by the enzyme orotate phosphoribosyl transferase appears to be a key first step. 5-FUMP is then subsequently converted to 5-fluoro-deoxyuridylate (5-FdUMP), a potent inhibitor of the enzyme thymidy-

late synthase, or to 5-fluorouracil triphosphate (5-FUTP); this
latter compound may be incorporated into RNA.

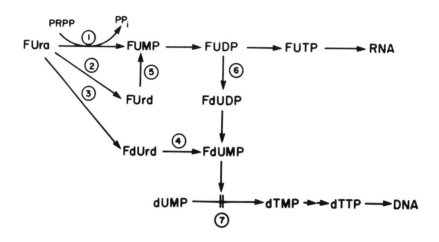

FIGURE 1   Metabolic activation and pharmacological actions of 5-FU.
Circled numbers refer to following enzymes: (1) orotate phosphoribosyltransferase; (2) uridine phosphorylase; (3) thymidine
phosphorylase; (4) thymidine kinase; (5) uridine kinase; (6)
ribonucleotide reductase; (7) thymidylate synthetase. Abbreviations used are: FUra, (5-FU), FUMP, FUDP, FUTP, 5-fluorouracil,
5-FU ribose monophosphate, diphosphate, and triphosphate, respectively; FUrd, 5-fluorouridine; FdUDP, 5-FU deoxyribose
diphosphate; FdUrd, 5-fluorodeoxyuridine.

5-FU has also been shown to be incorporated into DNA (4). Both 5-FU and MTX may also result in misincorporation of uracil into DNA (5). Any of these effects could then result in cell death.

How would pretreatment with MTX enhance 5-FU cell kill? MTX has been shown to increase 5-FU nucleotide levels in cells, presumably by the increase in intracellular levels of 5-phosphoribosyl-1- pyrophosphate (PRPP) that occurs as a consequence of inhibition of purine biosynthesis by MTX (6).

Formation of 5-FUMP appears to be limited by the availability of this cosubstrate (Fig. 1). Thus pretreatment with any drug that inhibits purine biosynthesis enhances 5-FU induced cell kill (7,8). MTX also increases the level of dihydrofolate polyglutamates in cells; this compound (s) increases binding of 5-FdUMP to thymidylate synthase (9), and could also contribute to the enhanced cell kill observed with the sequence MTX → 5-Fu.

3. STUDIES IN EXPERIMENTAL TUMORS

Studies of mice bearing the S-180 Sarcoma indicated that even a one hour interval between MTX and 5-FU administration was sufficient to cause synergistic antitumor effects without a corresponding increase in host toxicity (10). Subsequent studies of human breast and colon cells (11) propagated in vitro, show that a longer interval may be necessary for optimum cell kill (12-24h). However, increased levels of PRPP were found in intestinal mucosa as well as in human colon cancer cells propagated in immune deprived mice 24 hours after MTX treatment, indicating that administration of these drugs with a 24h interval might result in increased gastrointestinal toxicity as well as produce increased antitumor effects (12).

4. CLINICAL STUDIES

a. Head and Neck Cancer

MTX, followed by 5-FU, 1-2 hrs later, produced a high response rate in two Phase II studies (71 and 63%) (13,14), but not in a third (17%) (15). Of interest are two trials that compared simultaneous MTX and 5-FU with sequential treatment (1 hr interval), or the sequence MTX → FU with the reverse sequence, again with a one hour interval (Table 1). Both studies have not demonstrated an advantage to the sequence MTX → 5 FU over the other schedules, although the percentage of patients responding to the combination was high (16,17). Additional studies are needed, in particular of longer intervals between drug administration.

TABLE 1 Studies of the effect of sequence on tumor response in patients with cancer of the head and neck

Sequence	No. patients	% tumor response	References
a) MTX → 5-FU (1 hr)	13	69	(16)
5-FU → MTX (1 hr)	12	67	
b) MTX, 5-FU simultaneous*	39	61	(17)
MTX → 5-FU (1 hr)	34	32	

*MTX was administered first, followed immediately by 5-FU.

b. Breast Cancer

To date except for one study, Phase II trials of the MTX and
5-FU sequence in carcinoma of the breast have been limited to a
one hour interval between drug administration (18-22). Gewirtz
and Cadman reported a 53% response rate with minimal toxicity using
MTX (200 mg/m^2) and 5-FU (600 mg/m^2), some of the responses were
in patients previously treated with CMF (18). A 50% response rate
was noted by Herrmann et al. (23), in heavily pretreated patients,
utilizing a longer interval of administration (7 hr) and a higher
dose of 5-FU (900 mg/m^2).

The use of sequential MTX and 5-FU following "synchrony" by
pretreatment with tamoxifen and premarin produced an excellent
response rate (69%) in patients with advanced breast cancer (19).
Of great interest was the high percentage of complete remissions
(47%).

c. Colorectal Cancer

A large number of Phase II studies have been reported employing
sequential MTX and 5-FU in the treatment of advanced colorectal
cancer (reviewed in 1). MTX doses have varied between 40 mg/m^2
to 1500 mg/m^2 (with leucovorin rescue). 5-FU doses have ranged
between 600 to 1500 mg/m^2. Since, in addition to the relatively
small numbers in each group, the interval between drug administration has ranged from 1 to 27 hr, and the treatments repeated every
1-3 weeks, it is difficult to make definite conclusions concerning
the effect of timing on tumor response.

In studies utilizing moderate dose MTX (200-250 mg/m^2) and
standard dose 5-FU (600 mg/m^2) with a one hour interval, disap-

pointing response rates have been reported (22,24-26). Using a
4-7 hour interval between MTX and 5-FU administration, higher
response rates were obtained (27-30). Substantial hematologic
and gastrointestinal toxicity has been observed in one of these
studies (30). Longer intervals between MTX and 5-FU have also
been piloted: Kemeny, et al (31) used low dose MTX (40 mg/m^2)
without leucovorin rescue followed 24h later by 5-FU (600 mg/m^2)
at weeks 1 and 2 each month, and reported a 35% response role in
23 patients. Mehrotra, et al, using weekly moderate dose MTX
(100 mg/m^2) with LV rescue followed after 18h by 5-FU (600 mg/m^2)
reported no activity and unacceptable toxicity (29). A Phase I
trial at Yale, using a 24h interval between MTX and 5-FU demonstrated
that biweekly, but not weekly therapy is tolerable with these doses
of drugs (32). A multicenter group in Germany recently reported
results in 42 patients using a 7 hour time interval between MTX
and 5-FU (33). MTX (150 mg/m^2) was administered intravenously by
push injection, followed by MTX, 150 mg/m^2 intravenously over 4 hrs.
5-FU, 900 mg/m^2 was given intravenously 7 hrs after the MTX was
started. Leucovorin (22.5 mg) was given orally every 6 hrs for 8
doses beginning 24 hr after MTX. Sixteen of 42 evaluable patients
achieved an objective response. The median survival of patients
with response or stable disease was 13.5 and 16.5 months respectively, as compared to 9 months for patients with progressive
disease.

TABLE 2   Effect of interval between MTX and 5-FU on response
rate in metastatic colorectal cancer

MTX/5-FU Interval (hrs)	No Patients	Objective Responses	References
1	62	10%	(20),(22),(24),(25),(26)
4 - 7	103	37%	(27),(28),(29),(30),(34)
18 - 24	26	31%	(29),(31)

5.   CONCLUSIONS

Synergy in regard to antitumor effects has been clearly observed
in several experimental systems when MTX precedes 5-FU. The interactions between these drugs are complex, and the mechanism of
synergy may involve either a RNA effect, or DNA effect, and the
mechanism of cell kill may depend on the cell type and growth rate.

In the clinic, Phase I-II trials have shown some possible
synergy in patients with head and neck cancer, breast cancer, and
gastrointestinal cancer. In head and neck cancer, two studies
have not demonstrated the superiority of a one hour interval of
sequency of MTX and 5-FU to simultaneous use, or the reverse
sequence. Trials in patients with colorectal cancer support the
data obtained in the laboratory using colon cancer cells; namely
that longer intervals between drug administration result in more
cell kill. In all three solid tumor studies, additional trials are
needed to establish the optimum dosage of drugs, and the time between drug administration. Phase III studies will then be required
to compare this regimen to the best treatment for the three types
of cancer discussed.

REFERENCES

1. Bertino JR, Mini E. (1983) The use of sequential methotrexate and 5-fluorouracil in the treatment of human malignancies. In: Proc. 13th Int. Congress of Chemotherapy (eds) R Spitzy and R Handrouer, Vienna, Austria, 1983.

2. Mini E, Bertino JR. (1983) Sequential methotrexate and 5-fluorouracil: Biochemical pharmacology and therapeutic use. Chemotherapia 2: 147-162.

3. Heidelberger C, Danenberger PV, Moran RG. (1983) Fluorinated pyrimidines and their nucleotides. Adv Enzymol 54: 57-119.

4. Major PP, Egan E, Herrick D, Kufe DW. (1982) 5-fluorouracil incorporation in DNA of human breast carcinoma cells. Cancer Res 42: 3005-3009.

5. Goulian M, Bleile B, Tseng BY. (1980) Methotrexate-induced misincorporation of uracil into DNA. Proc Natl Acad Sci USA 77: 1956-1960.

6. Cadman E, Heimer R, Davis L. (1979) Enhanced 5-fluorouracil nucleotide formation after methotrexate administration: explanation for drug synergism. Science (Wash. D.C.) 205: 1135-1137.

7. Cadman E, Benz C, Heiman R, O'Shoughnessy J. (1981) Effects of de novo purine synthesis inhibitors on 5-fluorouracil metabolism and cytotoxicity. Biochem Pharmacol 30: 2049-2472.

8. Benz E, Cadman E. (1981) Modulation of 5-fluorouracil and cytotoxicity by antimetabolite pretreatment in human colo-rectal carcinoma. Cancer Res 41: 994-999.

9. Fernandes DJ, Bertino JR. (1980) 5-Fluorouracil-methotrexate synergy. Enhancement of 5-fluorodeoxyuridylate binding to thymidylate synthetase by dihydropteroylpolyglutamates. Proc Natl Acad Sci USA 77: 5663-5667.

10. Bertino JR, Sawicki WL, Lindquist CA, Gupta VS. (1977) Schedule-dependent antitumor effects of methotrexate and 5-fluorouracil. Cancer Res 37: 327-328.

11. Benz C, Schoenberg M, Choti M, Cadman E. (1980) Schedule-dependent cytotoxicity of methotrexate and 5-fluorouracil in human colon and breast tumor cell lines. J Clin Invest 66: 1162-1165.

12. Houghton JA, Tice AJ, Houghton PJ (1982) The selectivity of action of methotrexate in combination with 5-fluorouracil in xenografts of human colon adenocarcinomas. Mol Pharmacol 22: 771-778.

13. Pitman SW, Kowal CD, Bertino JR. (1983) Methotrexate and 5-fluorouracil in sequence in squamous head and neck cancer. Sem Oncol 10 (Suppl 2): 15-19.

14. Ringborg U, Ewert G, Kinnman J, et al. (1983) Methotrexate-5-fluorouracil in head and neck cancer. Sem Oncol 10: 20-22.

15. Jacobs C. (1982) Use of methotrexate and 5-FU for recurrent head and neck cancer. Cancer Treat Rep 66: 1925-1928.

16. Coates AS, Hedley D, Fox RM, et al. (1983) Randomized trial of sequential methotrexate (M) followed by 5-fluorouracil (F) versus F followed by M. Proc Am Assoc Cancer Res 24: 140.

17. Browman GF, Young JM, Archibold SD, et al. (1983) Prospective randomized trial of one hour sequential versus simultaneous methotrexate (MTX) + 5-fluorouracil (5-FU) in squamous carcinoma of head and meck. Proc Am Soc Clin Oncol 2: 158.

18. Gewirtz AM, Cadman E. (1981) Preliminary report on the efficacy of sequential methotrexate and 5-fluorouracil in advanced breast cancer. Cancer 47: 2552-2555.

19. Allegra JC. (1983) Methotrexate/5-fluorouracil following tamoxifen and premarin in advanced breast cancer. Sem Oncol 10 (Suppl 2): 23-28.

20. Tisman G, Wu SJG. (1980) Effectiveness of intermediate dose methotrexate and high dose 5-fluorouracil as sequential combination chemotherapy in refractory breast cancer and as primary therapy in metastatic adeno-carcinoma of the colon. Cancer Treat Rep 64: 829-835.

21. Plotkin D, Waugh WJ. (1982) Sequential methotrexate 5-fluorouracil (M→F) in advanced breast carcinoma. Proc Am Soc Clin Oncol 1: 80.

22. Panasci L, Margolese R (1982) Sequential methotrexate (MTX) and 5-fluorouracil (FU) in breast and colorectal cancer. Results of increasing the dose of FU. Proc Am Soc Clin Oncol 1: 101.

23. Herrmann R, Westerhausen M, Bruntsch U, et al. (1982) Sequential methotrexate (MTX) and 5-fluorouracil (FU) is effective in extensively pretreated breast cancer. Proc Am Soc Clin Oncol 1: 86.

24. Blumenreich MS, Woodcock TM, Allegra M, et al. (1982) Sequential therapy with methotrexate (MTX) and 5-fluorouracil (5-FU) for adenocarcinoma of the colon. Proc Am Soc Clin Oncol 1: 102.

25. Burnet R, Smith FP, Woolmi B, et al. (1981) Sequential
methotrexate-5-fluorouracil in advanced measurable colorectal
cancer: lack of appreciable therapeutic synergism. Proc
Am Assoc Cancer Res 22: 370.

26. Cantrell JE Jr, Brunet R, Lagarde C et al. (1982) Phase II
study of sequential methotrexate 5-FU therapy in advanced
measurable colorectal cancer. Cancer Treat Rep 66: 1563-1565.

27. Drapkin R, Griffiths E, McAloon E, et al. (1981) Sequential
methotrexate (MTX) and 5-fluorouracil (5_FU) in adenocarcinoma
of the colon and rectum. Proc Am Assoc Cancer Res 22: 453.

28. Herrmann R, Manegold C, Holzmann K, Fritze D. (1982)
Sequentielle verabreuchung von methotrexat und fluorouracil
bei metastasierenden kolorektalen karzinomen. Ergebnisse
einer phase-II-Pilotstudie. Dtsch Med Wochenschr 107: 491-493.

29. Mehrotra S, Rosenthal CJ, Gardner B. (1982) Biochemical modulation of antineoplastic response in colorectal carcinoma:
5-fluorouracil (F), high dose methotrexate (M) with calcium
leucovorin (L) rescue (FML) in two sequences of administration.
Proc Am Soc Clin Oncol 1: 100.

30. Weinerman B, Schachter B, Schipper H, et al. (1982) Sequential
methotrexate and 5-FU in the treatment of colorectal cancer.
Cancer Treat Rep 66: 1553-1555.

31. Kemeny N, Michaelson R. (1982) Phase II trial of low dose
methotrexate and sequential 5-fluorouracil in the treatment
of metastic colorectal carcinoma. Proc Am Soc Clin Oncol 1: 95.

32. Benz C, Schoenberg M, Cadman E. (1983) Use of high dose oral
methotrexate sequenced at 24 hours with 5-FU in clinical
toxicity study. Cancer Treat Rep 67: 297-299.

33. Herrmann R, Spehn J, Beyer JH, et al. (1983) Sequential methotrexate and 5-fluorouracil. Improved response rate in metastatic colorectal cancer. In: Proc 13th Int. Congress of
Chemotherapy (eds) R Spitzy and R. Handrouer, Vienna, Austria,
1983.

34. Solan A, Vogl SE, Kaplan BH, et al. (1982) Sequential chemotherapy of advanced colorectal cancer with standard or high-
dose methotrexate followed by 5-fluorouracil. Med Pediatr
Oncol 10: 145-149.

© 1984 Elsevier Science Publishers B.V.
Fluoropyrimidines in Cancer Therapy
K. Kimura, S. Fujii, M. Ogawa, G.P. Bodey, P. Alberto, eds.

A PHASE II STUDY OF SEQUENTIAL METHOTREXATE AND 5-FLUOROURACIL IN THE TREATMENT OF CANCER

Kazuo Ota

1. INTRODUCTION

The efficacy of sequential combination of methotrexate (MTX) and 5-fluorouracil (5-FU) has been demonstrated in animal experiments as well as in management of head and neck cancer by Bertino et al. (1, 2) and Cadman et al. (3). In order to evaluate the efficacy of sequential MTX and 5-FU in lung cancer, we performed a phase II study involving 32 institutions in Japan.

2. MATERIALS AND METHODS

2.1. Patients

Fifteen patients treated included seven lung cancers and one each of gallbladder, colon, esophagus, ovary, breast, rectum and primary unknown metastatic ovarian cancer, consisting of 5 males and 9 females with a median age of 58 years (range: 38 to 76). The median performance status was 2 (range: 0 to 4). Ten of the patients had received prior chemotherapy (Table 1).

2.2. Chemotherapy

MTX was administered in doses of 100 to 300 mg/m^2

given as an i.v. infusion for one hour, followed one hour

TABLE 1   Patients treated with sequential MTX and 5-FU
           therapy

Total patients		14
Male		5
Female		9
Age Median		57.5
Range	38 -	76
Performance status		
Median		2
Range	0 -	4
Prior chemotherapy		
Treated		10
Untreated		4

later by 5-FU of 600 mg/m^2, as an i.v. infusion for
one hour. Twenty-four hours after MTX administration,
leucovorin rescue in a dose of 15 mg p.o. was started
every 6 hours for 8 doses. The treatment was repeated
once weekly unless toxicity or disease progression
supervened. The dose levels of MTX were modified based
on achievement of response and tolerance. The dose
level of 5-FU was not altered. The mean total number of
MTX doses given was 6 (range: 3 to 10) and the mean
total dosage was 900 mg/m^2 (range: 300 to 1,900
mg/m^2) (Table 2).

3. RESULTS

   3.1. Response

   The patients treated with the sequential MTX and
5-FU therapy are shown in Table 3. Patient No. 6 had a

motastatic adenocarcinoma of primary unknown, probably of gastrointestinal origin. Initially the pathology was determined in a resected ovarian tumor, thereafter

TABLE 2 Method of sequential MTX and 5-FU therapy

MTX	$100 - 300$ mg/m^2 iv drip 1 hr	
	↓	1 hr interval
5-FU	600 mg/m^2 iv drip 1 hr	
	↓	at 24 hr
Leucovorin	15 mg po x 8 q 6 hr	
	weekly (for 4 doses) ⟶ q2w maintenance	
MTX	Mean	5.9 doses
	Range	3 - 10 doses
5-FU	Mean	897 mg/m^2
	Range	300 - 1,920 mg/m^2

TABLE 3 Sequential MTX and 5-FU in the treatment of cancer

No.	Pts.	Sex	Age	Primary	Prior CTR	MTX (mg/m^2)	Response	Side effect
1	AT	M	49	Gallbladder	+	120x4 240x6	NC	Nausea (LV)
2	FS	F	76	Colon	+	110x3 220x4 300x2	MR	–
3	IY	M	44	Esophagus	+	130x4 260x4	MR	–
4	KY	M	71	Lung (Ad)	–	100x7	PR	Diarrhea
5	OY	M	67	Lung (Sq)	–	130x7	NC	Fever
6	MT	F	40	Unknown meta. ovarian cancer (Ad)	+	150x4 220x2	Responded (Improvement of ileus)	–
7	KS	F	49	Lung (Ad)	+	140x4 210x2	NC	–
8	SM	F	43	Lung (Ad)	–	130x6	NC	Diarrhea
9	IY	F	58	Lung (Sq)	+	150x1 110x3	NC	Leukopenia (2300)
10	MI	F	63	Ovary	+	130x4	NC	Leukopenia (2300)
11	MM	F	57	Breast	–	130x4	MR	–
12	ON	F	38	Rectum	+	130x4	NC	Diarrhea
13	MK	F	63	Lung (Ad)	+	130x4	NC	–
14	NT	M	76	Lung (Lg)	+	100x3	PD	–

CTR: chemotherapy
LV: due to leucovorin

it was found disseminated in the abdominal cavity at laparotomy for ileus. She received therapy with 6 doses of 140 to 210 mg/m^2 MTX. Though she had been previously exposed to MFC combination consisting of mitomycin C, 5-FU and cytosine arabinoside (ara-C), and thereafter tegafur, a marked improvement of the ileus was observed with the current therapy. CEA level fell from 53.2 to 22.2 ng/ml, and a good remission continued for 8 months, and no side effect was observed. Patient No. 4 with adenocarcinoma of the lung was treated with 7 doses of 100 mg/m^2 MTX and achieved a partial response; however, the treatment was interrupted because of severe diarrhea.

A summary of the response is described in Table 4. Out of 7 patients with lung cancer one patient (14%) achieved a partial response. Out of total 14 patients including carcinoma of the esophagus, gallbladder, colon, rectum, breast, ovary and adenocarcinoma of the unknown primary, 2 patients described above (14%) achieved partial response, additional 3 patients (22%) achieved minor response, 8 (57%) had no change, and 1 (17%) was progressive disease. Out of 10 patients with prior chemotherapy, one (10%) achieved a partial response, and one of 4 patients (25%) without prior chemotherapy also achieved a partial response.

TABLE 4   Sequential MTX and 5-FU therapy

		No.	PR	MR	NC	PD (%)
Lung	Ad	4	1(25)		3	
	Sq	2			2	
	Lg	1				1
Subtotal		7	1(14)		5	1
Esophagus		1		1		
Gallbladder		1			1	
Colon		1		1		
Rectum		1			1	
Breast		1		1		
Ovary		1			1	
Unknown adenoca		1	1			
		14	2(14)	3(22)	8(57)	1(7)
Prior CTR	(+)	10	1(10)	2(20)	6(60)	1(10)
	(-)	4	1(25)	1(25)	2(50)	

3.2. Toxicity

Toxicity of the therapy was very mild: three patients (21%) manifested diarrhea, one (7%) had nausea due to leucovorin, one had fever, and two had mild leukopenia (Table 5). No mucositis due to MTX was observed.

TABLE 5   Toxicity of sequential MTX and 5-FU therapy

Diarrhea	3 (21%)
Fever	1 (7%)
Nausea (LV)*	1 (7%)
Leukopenia <3000	2 (14%)
No toxicity	7 (50%)

*due to leucovorin

Investigators have recently reported the results of sequential MTX and 5-FU therapy in carcinoma of the head and neck, breast and colorectum. Many of them have used dose schedules of approximately 200 mg/m^2 MTX and 600 mg/m^2 5-FU at one-hour interval. Some of them have used high-dose MTX of 800-1,500 mg/m^2 with a 7-hour interval between MTX and 5-FU. Response rates have varied between 16 (4) to 100% (2) in head and neck cancer, 14 (5) to 53% (6) in breast cancer, and 6 (7) to 80% (8) in colorectal cancer. In a randomized trial of one-hour sequential versus simultaneous MTX plus 5-FU in head and neck cancer reported by Browman et al. (9) sequential therapy was not superior to simultaneous combination. Another randomized trial of schedule of sequential MTX and 5-FU therapy conducted by Coates et al. (10) indicated that the combination was effective in head and neck cancer; however, the sequence of drug administration was not crucial.

In the present phase II study only two patients out of 14 achieved partial response. However, substantial antitumor activity was observed in one patient without prior chemotherapy out of four with adenocarcinoma of the lung, and it is noteworthy that disseminated adenocarcinoma of primary unknown cancer with prior chemotherapy including 5-FU also responded well to the therapy with a marked improvement in ileus. Toxicity, especially to the bone marrow was mild. Therefore, sequential MTX and 5-FU therapy appears to be promising. A large scale study in patients with adenocarcinoma of the lung and stomach is needed in order to better define the efficacy of this regimen.

REFERENCES

1. Bertino JR, Sawicki WL, Lindquist CA, et al. (1977) Schedule-dependent antitumor effects of methotrexate and 5-fluorouracil. Cancer Res 37: 327-328.

2. Pitman SW, Rowal CD, Papac RJ, Bertino JR. (1980) Sequential methotrexate-5-fluorouracil: a highly active drug combination in advanced squamous carcinoma of the head and neck. Proc Am Assoc Cancer Res 21: 607.

3. Cadman E, Heimer R, Davis L. (1979) Enhanced 5-fluorouracil nucleotide formation after methotrexate administration: explanation for drug synergism. Science 205, 14: 1135-1137.

4. Jacobs C. (1982) Use of methotrexate and 5-FU for recurrent head and neck cancer. Cancer Treat Rep 66: 1925-1928.

5. Plotkin D, Waugh WJ. (1982) Sequential methotrexate-5-fluorouracil in advanced breast cancer. Proc Am Soc Clin Oncol 1: 80.

6. Gewirtz AM, Cadman E. (1981) Preliminary report on the efficacy of sequential methotrexate and 5-fluorouracil in advanced breast cancer. Cancer 47: 2552-2555.

7. Cantrell JE, Jr, Brunet R, Lagarde C, et al. (1982) Phase II study of sequential methotrexate-5-FU therapy in advanced measurable colorectal cancer. Cancer Treat Rep 66: 1563-1565.

8. Mehrotra S, Rosenthal CJ, Gardner B. (1982) Biochemical modulation of antineoplastic response in colorectal carcinoma: 5-fluorouracil, high dose methotrexate with calcium leucovorin rescue in two sequences of administration. Proc Am Soc Clin Oncol 1: 100.

9. Browman GP, Young FEM, Archibald SD, et al. (1983) Prospective randomized trial of one hour sequential versus simultaneous methotrexate (MTX) + 5-fluorouracil (5-FU) in squamous carcinoma of head and neck (SCHN). Proc Am Soc Clin Oncol 1: 616.

10. Coates AS, Headley D, Fox RM, et al. (1983) Randomized trial of sequential methotrexate (M) followed by 5-fluorouracil (F) versus F followed by M. Proc Am Assoc Cancer Res 24: 555.

Fluoropyrimidines in Cancer Therapy
K. Kimura, S. Fujii, M. Ogawa, G.P. Bodey, P. Alberto, eds.

LOW DOSE METHOTREXATE AND SEQUENTIAL 5-FLUOROURACIL IN ADVANCED GASTRIC CANCER

Tsuneo Sasaki

1. INTRODUCTION

5FU is one of the most active drugs for adeno-carcinoma in gastric cancer, colorectal cancer and breast cancer. However its effectiveness is far from satisfactory. According to experimental data, it strongly suggests a synergistic cytotoxic effect when methotrexate and 5FU are administered sequentially. The proposed mechanisms are as follows: 1) by increased cell uptake of 5FU, and 2) by increased binding of FdUMP to thymidilate synthetase (1, 2). In this paper, we present our findings with sequential low dose of methotrexate and 5FU therapy on experimental animals and in clinical studies.

2. MATERIALS AND METHODS

Experimental study

Female BDF_1 mice weighing 19 to 21 grams were used for survival studies. Three L1210 cell lines were used, one sensitive to many drugs, one resistant to methotrexate and the other resistant to 5FU. Each was inoculated into each mouse (10^5 cells/mouse). These three L1210

cell lines were obtained from Dr. Fujimoto of the Cancer
Institute Hospital, and of the Division of Clinical
Chemotherapy at the Cancer Chemotherapy Center.

Clinical study

Sixteen patients with advanced gastric cancer were
admitted to the trial. The pretreatment characteristics
are summarized in Table 1. The median age of the
patients was 55 years, with a range of ages from 28 to 87.

TABLE 1   Characteristics of treated patients

Characteristics	No. of patients
Sex Males/Females	11/5
Median age in yrs (range)	55.1 (28–87)
Site of measurable disease	
Stomach	7
Abdomen and peritoneum	7
Lung	2
Liver	3
Prior therapy	
Surgery (Gastrectomy)	3
Chemotherapy	8
Performance status	0-1 : 0
(ECOG scale)	2 : 3
	3 : 8
	4 : 5

All of the patients were completely or partially bedridden. The anatomical sites of their main tumors were the stomach in 7 patients, the abdomen and peritoneum in 7 patients, and the lung in 2 patients. Only 3 patients had recurrences after previous operations and the others were inoperable. Seven patients received prior chemotherapy with a combination including 5FU.

Treatment regimen: methotrexate 30 mg/m^2, followed 3 hours later with 5FU 750 mg and 24 hours later with leucovorin 30 mg/m^2. Each drug was administered as an iv bolus. Treatments were repeated weekly.

The response was assessed by clinical examinations, serial x-rays, CT scans and endoscopies.

The response evaluation to therapy was classified as complete response (CR), partial response (PR), minor response (MR), no change (NC), and progressive disease (PD). CR is defined as complete disappearance of all measurable lesions for at least one month. PR is a reduction in the products of 2 perpendicular diameters of each measurable lesion by more than 50 % for one month. MR is a tumor regression greater than 25 % but less than 50 %. NC is defined as either a reduction of less than 25 %, or an increase of less than 25 % of in tumor size. PD is an increase in tumor size of more than 25 %.

3. RESULTS

Experimental study

15 mg/kg of methotrexate were administered intraperitoneally 3 hours before, at the same time, and 3 hours
after 50 mg/kg of 5FU were injected. Pretreatment with
methotrexate obtained the best therapeutic results in
L1210 sensitive cell lines, as compared to any other
treatment sequence (see Fig. 1). The difference between
pretreatment with methotrexate in L1210 sensitive cell
lines versus the other groups was significant at 0.01
level. In the L1210 cell line resistant to methotrexate
and the cell line resistant to 5FU, pretreatment with
methotrexate was somewhat better than treatment with
other groups.

When the dose of methotrexate was decreased from 5
mg/kg to 1 mg/kg in the L1210 sensitive cell line,
pretreatment with methotrexate was better than treatment
with methotrexate and 5FU used simultaneously (Fig. 2).

Clinical study

Table 2 illustrates a summary of 16 patients with
gastric cancer. Of these 16 patients who were evaluated,
four had a PR and 5 had an MR. These response rate was
25 %. The remission duration in the 4PR patients were 5
months in one case, more than 4 months in one case and
more than 2 months in 2 cases. The histology in the 4PR
patients was mucocellular adenocarcinoma in 2 cases and
tubular adenocarcinoma in 2 cases. Of the 7 patients

who had been previously treated with a combination of chemotherapy including 5FU, there were 2PR and 3 MR patients.

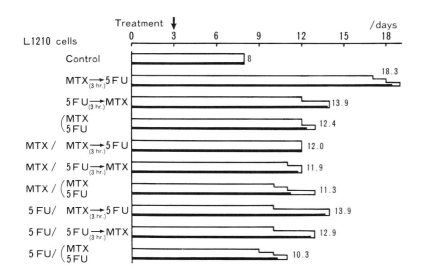

FIGURE 1 Effect of sequence administration of methotrexate and 5FU on survival of mice with L1210 cells. Treatment was administered on the 3rd day after animals were inoculated with 10^5 cells. The dose of methotrexate used was 15 mg/kg, the dose of 5FU was 50 mg/kg. The control group of animals received no treatment. There were six animals in each group. MTX/:resistant to methotrexate. 5FU/:resistant to 5FU.

These 16 patients have received 105 cycles of the therapy thus far. This regimen has been well tolerated by the patients. Mild nausea and vomiting were seen in 8 of the patients. No patient had a WBC nadir of less than 2000 cells/mm^3, and no patient had a platelet count nadir of less than one hundred thousand platelets/mm^3. No other toxicity was detected.

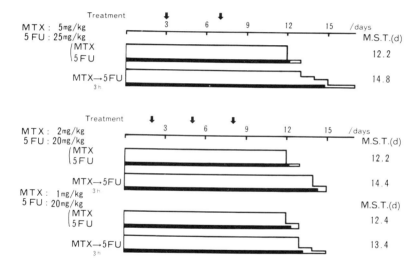

FIGURE 2 Effect of low dose of methotrexate and 5FU on survival of mice with L1210 cells. Each mouse was inoculated with 10^5 cells. The dose of methotrexate was decreased from 5 mg/kg to 1 mg/kg.

TABLE 2　Low dose methotrexate and sequential 5FU in gastric cancer.

case	sex/age	histology	main tumor site	P.S.	prior chemotherapy	effect
1. KS	M72	anaplastic c.	abdomen	4	ADM·VCR·EX	MR
2. IM	M42	mucocell. ad.	lung	3	FAM, CDDP·EX·VCR	PR
3. MK	F35	tubular ad.	abdomen	4		NC
4. YY	F30	mucocell. ad.	abdomen	3	FAM, FT207	PD
5. TC	F60	mucocell. ad.	stomach	2		PR
6. OK	M58	mucocell. ad.	abdomen	3	FAM	MR
7. AY	M73	papillotub. ad.	stomach	3		NC
8. IG	M81	papillotub. ad.	stomach	2	5FU	MR
9. SA	M56	anaplastic c.	abdomen	4		MR
10. CR	M59	papillotub. ad.	stomach	3		NC
11. OY	F35	poorly diff. ad.	stomach	3		NC
12. MS	F48	mucocell. ad.	abdomen	3	FAM	PR
13. SH	M28	tubular ad.	stomach	3		MR
14. TM	M72	tubular ad.	stomach	2	5FU	MR
15. MT	M87	tubular ad.	lung	4		PD
16. AK	M46	tubular ad.	abdomen	4	FAM	PR

ADM ： Adriamycin　　　VCR ： vincristine　　　EX ： cyclophosphamide

FAM ： combination of 5FU, Adriamycin and mitomycin C.

CDDP ： cis-platinum

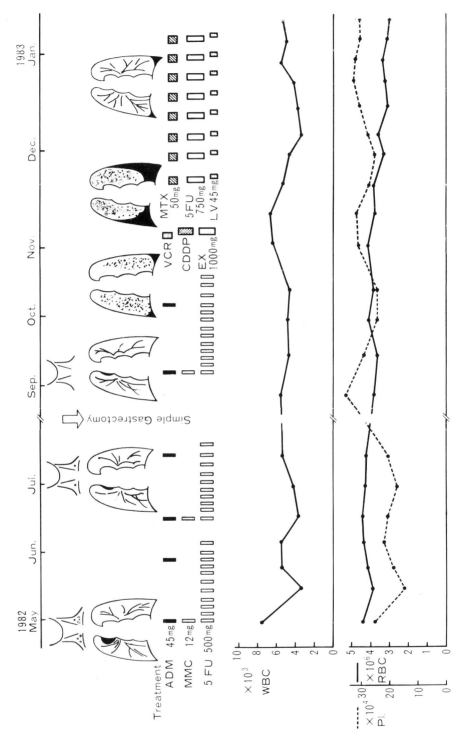

FIGURE 3 Details of clinical history of the patient.

276

Case report (in Fig. 3)

I.M. - a 42-year old male. When he visited our hospital on April 28th, 1982, gastric cancer had already spread to his bilateral neck lymphnodes and upper right mediastinum. His histology was defined by a biopsy as mucocellular adenocarcinoma. He was treated with FAM therapy, which is a combination of 5FU, Adriamycin and mitomycin C. After 2 courses of FAM therapy, his bilateral neck lymphnodes were diminished and his upper right mediastinal tumor was decreased. However the primary site was not changed endoscopically. He was then operated on for a simple gastrectomy on August 18th. About three weeks after the operation, the patient started FAM therapy again. Lung metastasis and pleural effusion occurred in the patient toward the end of September, in spite of the FAM therapy. The FAM therapy failed and its use was terminated on October 10th. A combination of vincristine, cisplatinum and cyclophosphamide was then used on the patient, but this also proved ineffective. Dyspnea and coughing in the patient increased, he could not move in bed and needed O_2 inhalation. Cytology of sputum and pleural effusion were class 5 in a Papanicolaou stain. His chest x-ray showed that his condition was worsening. Sequential methotrexate and 5FU therapy began on November 19th. Two weeks later, dyspnea and coughing became less serious, and one week after this, O_2 inhalation was not necessary. The patient's chest x-ray films became clear and ploural effusion was decreased. Two months later the patient was discharged from the hospital.

4. DISCUSSION

On experimental animals, we found that a synergistic effect was obtained not only with a high dose, but also with a low dose of methotrexate in L1210 sensitive cell lines, when methotrexate was used 3 hours before the 5FU treatment.

Based on this study, we began a pilot trial employing low doses of methotrexate and sequential 5FU therapy in cases of advanced gastric cancer. A synergistic effect was observable at only 30 mg/m^2 of methotrexate. Kemeny had reported that a 34 % response rate was obtained utilizing low dose of methotrexate (40 mg/m^2) in colorectal cancer (3).

We believe that sequential methotrexate and 5FU therapy can be effective against gastric cancer in patients who are already refractory to 5FU. It is also important to note that our regimen had minimal toxicity. This lack of toxicity will allow us to develop additional treatment protocols, utilizing new agents with this regimen.

REFERENCES

1. Cadman E, Heimer R, et al. (1981) The influence of methotrexate pretreatment on 5-fluorouracil metabolism in L1210 cells. J Biol Chem 256(4): 1695-1704.

2. Fernandes DJ, Moroson BA, Bertino JR. (1981)
The role of methotrexate and dihydrofolate polyglutamates in the enhancement of fluorouracil action by
methotrexate. Cancer Treat Rep 65 (supp. 1): 29-35.

3. Kemeny N, Michaelson R. (1982) Phase II trial of
low dose methotrexate and sequential 5-fluorouracil in
the treatment of metastatic colorectal carcinoma.
Proc Soc Clin Oncol 1: 95.

© 1984 Elsevier Science Publishers B.V.
Fluoropyrimidines in Cancer Therapy
K. Kimura, S. Fujii, M. Ogawa, G.P. Bodey, P. Alberto, eds.

5-FLUOROURACIL, ADRIAMYCIN AND METHOTREXATE: A COMBINATION PROTOCOL (FAMETH) FOR THE TREATMENT OF METASTASIZED STOMACH CANCER

Hans O. Klein, Premaratne Dias Wickramanayake, Volker Schulz
Rüdiger Mohr, Hans Oerkermann and Gholam-Reza Farrokh

In a phase II trial we tried to evaluate the efficacy of a sequential combination of high-dose (HD) MTX and 5-FU combined with Adriamycin (ADM). In a pilot study we found HDMTX effective as a single agent in gastric cancer. MTX and 5-FU were combined sequentially because Cadman and Bertino had shown synergism for this combination. The therapy protocol consisted of HDMTX, 1.5 g/m² of body surface, and HD5-FU, 1.5 g/m². MTX was administered 1 hour prior to 5-FU. Both drugs were given as a bolus. Twenty-four hours after MTX administration, citrovorum factor rescue was started, 15 mg/m², q6h x 12, orally. Forty-eight hours after MTX administration, serum concentration of the drug was measured by HPLC and an enzyme-immuno-assay. Fourteen days after MTX was given, ADM, 30 mg/m², was injected as a bolus. This protocol was repeated every 28 days. Patients eligible for this treatment should have a creatinine clearance of >60 ml/min. The study included 65 patients with metastasizing gastric cancer and performance status between 40 and 70%. The response rate was 68 (44 of 65 patients). Four of 65 patients had complete remission, which are still maintained. The median survival for responders is 18 months: 48% are still living after 31+ months. The median survival for nonresponders was only 4 months. The difference in survival curves is significant at a level of $P \leq 0.001$. Cytostatic treatment was well tolerated. Thirty-two percent of the patients could be treated on an outpatient basis. Patched alopecia was observed in only 72% of the patients. Severe leukopenia, thrombocytopenia, and kidney disorders were observed in 11%, 6% and 3% respectively.

Based on experimental studies performed by Bertino and his group (1), we developed a cytostatic protocol for treatment of metastasizing stomach cancer using high dose methotrexate and high dose 5-fluorouracil sequentially. The reasons we administered these drugs at a high dose were, first, because pilot studies in patients with stomach cancer, peritonitis carcinomatosa and ascites had shown increasing tumor cell reduction after each drug had been injected alone intraperitoneally, using increasing doses (unpublished data). Secondly, from a theoretical point of view, administration of a high dose of cytostatic drug may enhance permeation of the drug in the central areas of poorly vascularized tumor nodules (3,4,5). Furthermore, autoradiographic analyses of tumor cell proliferation, as well as flow cytophotometry measurements of DNS histograms as a function of time after methotrexate-fluorouracil treatment in patients with neoplastic ascites, had revealed recruitment phenomena of tumor cells starting in general between the 10th and 14th day after cytostatic treatment (unpublished data). In order to prevent this reaction, adriamycin, a powerful drug against stomach cancer, was added to the protocol.

We tested this combination treatment in a phase II trial. Of 65 evaluable patients, 48 (74%) were male and 17 (26%) were female. The median agee was 53,7 years with a range of 23 to 80 years. The Karnofsky status of these patients was poor. Ten scored between 40 and 49% and 36 patients were between 50 and 59%.

Metastasizing Stomach Cancer
Patients'Characteristics (Continued)

Operation

no Operation	n=10	15%
Laparotomy	n=21	32%
Gastroenteroanastomosis	n= 2	4 %
Subtotal Gastrectomy	n=24	37%
Total Gastrectomy	n= 8	12%

Localisation of Metastasis *)

Liver	n=25	38 %
Omentum major and minor	n=23	35 %
Lymphnodes	n=41	63 %
Peritoneal Carcinosis	n=14	22 %
Ascites	n=14	22 %
Bone	n= 3	5 %
Skin	n= 2	3 %
Lung	n= 3	5%
Brain	n= 2	3%

*) Each Patient had more than one Organ involved.

FIGURE 1

282

Figure 1 lists the pretreatment of these patients. While only 10 patients had no prior surgery, 21 of 65 (32%) had exploratory laparotomy. All patients displayed metastasis in more than one organ and most of these were to the lymphnodes (63%) or liver (38%). Histology showed well-differentiated adenocarcinoma in 36 patients (55%) and mucus producing adenocarcinoma in 29 (45%). Cytostatic treatment was performed on an outpatient basis in 21 of 65 patients.

Metastasizing Stomach Cancer

Therapy Protocol

Day1 T=0 $1500\,mg/m^2$ MTX   i.v. Injection
           +1 Amp. Metoclopramide
      T=1H $1500\,mg/m^2$ 5 - FU   i.v. Injection
           + 1Amp. Metoclopramide

Day 2 T=24H
              $15\,mg/m^2$ Leucovorin Tabl. Q 6H x12

Day14 $30\,mg/m^2$ Adriamycin   i.v. Injection
Cycle is repeated after 28 Days

FIGURE 2

Figure 2 outlines the protocol. On day one, methotrexate 1500 mg/m² was given as a push injection followed one hour later by 5-fluorouracil 1500 mg/m². Twenty-four hours after methotrexate administration, we started oral leucovorin rescue at 15 mg/m² every six hours for 72 hours. On day 14, in order to prevent recruitment, 30 mg/m² adriamycin was injected as an infusion over 30 minutes and the cycle was repeated every 28 days. Patients eligible for this treatment should have a 24-hour-creatinine-clearance of $>$ 60 ml/min. Using a HPLC method (2), we measured methotrexate concentration in the serum of all patients at hour 48 following initial infusion. The concentration of methotrexate is shown in FIGURE 3.

Metastasizing Stomach Cancer

Concentration of Methotrexate in the Serum.
HPLC - Method

Patients with	Therapy Cycles (n)	MTX Concentration 48 Hrs. after Therapy (nmol/ml)	
normal Kidney Function	90	$\bar{x}$ SD$\pm$ Range	0,051 0,059 0 -0,252
Kidney Disturbances	5	$\bar{x}$ SD$\pm$ Range	2,7 3,886 0,528-9,571
	Enzyme- Immuno- Assay (EMIT [R])		
Patients with	Therapy Cycles (n)	MTX Concentration 48 Hrs. after Therapy (nmol/ml)	
normal Kidney Function	141	$\bar{x}$ SD$\pm$ Range	0,489 1,22 0,073 -1,71

FIGURE 3

284

In five patients who had creatinine-clearance smaller than 60 ml/min, the concentration of methotrexate in the serum was high (2,7 nmol/ml). Dialysis and forced diuresis rescue were used in all four cases effectively.

Overall response rate was 68% (44/65), with four patients in complete remission. Two patients had two-third resection prior to cytostatic treatment and a Karnofsky scale of 70% and 60% respectively. Histology was adenocarcinoma in both. One patient had no operation (Karnofsky index 60%) and the fourth patient had a laparotomy (Karnofsky index 60%). Survival probability is listed in figure 4.

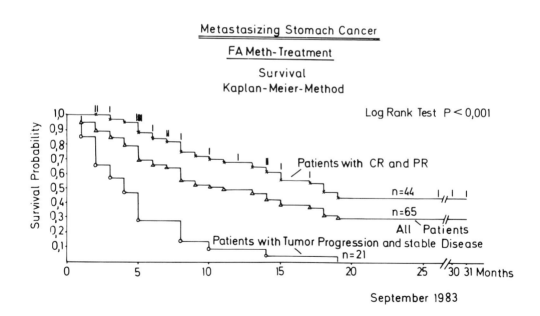

FIGURE 4

285

The median survival time for responders is 10 months, but for those patients who did not respond to therapy or had stable disease, it is four months. The difference between the curves is highly significant at a level of < 0.001. It is important to note that under our protocol, those patients who failed to respond to methotrexate-fluorouracil-adriamycin regimen or who relapsed were to be treated according to the FAM (5-fluorouracil, adriamycin, mitomycin C) protocol (7). No patient who went on the FAM protocol responded, so we can state that, at least according to this data, there is a cross resistance between both protocols. Toxicity was listed according to the WHO classification.

Metastasizing Stomach Cancer
FAMeth Treatment
Acute and Subacute Toxicity[*]

Side Effects	Toxicity Grades									
	0		1		2		3		4	
	n	%	n	%	n	%	n	%	n	%
Leucopenia	23	35	7	11	23	35	5	8	7	11
Thrombocytopenia	44	68	6	9	5	8	6	9	4	6
Stomatitis GI Toxicity	36	55	25	38	4	6	0		0	
Alopecia	8	12	10	15	47	72	0		0	
Kidney Failure	53	82	8	12	0		2	3	2	3
CNS Disturbances	61	94	4	6	0		0		0	
Occular Irritation	55	85	10	15	0		0		0	
Erythema	50	77	15	23	0		0		0	
Vascular Disord. (Thrombosis)	64	98	1	2	0		0		0	
Priapismus	63	97	2	3	0		0		0	

[*]WHO Classification

FIGURE 5

286

Only thirteen patients (20%) had evidence of grade IV
toxicity. Patched hair loss was observed in 72% of the
patients. Therapy-induced anemia was only seen rarely.

REFERENCES

1. Bertino, JR, Sawicki, WL, Lindquist, CA, et al.(1977)
    Schedule-dependent antitumor effects of methotrexate
    and 5-fluorouracil. Cancer Res 37: 327

2. Cansell, C., Sadée, W.(1980) Methotrexate and 7-hy-
    droxy-methotrexate serum level monitoring by high
    performance liquid chromatography. Cancer Treat Rep
    64: 165

3. Donelli, MG, Garattini, S.(1977) Differential accu-
    mulation of anticancer agents in metastases compared
    with primary tumors in pxperimental models. In: Re-
    cent Advances in Cancer Treatment (eds) HJ Tagnon and
    MJ Staquet. New York, Ravens Press, p. 177

4. Druckrey, H, Kuk, BT, Schmähl, D, Steinhoff, D.(1958)
    Kombination von Operation und Chemotherapie beim
    Krebs. Modellvergleich an einem resistenten Tumor der
    Ratte. Münch Med. Wschr 100: 1913

5. Druckrey, H, Steinhoff, D, Nakayama, M, et al.(1963)
    Experimentelle Beiträge zum Dosisproblem in der
    Krebschemotherapie und zur Wirkungsweise von Endoxan.
    Dtsch Med Wschr 88: 651

6. Klein, HO, Dias Wickramanayake, P, et al. (1982)
    Chemotherapieprotokoll zur Behandlung des metasta-
    sierenden Magen-Carcinoms. Dtsch Med Wschr 107: 1708

7. McDonald, JS, Woolley, PK, Smythe, T, et al. (1979)
    5-Fluorouracil, adriamycin, and mitomicin C (FAM)
    combination chemotherapy in the treatment of advanced
    gastric cancer. Cancer 44: 42

© 1984 Elsevier Science Publishers B.V.
Fluoropyrimidines in Cancer Therapy
K. Kimura, S. Fujii, M. Ogawa, G.P. Bodey, P. Alberto, eds.

DISCUSSION

Holyoke: Dr. Konda, do you have information on the variability of blood levels from rectal route under clinical conditions? Another question is, how do you measure lymph node response?

Konda: Measurement of the tegafur concentration in lymph nodes was done by Japanese investigators. Concentrations of tegafur in the lymph nodes were higher than in other tissues. There is a correlation between concentration and effect. Response in superficial lymph nodes means complete disappearance, whereas regression of lymph nodes inside of the abdomen is measured by using echography.

Holyoke: How about the variability of blood levels under clinical conditions? Is it a factor of two or three? Is there a large standard deviation? Do you have that information?

Konda: According to our investigations, if the patient has a liver metastasis, the blood level is low for tegafur and 5-FU.

Sadée: This is also a question to Dr. Konda. I was impressed by the high variability of tegafur from suppositories. I wonder if anyone has given any thought to including UFT, the combination of uracil with tegafur, in suppositories, because this would provide a real difference. As you have shown, the tegafur bypasses the liver, and uracil given in any other form, orally, will go through the liver and will be largely removed. So if you give a combination UFT, you will have a very different situation. You will get much more uracil into the body, and that may change the response rates. Has there been any consideration of that?

Konda: I also have a question for you. Do tegafur and uracil have equal absorption ratios in rectal administration?

Sadée: I don't know. If uracil would be absorbed as well as tegafur and it would bypass the liver, you might need less uracil. On the other hand, it is possible that you have an absolute limit as to how much uracil you can get into the body by tablet form. Thus, you may be able to load up much more uracil, which may change your response pattern. So you can try either less uracil, or you can try as much ura-

...cil as in the other dosages and see what the difference is.

Yan Sun: Dr. Konda, you mentioned bleeding in about 6-8%. Was bleeding a severe complication of chemotherapy? Another question is to Dr. Kurihara. You did a large comparative study of rectal and oral administration. What is your idea about those types of administration?

Konda: The incidence of bleeding following oral administration or rectal administration is not much different. The degree of bleeding is not much different either. Local and rectal bleeding are not severe. Cessation of administration for a short time causes disappearance.

Yan Sun: Do you mean rectal bleeding?

Konda: I don't really know if it is rectal bleeding or systemic bleeding. The degree of systemic bleeding is not severe. It is very mild.

Kurihara: I will comment on the tegafur suppository. I have had experience with more than 60 cases of GI cancer treated with tegafur suppository. Among them, there were no severe side effects in terms of myelosuppression or rectal bleeding. Dr. Yan Sun, as regards your question about oral and rectal administration of 5-FU, I do not have experience with rectal administration of 5-FU. We did a few phase I studies, but severe side effects of rectal bleeding caused us to discontinue our study.

Majima: I have a question for Dr. Kurihara. I am wondering about the duration of administration of 5-FU. As far as I know, absorption of this compound is extremely variable from patient to patient and even in the same patient. When administration is maintained over a prolonged period of time (more than four or five weeks), the microvilli of the intestine get atrophic and absorption gets worse. If you aim at local effects, this is a different story; but if you think about systemic absorption and expected effect, what kind of consideration do you give to your patients?

Kurihara: This is a very difficult question. 5-FU tablets are dissolved in a few minutes in the stomach and expected to have direct effects on gastric cancer. Compared with the syrup form, they are sustained in the stomach much longer and gradually move to the small intestine. As a result, it is considered to be less toxic to the small intestinal membrane compared to 5-FU syrup. This is my hypothesis.

Kimura: I have a few comments as to the questions from our foreign guests. In general, stomach cancer patients cannot take any food. How then can such stomach cancer patients be treated? This is a very difficult problem for us. Therefore, we developed a suppository more than ten years ago. Now this kind of therapy is popular in Japan, and we have extended its use to patients with metastatic colon cancer.

Ota: I would like to comment on the differences between oral and rectal administration of 5-FU or tegafur. In direct antitumor activity such as in stomach or lower rectal cancer, 5-FU is much greater than tegafur because a direct effect appears with 5-FU. But, when we use tegafur, the systemic effects are much greater than 5-FU because tegafur is activated to 5-FU mainly through the liver.

Bertino: I must say that in contrast to the United States where we use either weekly or 5-day schedules of 5-FU, it seems that the most popular schedule here in Japan is daily oral doses for many days. Dr. Lokich in Boston has been administering 5-FU by continuous infusion in low doses for long periods of time. The optimum way of giving 5-FU, it seems to me, is almost determined by the convenience of administration and the type of patient. Would you agree with that, Dr. Kimura; or is there a recommended method of giving 5-FU; or does this depend upon the patient?

Kimura: In Japan, we have many patients with stomach cancer. For them we need a treatment of long duration on an outpatient basis. Further, I have already reported that tegafur and 5-FU are time-dependent drugs, so time is very important in obtaining a significant effect. Therefore, oral use of tegafur has been preferred.

Ogawa: I was very impressed by the presentation by Dr. Klein because, to my knowledge, his response rate is the highest in the world, and the duration of survival is the longest - 18 months. However, I would like to know the role of adriamycin in this regimen. You mentioned that approximately ten to fourteen days later there is a recruitment of cancer cells. That is the reason you used adriamycin in a rather small dose. What would happen in your regimen without adriamycin? Secondly, we feel that to assess complete response in gastric cancer is extremely difficult. In the four complete responders that you listed, there are three patients with responses at the primary site. What is the method used to assess complete response in primary gastric lesions?

Klein: As to the first question, it is correct that recruitment takes place between days 10 and 14. We used adriamycin in order to prevent toxicity of methotrexate and 5-FU to the gastrointestinal tract. In the pilot study we studied the single-agent activity of methotrexate and 5-FU, and in four of 5 patients treated we observed a partial response with methotrexate and also with 5-FU in sequence. But when we repeated the sequence a fortnight later, these patients developed diarrhea, as Dr. Bertino has already mentioned. To avoid these side effects on the gastrointestinal tract, we thought it was necessary to use a drug which does not have such a broad side effect spectrum like the methotrexate and 5-FU sequence. This is the reason for administering adriamycin. The dosage is low, of course, but in the

pattern of leukocyte values after adriamycin, there is a
fall of leukocytes to levels around 1,000 cells per μl
blood. That means that if we use a higher dose, we will
get myelosuppression. To your second question, we stopped
therapy after we got confirmation that these patients
were in complete remission. They are still alive, as I
have shown. All these patients had not only gastric prim-
aries but also secondaries in lymph nodes. The patients
with two-thirds stomach resections had, histologically,
infiltrations in the resection margin. All these patients
were checked every three months by endoscopy, biopsy, CAT
scan, and ultrasonography. The study parameters were
survival and these clinical parameters in order to check
whether the patients were free of disease.

Woolley: I would like to congratulate Dr. Klein on his
presentation and his work. I hope that this work is
confirmed by other investigators because, if so, it is
the first significant improvement on the treatment of
gastric cancer since we described the 5-FU+adriamycin+
mitomycin combination. I would like to ask two questions
and make a comment. Is your criterion for partial response
a 50% reduction in perpendicular diameters of the tumors?

Klein: Yes.

Woolley: Good. My second question is whether you can tell
us what is the minimum median survival that is possible in
your patient population at this point?

Klein: We have lost patients who responded to therapy after
six weeks. These were two patients. One had a heart attack
and died suddenly; this was proven by autopsy. But tumor
shrinkage was more than 50% and he had this attack during
a visit to the hospital for a check-up. The other patient
was one who died after eight weeks and had, at autopsy, a
partial remission; but the immediate cause of death remained unknown. Consequently, minimum survival in patients who
responded is six weeks.

Woolley: I believe the minimum median survival is longer
than six weeks. Finally, I would like to make a comment.
The subject of protein-ligand interactions has been one of
considerable interest to me for several years. I have yet
to be convinced that interaction between methotrexate and
serum albumin or any other protein is sufficiently tight
and results in high proportion of methotrexate actually
being bound that drug-drug interactions are truly a
significant clinical problem. It is my feeling that it
mostly applies to drugs that are very tightly bound to
protein and are perhaps greater than 90% transported in
protein complex. Under these circumstances if you add a
competing drug, you get a very high relative increase in
the proportion of free-circulating drug. I would be interested to know if that is really a significant interaction
or not.

291

Bertino: I think you are right. I think the binding of methotrexate-albumin is very loose. It is on the order of 10^{-5} molar; so it doesn't really interfere with the action of the drug. I think Dr. Klein may wish to comment on this. I think the reason why he probably did not use allopurinol was because he did not want elevated hypoxanthine levels to counteract the effect of the sequence. I think the salicylate avoidance was not only because of displacement from protein binding but because he did not want to acidify the urine.

Klein: The EORTC has started a trial on this sequence in gastric cancer. They observed toxicity in patients having a very low albumin fraction in electrophoresis. So it might be that the binding capacity of protein is a little bit responsible for toxicity, but I have no firm data to confirm this.

Vidal (Hospital Paula Jaraquemada, Santiago): We are using, in advanced gastric cancer with measurable disease, the same regimen of methotrexate, 5-FU, and adriamycin, but in low doses. We are using methotrexate 15 mg/m^2 on days 1 and 8, 5-FU 600 mg/m^2 on the same days, and adriamycin 30 mg/m^2 on day 1. The courses are repeated every 28 days, and the interval between methotrexate and 5-FU is two hours. In less than 20 patients with measurable disease, the response rate was about 40%. The median survival period was about twelve months for those patients who responded and 3.5 months for those patients with no response.

H. Fujita: Is there any experimental data whether or not thymidine can rescue the toxicity of methotrexate and 5-FU instead of leucovorin?

Bertino: We don't have that particular data, but there are some data. In some cell lines thymidine does not rescue 5-FU which might indicate that 5-FU was killing by more of an RNA effect.

Blokhina: I would like to say a few words about the treatment of cancer of the stomach. I have studied this question for 20 years and have tried many combinations. I must say that unfortunately I have had no success - especially concerning patients who have a performance status below 40% or 60%. It seems to me that it is not useful to treat them, because they probably live longer than when we use some treatments.

Bertino: Another theoretical reason for using the alternating combination that Dr. Klein mentioned is the avoidance of drug resistance. As some of you know, Drs. Goldie and Coldman have made some theoretical calculations based upon the earlier studies of Drs. Lurie and Delbruck in experimental bacterial systems and have come up with the observation that alternating drug combinations may be the best way to use drug combinations. So that an alternating sequence may not only do what Dr. Klein thought it would do in terms of the recruitment but also cut down the number of drug-resistant cells. That may be another reason for the efficacy of the program.

Woolley: I would like to ask Dr. Bertino if he or anybody else has experience with methotrexate followed by 5-FU infusions. If so, do you have any comment about the timing of leucovorin rescue, and whether or not it is possible to repeat the dose of methotrexate during a 5-FU infusion.

Bertino: We don't have any information on that. I think it is reasonable to give a longer duration of 5-FU than we do by rapid bolus. By using a very large dose, Dr. Klein has prolonged the serum level because even though the half-life is short, there is an effective half-life for a longer period of time. The other alternative would be to give an infusion of 5-FU for 12-24 hours. There are many variables and it is hard to know exactly where to start.

Tattersall: I would like to ask Dr. Klein about his studies with flow cytometry. You mentioned that you had shown tumor recruitment at about day 14, and I wonder if you have done any studies of normal bone marrow. Have you looked at the effect on the tumor with methotrexate alone?

Klein: Yes, we did. In the pilot study, among these five patients there was one with ascites. We obtained samples of bone marrow, ascites fluid, and biopsies from the primary corrected by endoscopy. What is interesting is that after methotrexate we saw the same thing that Dr. Bertino showed with flow cytometry. There is an accumulation of cells in the early part of the S phase that later disappeared. We observed the same phenomenon in the bone marrow as the primary tumor, but recovery came much earlier than in the tumor cells. We observed recovery after the eighth day, and this corresponded very well to the leucocyte recovery in the blood. I think that this depends upon the proliferation of these cells. Normal tissue cells like hemopoietic cells usually have a shorter regeneration time than the stomach cancer cells. It might be that that makes the difference. I believe that these kinetic differences in normal tissues and in neoplastic tissues provide some advantages to the use of sequential therapy, not only the biochemical aspects, but also these proliferation kinetics may play a role in tolerability, feasibility, and maybe also response.

Tattersall: You didn't quite answer my question about whether the addition of 5-FU alters the phenomenon.

Klein: From the patients treated with methotrexate-5-FU sequence one accepted many biopsies. In one patient following the administration of 5-FU after methotrexate there was a complete disappearance of cells in the DNA synthesis phase starting one hour after the administration of 5-FU. It was a direct lysis of cells piled up in the early part of the S phase. This lasted for a very long time, and after ten days (between ten and fourteen days) cells progressed again into the S phase. This was also shown by autoradio-graphy, the single-cell methods (that means thymidine incorporation). We also measured the DNA synthesis phase by the double-labeling technique.

Kimura: Dr. Bertino, in your sequential schedule, can we consider the collateral sensitivity between methotrexate and 5-FU?

Bertino: We have looked at 3 or 4 methotrexate-resistant cell lines for sensitivity to 5-FU, and we have not seen any increased or decreased sensitivity. I don't think that we are getting collateral sensitivity in the usual sense of that phrase. But we think it is a biochemical synergy.

Ota: In closing this session, I would like to make a short comment. Methotrexate and 5-FU sequential therapy is very interesting. I attended a symposium last September under Dr. Bertino's chairmanship and I was very stimulated by the data. In Japan, Dr. Sasaki and the doctors of Tohoku University are now studying this combination. Many results have been reported, but the efficacy is extremely variable. In Japan, where stomach cancer is frequent, we have to examine the dose schedule of methotrexate and 5-FU treatment for this tumor. This sequential combination of methotrexate and 5-FU should be evaluated for the adeno-carcinomas of the lung, the colon and the rectum as well.

CHEMOTHERAPY FOR ADVANCED CANCER: GASTROINTESTINAL TUMORS

© 1984 Elsevier Science Publishers B.V.
Fluoropyrimidines in Cancer Therapy
K. Kimura, S. Fujii, M. Ogawa, G.P. Bodey, P. Alberto, eds.

CHEMOTHERAPY FOR ADVANCED GASTROINTESTINAL TUMORS IN AUSTRALIA

Martin H.N. Tattersall

INTRODUCTION

Chemotherapy is not used routinely in the management of advanced gastrointestinal tumours in Australia. In comparison with the USA, Australia has few medical oncologists outside the major institutions in the state capitals, and the majority of the colorectal tumours, the most numerous GI cancer in Australia, is managed in the community hospitals by general surgeons. In the past five years a few multi-institutional studies of different management approaches in GI cancer have been commenced, but only one of these has accrued large numbers of cases.

5-Fluorouracil (FU) is the most widely used drug in advanced GI cancers. In colorectal cancers, FU is most often administered as a single agent, either by weekly intravenous injection, or as a five day intravenous infusion repeated at monthly intervals. A few institutions have developed an interest in regional FU administration most commonly by hepatic arterial infusion for patients with liver metastases. There is a growing interest in the umbilical vein as a route of

297

FU administration, and a multi-institutional study in operable colorectal cancers has been commenced recently. FU is occasionally given intraperitoneally in patients with malignant ascites, but the "belly bath" method is not utilised. FU is rarely given orally, and Australian studies have documented erratic absorption[1]. The notion that some changes in FU formulation might improve the absorption is being investigated currently.

FU is commonly used in combination with other agents in management of advanced gastric cancer patients. The reports that Adriamycin had antitumour activity in gastric cancer led one group to pilot a combination of FU, Adriamycin and BCNU in 35 gastric cancer patients[2]. An objective tumour response was reported in 52%, with the survival of responding patients being three fold longer than that of patients having no tumour regression. A multi-institutional study of this regimen compared to Adriamycin as a single agent has accrued over 200 patients. The trial end points are tumour response rates, time to disease progression, and survival, but no results have been published at this juncture.

There is current interest in the reports of combined FU-Mitomycin and irradiation having impressive effects in anal and oesophageal cancer[3,4]. Preliminary experience in Australia with this combined modality therapy has been

298

most promising, and this approach is likely to be pursued enthusiastically if the initial experience is confirmed. It is possible that this approach may be applied in the management of locally advanced rectal and gastric cancers but there are no facilities in Australia for intra operative external radiotherapy.

Modulation of Fluorouracil Activity
Nucleosides

Considerable interest has recently developed on the possibility of modulating FU therapy by nucleosides and methotrexate[5,6,7]. This approach is based on the complexity of the biochemical pathways of FU metabolism, and the possibility that FU may interfere with the synthesis of DNA and or RNA in different tissues. An understanding of the molecular bases of normal tissue toxicity of FU may emerge from these studies potentially opening the way to the design of more selective FU analogues and methods of enhancing tumour selectivity.

Different pathways of FU anabolism have been demonstrated in a variety of cultured cell lines. FU can be activated to fluorodeoxyuridine monophosphate (FdUMP), by three (potential) enzymatic pathways: (I) orotate phosphoribosyl transferase (OPRT ase); (II) uridine phosphorylase; or (III) thymidine phosphorylase (Fig.I). Piper et al[8] in this laboratory have demonstrated that in the human leukaemic T cell line CCRF-CEM, the major pathway of FU anabolism is OPRTase, while in the human B cell line LAZ007 thymidine and uridine phosphorylase are major pathways (Table I). Differential effects of

TABLE I   Activities of FU activating enzymes in CCRF-CEM and LAZ007 cells

Enzyme	Substrate	Activity (nmol/hr/mg protein)[a]	
		CEM	LAZ
OPRT ase	orotic acid	52 ± 12	34 ± 5
	FU	75 ± 16	33 ± 7
UR phosphorylase	Uracil	3[b]	74 ± 21
	FU	3	139 ± 30
TdR phosphorylase	Thymine	3	1454 ± 103
	FU	3	1610 ± 97

a. The figures are the means and range of the values obtained in 4 separate experiments.

b. The limit of detection is 3nmol/hr/mg protein.

modulators of these anabolic pathways have been demonstrated in vitro. In particular, allopurinol and hypoxanthine both reduce the metabolic and growth inhibitory effects of FU in CEM cells without significant effects on LAZ cells (Table II).   Schwartz et al[9] have

TABLE II   Effect of Allopurinol and Hypoxanthine on the
           inhibition by FU of Deoxyuridine conversion to
           Thymidine nucleotides in CCRF-CEM and LAZ 007
           cells

	% inhibition of Deoxyuridine conversion in the presence of FU plus Imm		
FU (M)	Control	Allopurinol	Hypoxanthine
CCRF-CEM cells			
5×10^{-5}	71	0	0
5×10^{-4}	96	7	46
LAZ 007			
1×10^{-6}	63	34	12
5×10^{-6}	94	94	92

shown that allopurinol can prevent FU toxicity in mice.

One potential mechanism relates to the metabolism of

allopurinol and oxipurinol to nucleotides by OPRTase and

hypoxanthine   guanine   phosphoribosyl   transferase

(HGPRTase), both of which are strong inhibitors of

ODCase.   The   subsequent   accumulation   of   orotidine

monophosphate (OMP) and elevation of orotic acid compete

with FU activation by OPRTase.

    Changes in purine levels in the serum caused by

allopurinol, or regional variations may also have

important modulating effects on FU activation[10] (Table III). Prevention by allopurinol of FU toxicity in

TABLE III Extra cellular purine levels in plasma (P) and bone marrow aspirates(BM).

Subjects	Xanthine/ Hypoxanthine		Inosine		Adenosine		Total	
	P	BM	P	BM	P	BM	P	BM
1	0.7	16.2	nd	0.4	1.9	5.3	2.6	21.9
2	1.5	15.0	0.7	7.7	1.6	6.9	3.9	29.6
3	3.0	28.0	0.1	10.0	8.8	54.	11.9	92.0
4	0.7	4.5	0.3	2.0	2.5	10.8	3.5	17.3
5	1.1	36.0	0.4	11.0	6.6	60.0	11.1	107.4

Purine levels (uM)

mice presumably reflects inhibition of FU activation in normal tissues[9]. We undertook clinical and pharmacological studies of allopurinol modulation of five day intravenous infusion of FU in patients with advanced cancers[11]. Among 26 colorectal cancer patients assessable for tumour response, there was a 15.4% response rate, and two of four patients with metastatic gastric cancer responded. The daily FU dose ($2-2.25gm/m^2$/day) is approximately twice the maximum tolerated dose in patients not taking allopurinol. The predominant form of toxicity was mucosal which contrasts with the usual myelosuppresion seen as the dose limiting toxicity of FU when it is given by intravenous push or in conjunction with thymidine. These results suggest that allopurinol and or hypoxanthine reduce the toxicity of FU treatment in vivo, but do not necessarily modify the expected antitumour activity. More detailed understanding of the mechanism of FU action in normal bone marrow and gut cells is required before more rational attempts to modulate FU action in vivo can be determined.

Methotrexate

Combination chemotherapy regimens containing FU and methotrexate (MTX) have been in clinical use for many years. Concern about the optimum method of scheduling MTX and FU in cancer treatment has arisen from reports that the combination may show antagonistic or synergistic toxicity depending upon the sequence of drug administration[6,7,12]. Synergistic effects observed when MTX precedes FU have been ascribed either to enhanced binding of FdUMP to thymidylate synthetase in the presence of increased levels of dihydropteroyl polyglutamates[13], or to enhanced FU-nucleotide formation with resultant increased incorporation into

RNA. The latter mechanism is dependent upon accumulation of phosphoribosyl pyrophosphate (PRPP) in cells exposed to MTX. Antagonistic effects observed when FU precedes MTX have been ascribed to sparing effects of thymidylate synthetase inhibition on the utilisation of reduced folates for purine biosynthesis[6]. We have reported that treatment of murine L1210 cells with MTX followed by FU produced synergistic cytotoxicity only in medium containing low concentrations of hypoxanthine (eg. horse serum or dialysed foetal calf serum)[14]. Addition of 1-10uM hypoxanthine reduced the synergism of sequential MTX (1-100uM) - FU (30-300uM) treatment (Table IV).

TABLE IV Prevention by Hypoxanthine of sequential MTX-FU synergy in LI210 cells growing in dialysed foetal calf serum

Variation with MTX concentration			
	% MTX-FU compared to MTX		
Hypoxanthine (uM)	MTX (uM)		
	1	10	100
0	0.5	1.2	0.6
1	47.6	9.6	0.9
3	119.3	60.9	56.7

The reduction of synergy by hypoxanthine varied with the MTX concentration employed, higher hypoxanthine concentrations being required to prevent synergy at higher MTX concentrations. The cytotoxicity produced by sequential MTX (10uM) - FU (30-300uM) treatment was also reduced by thymidine (> 0.5uM). Thymidine concentrations in human peripheral plasma are 0.5-1.5uM[15] and thus both thymidine and hypoxanthine concentrations in human plasma call into question the clinical relevance of MTX/FU synergy observed in in vitro experiments in the presence of horse serum, and in vivo experiments in mice.

Clinical Studies of Sequential MTX and Fluorouracil

Because of biochemical evidence casting doubt on the physiological relevance of reported synergy afforded by sequential MTX followed by FU, we are conducting a randomised controlled clinical trial in which patients with colorectal, gastric or head and neck cancer are randomised to receive these drugs at an interval of one hour, either in the above or in the reversed sequence. To date 75 patients have been entered on this trial, including 50 patients with head and neck cancer, 19 patients with colorectal cancer and four patients with gastric cancer. The dose of MTX was $250mg/m^2$ and of FU $600mg/m^2$. Patients received oral or intravenous bicarbonate to ensure a urine pH > 7 at the time of MTX administration, and for 24 hours thereafter then oral citrovorum factor rescue for eight doses of 15mg each six hours commenced 24 hours after the MTX. The treatment regimens were well tolerated in most patients with a low incidence of haematologic and no significant renal toxicity, but occasional several diarrhoea or mucositis in spite of normal renal function and administration of citrovorum factor acid rescue. No differences in toxicity according to the treatment sequence has been observed (Table V). Plasma purine levels have been

TABLE V   Toxicity of sequential Methotrexate-Fluorouracil

		Treatment sequence	
No. eval.		M F 34	F M 34
Toxicity grades			
WBC	2	3	7
Mucositis	2	8	8
Nausea & vomiting	2	8	9
Diarrhoea	2	6	4
Treatment rel. Death		2	2

monitored in some patient immediately before and one hour

after the first drug administration (Table VI). There

TABLE VI Plasma purine levels (uM) in first treatment
cycle

Treatment sequence

MF	No.	Xanthine/ Hypoxanthine	Inosine/ Adenosine	Total
Pretreatment	6	1.3 ± 0.5	1.8 ± 0.6	3.1 ± 0.9
1hr after MTX	6	1.3 ± 0.5	1.5 ± 1.1	2.8 ± 1.3
FM				
Pretreatment	6	1.7 ± 0.9	2.9 ± 1.8	4.6 ± 2.4
1hr after FU	6	1.5 ± 1.0	2.4 ± 1.0	3.9 ± 1.5

is no significant difference between the two sequence
regimens in the changes observed, nor is there any
apparent correlation between plasma purine change and
response to treatment. Both treatment sequences were
effective in colorectal and head and neck cancers. A
response rate of 38% (95% cl 15-65%) was seen in
colorectal cancer, and there was no difference between
the two treatment sequences. In head and neck cancer,
the overall tumour response rate was 52% (95% cl 37-67%)
with a survival exceeding 13 months but the order of drug
administration was not important. These results do not
support sequence dependent synergy between MTX and FU in
clinical practice.

CONCLUSIONS

Chemotherapy currently plays a minor role in the management of gastrointestinal cancers in Australia. A number of new approaches our being pursued and it is likely that some of the present clinical and laboratory slides will lead to an improved outcome for some patients, and perhaps a reduction in toxicity associated with chemotherapy to others.

ACKNOWLEDGEMENTS

I am grateful to my colleagues Professor R.M. Fox and Drs. A.S. Coates and A.A. Piper, and to P. Slowiaczek and many others for their help undertaking these investigations.

REFERENCES

1. Christophidis N, Vajda FJ, Louis WT, Moon W. (1978) Flourouracil therapy in patients with cancer of large bowel and pharmacokinetics of various rates and routes of administration. Clin Pharmacokinetics 3: 330-336.

2. Levi JA, Dalley DN, Aroney RS. (1979) Improved combination chemotherapy in advanced gastric cancer. Brit Med J 2: 1471-3.

3. Buroker T, Nigro N, Carsidine B, et al. (1979) Mitomycin C, 5-Fluorouracil and radiation therapy in squamous cell carcinoma of the anal canal. In: Mitomycin C (eds) Carter and Crook. Adacemic Press, pp.183-188.

4. Franklin R, Steiger Z, Vaishampayan G, Asfaw I, Rosenberg J, Loh J, Hoschner J, Miller P (1983) Cobmined modality therapy for esophageal squamous cell cancer. Cancer 51: 1062-1072.

5. Yoshida M, Hashi A, Kuretani K. (1978) Prevention of antitumor effect of 5-Fluorouracil by hypoxanthine. Biochem Pharmacol 27: 2979-82.

6. Tattersall MHN, Jackson RC, Connors TA, et al. (1973) Combination chemotherapy : the interaction of methotrexate and fluorouracil. Europ J Cancer 9: 733-739.

7. Bertino JR, Sawicki WL, Lindquist CA, et al. (1977) Schedule dependent antitumour effects of methotrexate and fluorouracil. Cancer Res 7: 327-328.

8. Piper AA, Fox RM. (1981) Differential metabolism of Fluorouracil in cultured human T and B cell lines. In: Nucleosides and Cancer Treatment (eds) MHN Tattersall and RM Fox. Academic Press, pp.251-265.

9. Schwartz PR, Dunigan JM, Marsh JC, Handschumacher RE. (1979) Allopurinol modification of the toxicity and antitumor activity of Fluorouracil. Cancer Res 40: 1885-1889.

10. Tattersall MHN, Slowiaczek P, De Fazio A. (1983) Regional variation in human extracellular purine levels. J Lab Clin Med (in press).

11. Fox RM, Woods RL, Tattersall MHN, et al. (1981) Allopurinol modulation of Fluorouracil toxicity. Cancer Chemother Pharmacol 5: 151-155.

12. Cadman ED, Heimer R, Benz C. (1981) The influence of methotrexate pretreatment on 5-fluorouracil metabolism in L1210 cells. J Biol Chem 256: 1695-1704.

13. Fernandes DJ, Bertino JR. (1980) 5-Fluorouracil-methotrexate synergy: Enhancement of 5-fluorodeoxyuridylate binding to thymidylate synthase by dihyropteroylpolyglutamates. Proc Natl Acad Sci 77: 5663-5676.

14. Piper AA, Nott SE, MacKinnon WB, Tattersall MHN. (1983) Sequential methotrexate-5-fluorouracil synergism in murine L1210 cells: Critical modulation by thymidine and hypoxanthine. Cancer Res (in press).

15.   Holden L, Hoffbrand AV, Tattersall MHN. (1980) Thymidine concentrations in human sera. Europ J Cancer 16: 115-120.

16.   Coates AS, Tattersall MHN, Slowiaczek P, et al. (1983) Sequential versus reversed methotrexate and 5-fluorouracil. A prospective randomized clinical trial of order of administration. J Clin Oncol (in press).

© 1984 Elsevier Science Publishers B.V.
Fluoropyrimidines in Cancer Therapy
K. Kimura, S. Fujii, M. Ogawa, G.P. Bodey, P. Alberto, eds.

UFTM CHEMOTHERAPY FOR GASTRIC CANCER: EFFECTIVENESS AND COMPARISON OF SURVIVAL BETWEEN UFTM AND SURGICAL TREATMENT IN PATIENTS WITH BORRMANN TYPE 4 GASTRIC CANCER

Shoji Suga, Kiyoji Kimura, Yuichi Yoshida, Tadashi Horiuchi
and Yasuhisa Yokoyama

1. INTRODUCTION

In a previous paper, it was reported that the uracil (U) - tegafur(FT) combination with a U/FT molar ratio of 4 (UFT), could produce an effective 5-fluorouracil (5-FU) level in tumour tissues of cancer patients and that UFT chemotherapy, daily oral administration of UFT at a dose of $200mg/m^2$ twice a day, is one of the most recommendable (effective and less toxic) types of chemotherapy for gastric cancer (1,2). In UFTM chemotherapy, mitomycin C was administered to the patients intravenously in addition to the UFT chemotherapy. It was also demonstrated that patients with gastric cancer experienced clinical responses at a considerably high (over 50%) rate with the UFTM chemotherapy(2). Thereafter, effectiveness of UFTM therapy was reconfirmed in an increased number of patients with Borrmann type 4 diffuse gastric cancer. In this paper, comparison of patients survival between UFTM and surgical treatment in patients with Borrmann type 4 gastric cancer is also presented.

2. PATIENTS AND METHODS

2.1. Patients

A total of 22 patients with Borrmann type 4 gastric cancer were treated with UFTM chemotherapy. Another 74 patients with Borrmann type 4 gastric cancer were treated surgically; 57 out of 74 patients were surgically resectable and the rest of 17 cases were non-resectable.

2.2. Patients survival

Patients survival was expressed as a survival rate by the duration of follow-up.

2.3. UFTM chemotherapy

First, the protocol of UFT chemotherapy was as follows; patents were given 200mg/m^2 of UFT orally twice a day before meals. In UFTM chemotherapy, mitomycin C was administered to the patients intravenously once a week at a dose of 4.0-5.3mg/m^2 (disolved in 20ml of saline solution) by the one-shot method, in addition to UFT chemotherapy. As a maintenance schedule, UFT was in some cases reduced to a dose of 133mg/m^2 twice a day and mitomycin C was in most cases given at a dose of 5.0-7.0mg/m^2 every two to four weeks, depending mainly on the degree of hematologic toxicity (2). UFT alone was usually administered to the patients during the period of leucocytopenia less than 2,000-3,000/mm^3 and/or thrombocytopenia less than 50,000-70,000/mm^3, because of the scarce hematological side effects of UFT. The main toxic reactions with UFT alone were diarrhoea, appetite loss and nausea which occurred in 10 to 20% of the patients. In Fig. 1, protocol of UFTM chemotherapy was presented, in which it was shown that the 4th administration of mitomycin C might have been skipped to avoid a possible hematological toxicity at the later time of therapy.

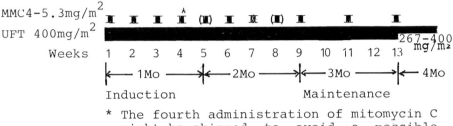

* The fourth administration of mitomycin C might be skipped to avoid a possible hematological toxicity at the later time of therapy.

Fig. 1. Protocol of UFTM chemotherapy.

3. RESULTS

3.1. Effectiveness and toxicity of UFTM chemotherapy

With UFTM chemotherapy, objective responses occurred in fifteen out of all 22 patients with Borrmann type 4 gastric cancer(68.2% response rate), i.e. disappearance of ascites due to peritonitis carcinomatosa and a decrease in size of metastatic tumours were observed in association with improvement of extensibility of the stomach wall.

With regard to the toxicity of the treatment, leuco-cytopenia and/or thrombocytopenia were major side effects of UFTM chemotherapy. Besides, diarrhoea and appetite loss or nausea occurred in 10 to 20% of the patients.

Phlebitis was also occationally induced with mitomycin C
in the cases of long term administration.

3.2. Survival time of the patients with Borrmann type 4
gastric cancer treated with UFTM chemotherapy

Patients survival with UFTM therapy was shown in Fig.
2. Fifty per cent survival time of all 22 patients was 8.4
months from the initiation of therapy. Duration of 50%
survival was 11.0 months in the responding group and 5.7
months in the non-responding patients.

3.3 Survival time of the patients with Borrmann type 4
gastric cancer treated surgically.

As shown in Fig. 3, fifty per cent survival time of
all 74 cases with surgical treatment was 7.6 months after
operation. Duration of 50% survival was 9.6 months in the
resectable cases and 2.4 months in the non-resectable
patients.

3.4. Comparison of patients survival between UFTM and
surgical treatment in the patients with Borrmann type 4
gastric cancer

Comparing the results in Fig. 2 and 3, no difference
was observed between UFTM and surgical treatment on the
survival time of the patients with Borrmann type 4 gastric
cancer.

314

Tablo 1. Clinical results of UFTM chemotherapy for patients with Borrmann type 4 gastric cancer

Total number of patients	Responders	Response rate(%)
22	15	68.2

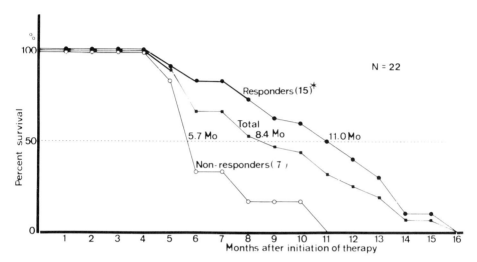

Fig. 2. Survival curve of patients with Borrmann type 4 gastric cancer treated with UFTM chemotherapy. *Operation was performed in one patient of the responders 7 months after therapy.

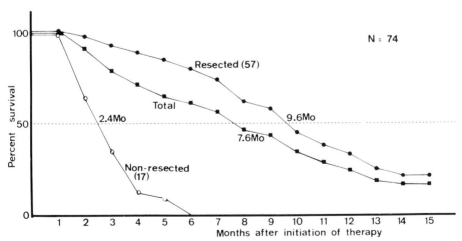

Fig. 3. Survival curve of patients with Borrmann type 4 gastric cancer treated surgically.

315

3.5. Case report

Y.O. 73 year-old female with the primary gastric cancer of Borrmann type 4 and peritonitis carcinomatosa. On Jun. 1, 1983, she visited our hospital with the complaints of distended abdomen and poor appetite or nausea. Ascites examination revealed the presence of malignant cells. Fluoroscopic findings of the stomach were presented in Fig. 4-a. A remarkable impairment of extensibility of the stomach wall which covered widely the upper two-thirds of the whole stomach was observed in association with the defective appearance of the cardia and fornix portion. Three weeks after initiation of UFTM chemotherapy, ascites disappeared, and the original lesions of the stomach were remarkably improved; i.e. disappearance of the defective finding of the upper stomach and an apparent improvement of extensibility of the stomach wall were observed (Fig. 4-b) at two months from the initiation of UFTM treatment. She has been alive in good health (Oct. 15, 1983).

4. DISCUSSION

In the previous studies on the pharmacokinetics of tegafur (FT) and UFT in patients with gastric cancer, it was demonstrated that UFT produced and maintained a higher (effective) level of 5-FU in tumour tissues than FT, and that 5-FU level was highest in tumour tissue, the value being decreased in the normal tissues and lowest in the blood. Such observations would be related to the more

316

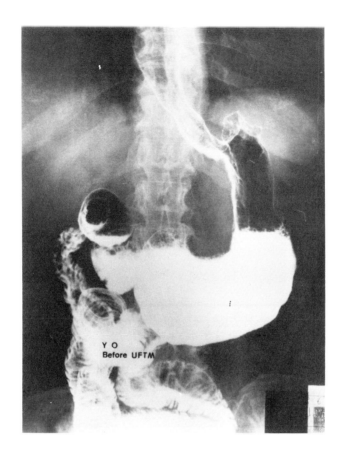

a) Before therapy

Fig. 4. Fluoroscopic findings of Case Y.O.

anticancer activity with less toxic effects of UFT to the hosts. It was further demonstrated that *in Situ* (more efficient in tumour tissue) activation of FT to 5-FU would participate in the high concentration of 5-FU in tumour tissues(3).

Recently, it was reconfirmed *in Vitro* that 5-FU exerts its anticancer activity with the administration schedule of lower doses for longer time periods. UFT chemotherapy

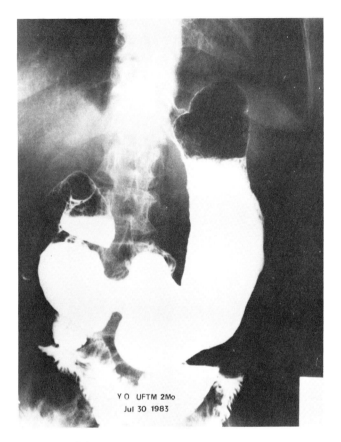

Y O UFTM 2Mo
Jul 30 1983

b)   2 Mo. after UFTM

is actually based on such fundumental experiments(4).

In UFTM chemotherapy, mitomycin C, a dose dependent and one of the major anticancer agents of clinical use, was combined with UFT which is one of the time dependent antimetabolite anticancer agents. It was demonstrated in the present paper that 68.2% response rate (15 out of 22) was obtained with UFTM chemotherapy for the patients with Borrmann type 4 gasric cancer.

As illustrated in Fig. 2 and 3, there was no difference between UFTM and surgical treatment in the survivals
of the patients with Borrmann type 4 gastric cancer.
Accordingly, it was concluded that except for the patients
of far-advanced gastric cancer, there was no particular
evidence which supports an alternative treatment of UFTM
or surgical operation for the patients with Borrmann type
4 gastric cancer.

ACKNOWLEDGEMENTS

This work was supported in part by a Grant-in-Aid for
Cancer Research (57-6) from the Ministry of Health and
Welfare.

REFERENCES

1. Kimura K, Suga S, Shimaji T, et al. (1980) Clinical
   basis of chemotherapy for gastric cancer with uracil
   and 1-(2'-tetrahydrofuryl)-5-fluorouracil. Gastroent
   Jpn 15: 324-329

2. Suga S, Kimura K, Yokoyama Y, et al. (1983) UFT and
   UFTM treatment for gastric cancer. Drugs Exptl Clin
   Res 9(1): 101-108

3. Suga S, Kimura K, Yokoyama Y, et al. (1983) Comparative studies on the pharmacodynamics of ftorafur (FT)
   and its metabolite-antimetabolite combination(UFT) in
   cancer patients. Proceedings of 13th International Congress of Chemotherapy (Vienna)

4. Calabro-Jones PM, Byfield JE, Ward JF, et al. (1982)
   Time-dose relationships for 5-fluorouracil cytotoxi-
   city against human epithelial cancer cells in Vitro.
   Cancer Res 42: 4413-4420

CLINICAL OVERVIEW OF TREATMENT FOR GASTROINTESTINAL TUMORS

Paul V. Woolley, III, Frederick P. Smith, John R. Neefe
James D. Ahlgren, Patrick J. Byrne and Philip S. Schein

1.   INTRODUCTION

The first cytotoxic drugs that were shown to have reliable activity in gastrointestinal cancer were the fluorinated pyrimidines. Extensive studies of 5-fluorouracil deoxyribonucleotide (5-FUdR) and 5-fluorouracil (5-FU) as single agents were performed during the 1960's and early 1970's. At that point the focus of clinical research changed to the investigation of combinations of fluorinated pyrimidines with other active drugs. At the present time we treat gastric and pancreatic cancer with drug combinations that invariably include fluorinated pyrimidines. For colon cancer, it is still difficult to identify agents more effective than 5-FU alone. There is now considerable interest in treating regional hepatic metastases with fluorinated pyrimidines infused through an implantable pump into the hepatic artery. Other topics of current interest include the modulation of 5-FU by allopurinol or methotrexate and the possibility of synergistic interaction between 5-FU and interferon.

The approach to gastrointestinal malignancies can be compartmentalized by considering three specific clinical situations:

1) the disease is advanced and metastatic

2) the disease is localized but incapable of
    surgical resection

3) the disease has been totally resected surgically

The significance of this approach is that in the first case,
treatment is with systemic chemotherapy. In the second case
treatment with local radiation to encompass the tumor, as well
as systemic chemotherapy, can be considered. The third case is
the surgical adjuvant situation and the question needs to be
asked as to whether immediate postoperative chemotherapy will
delay or prevent disease relapse.

Since 1974 we have treated advanced gastric cancer with
the combination of 5-FU, doxorubicin and mitomycin-C (FAM).

FIGURE I: The FAM Regimen

	WEEK	1	2	3	4	5	6	7	8	9
5-Fluororuacil	600 mg/m^2	X	X			X	X			R
Doxorubicin	30 mg/m^2	X				X				E
Mitomycin C	10 mg/m^2	X								P
										E
										A
										T

In a group of 62 gastric cancer patients reported from
Georgetown (1) the response rate was 42%, the median duration of
response was 9 months and the median survival of responders was

over 12 months. Responses occurred in primary local tumor masses and also in disease metastatic to liver, lung, lymph nodes and skin. Non-responders, by contrast, lived only 2-3 months. These results have now been confirmed by various investigators, including the Southwest Oncology Group, the Eastern Cooperative Oncology Group) and the University of Chicago. FAM has also been compared to combinations of 5-FU and methyl-CCNU by the Gastrointestinal Tumor Study Group and is superior to the two drug combinations.

After identifying the activity of FAM in gastric cancer, we made several attempts to improve the regimen by modifying its components or adding to the combination. The substitution of Tegafur for 5-FU seemed only to add to the toxicity without improving the rate or duration of response (2). The addition of the nitrosourea chlorozotocin to FAM also failed to improve therapeutic results (3). Substitution of the compound cisplatin for the mitomycin produced a regimen slightly inferior to FAM (4). Present attempts to schedule the antifolate triazinate have also not improved the response rate. Consequently FAM has yet to be surpassed as a therapy for advanced gastric cancer, although data reported for the combination of 5-FU, doxorubicin and BCNU may be equivalent (5).

Based on experience with FAM in advanced gastric cancer, we have also used it in less advanced disease. One particular situation is the locally advanced case in which tumor does not extend beyond the local primary site, but is unresectable. An early trial by the Gastrointestinal Tumor Study Group in this situation compared chemotherapy alone with 5-FU and methyl-CCNU to a combination of radiation therapy and chemotherapy. There were some early deaths in the combined modality arm, suggesting that it was too toxic. With subsequent experience, we have learned that such toxicity is not necessary in combina- tions of chemotherapy and radiation. We have treated locally unresectable gastric and pancreatic cancer with one cycle of FAM, followed by radiation to the primary site and then followed with further FAM treatment.

FIGURE 2: Sequential Use of FAM and Radiation for Locally
         Advanced Gastric and Pancreas Cancer

Time in Weeks	1-6	8-10		12-14	16
Treatment	FAM	Radiation 2250 R		Radiation 2250	FAM
	1 Cycle	RAD	E	RAD	for 6
		***	S	***	cycles
			T		

*5-FU 350 mg/m^2 IV on first 3 days of radiation.

When treatment is performed in this fashion, patient tolerance is excellent. Excessive myelosuppression is not encountered and there have been no treatment-related deaths. We have presently treated 26 patients with gastric cancer and 25 patients with pancreatic cancer with this regimen. The median survival of the gastric cancer patients is between 14 and 15 months while that of the pancreas patients is 12 months. Causes of failure have been both local and systemic disease progression.

Another approach to localized therapy of upper gastrointestinal malignancy is use of fast neutrons. We have used this in conjunction with 5-fluorouracil for both gastric and pancreatic malignancies (6). Rather severe myelosupression can be seen with this modality and is dependent upon the 5-fluorouracil dose. In addition liver tolerance of neutron radiation is poor and we have encountered several cases of anicteric hepatitis with defects in liver scan conforming to the region of overlap radiation. The survival data in these patients are somewhat less favorable than for FAM and radiation.

Surgical Adjuvant Treatment of Gastric Cancer: gastric cancer has a poor prognosis, even after complete surgical resection. Recurrence rates are high and an important question is whether the immediate institution of chemotherapy after surgery can delay or prevent disease relapse. The most recent prospective trials in this area have used either 5-FU plus methyl-CCNU or FAM as post-operative chemotherapy. A trial by the Gastrointestinal Tumor Study Group showed a survival benefit to treatment with 5-FU and methyl-CCNU (7). This group has now gone on to a trial comparing 5-FU plus methyl-CCNU to a similar regimen with doxorubicin added. At the same time trials by both the Veterans Administration Surgical Oncology Group and the Eastern Cooperative Oncology Group have failed to confirm the value of post-operative 5-FU and methyl-CCNU. Hence no firm conclusion can be drawn that this form of adjuvant therapy is really beneficial. The most important question at this point is whether FAM is an effective post-operative adjuvant therapy.

Two trials, one a multi-institutional international study and the other by the Southwest Oncology Group, are ongoing. Each compares immediate treatment with FAM to observation to the time of relapse. Definitive conclusions cannot be drawn from either of these trials at this time.

CARCINOMA OF THE PANCREAS

The group at Georgetown has described two combinations of drugs with activity in advanced carcinoma of the pancreas. These are FAM and SMF (streptozotocin, mitomycin-C and 5-FU). Each produced approximately a 40% objective partial response rate in trials conducted at Georgetown. However the median survival of responders was greater in the group treated with FAM. The same regimen of sequential FAM and radiation has been used for both localized gastric and localized pancreas cancer.

CARCINOMA OF THE COLON

The traditional treatment for colon cancer is a fluorinated pyrimidine, usually 5-fluorouracil. This drug may be administered on various dose schedules, including intermittent bolus injection, five day loading course or continuous infusion. The five day loading course has been regarded by some as the optimum method of using the drug as a single agent (8). While the intermittent dose schedule has been useful in our experience when the 5-FU is used in combination with other agents. The overall objective response rate for 5-FU in colon cancer is still about 20%.

There was hope during the mid 1970's that it would prove possible to combine 5-FU with other drugs such as nitrosoureas to improve response rates and survival. Despite initial encouraging data in this regard, recent work indicates that it is very difficult to improve on the efficacy of 5-FU alone by adding drugs such as hydroxyurea, DTIC or nitrosoureas. In addition, empiric drug testing has failed in recent years to identify new drugs active against colon cancer. Although virtually all drugs that come into Phase II trial through the National Cancer Institute's Decision Network are tested in colon cancer, the yield of this testing has been very low. Some of the agents that have been studied at Georgetown are the nitrosourea PCNU (9), methylglyoxal bis-guanylhydrazone (10) and mitoxantrone (11). None of these has produced any objective responses. The three drug combination 5-FU, doxorubicin and mitomycin-C (FAM) gave a response rate of 17% (12), similar to that of 5-FU alone. Studies with cloned leukocyte interferon A showed no responses in 26 patients.

The failure to develop new drugs has made the search for optimum use of 5-FU important. One approach to this problem is biochemical modulation of the effects of 5-FU by other agents. Two examples of this are the combinations of allopurinol/5-FU and of methotrexate/5-FU that have recently been studied. We have had a particular interest in the allopurinol/5-FU combination at Georgetown. In a recent Phase I trial (13), we showed that if allopurinol is given in a dose of 600 mg - 900 mg per day for four days, starting one day before a bolus dose of 5-FU, it can

326

markedly diminish the granulocytopenia produced by the 5-FU. As a consequence, doses of 1600-1800 mg/m^2 5-FU given with allopurinol are no more myelosuppressive than are doses of 1200-1800 mg/m^2 given without allopurinol. This study confirms previous studies showing that allopurinol can protect against the toxicity of infusional 5-FU also. The method will be of value if the protection of the marrow is selective, so that the 5-FU retains its antitumor activity. This will be determined by randomized trials of 5-FU with or without 5-FU in colon cancer, such as are presently being conducted by the Southeastern Cancer Study Group and by the Pan American Health Organization.

Another area of current interest is the direct infusion of fluorinated pyrimidines into the hepatic arterial circulation for treatment of liver metastases. Colon cancer is frequently treated in this manner because it is one disease that may metastasize to liver alone without other areas of involvement. The method has received recent new enthusiasm because of improvements in technology such as the implantable continuous infusion pump. Infusions of 5-FUdR for two weeks or more at doses of 0.1-0.3 mg/kg/day are feasible in this manner. The response rate increases over that seen with peripherally admini-stered 5-FU, and in properly selected patients survival appears prolonged, although that subject remains controversial.

The adjuvant therapy of surgically resected colon cancer is another important issue. Some trials, notably those of the Veterans Administration Surgical Oncology Group, suggest a benefit for post-operative 5-FU. Other trials have failed to confirm this finding. Our group at Georgetown presently has the attitude that there are no well defined adjuvant therapies for colon cancer and that consequently randomized trials utilizing an observation-only control arm are still critical. Our current study is one by the Gastrointestinal Tumor Study Group involving hepatic irradiation plus 5-FU.

The difficulty of identifying effective new treatments for colon cancer either by combining existing drugs or developing new ones through empiric testing suggests that the colon cancer cell is inherently more resistant to drugs than are cells of other lineages. A recent examination of stem cell cloning data supplied by Dr. D. Von Hoff supported the view that colon cancer cells are more resistant to billing by a variety of drugs and by radiation than are breast, ovary or lymphoma cells. The basis of this resistance is not known but it could lie at the level of the cell membrane, of DNA repair or other sites within the cell. In view of the frequency of large bowel cancer and the problems in its treatment, it would seem important to couple further efforts at drug development with studies of the biology of the colon cancer in order to understand the basis of this resistance.

REFERENCES

1. Macdonald JS, Schein PS, Woolley PV, Smythe TA, Ueno WM, Hoth DF, Smith FP, Boiron M, Gisselbrecht LW, Brunet R. and Lagarde C. (1980) 5-Fluorouracil, doxorubicin and mitomycin (FAM) combination for advanced gastric cancer. Ann Int Med 93: 533-536.

2. Woolley PV, Macdonald JS, Haller DG, Hoth DF, Smythe T. and Schein PS. (1979) Phase II trial of ftorafur, adriamycin and mitomycin in gastric cancer. Cancer 44: 1211-1214.

3.   Gisselbrecht C, Smith FP, Macdonald JS, Korsmeyer SJ, Boiron
      M, Woolley PV. and Schein PS. (1983) The effect of sequential
      addition of the nitrosourea, chlorozotocin, to the FAM com-
      bination in advanced gastric cancer. Cancer 51: 1792-1794.

4.   Woolley P, Smith F, Estevez R, Gisselbrecht C, Alvarez C,
      Boiron M, Machado C, Lagarde C. and Schein P. (1981) A phase
      II trial of 5-FU, adriamycin and cisplatin (FAP) in advanced
      gastric cancer. Proc Am Soc Clin Onc 22: 481.

5.   Levi JA, Dalley DN. and Aroney RS. (1979) Improved combination
      chemotherapy in advanced gastric cancer. Br Med J 2: 1471-1473.

6.   Smith FP, Schein PS, Macdonald JS, Woolley PV, Ornitz R. and
      Rogers C. (1981) Fast neutron irradiation for locally advanced
      pancreatic cancer. Int Rad Onc 7: 1527-1531.

7.   Gastrointestinal Tumor Study Group (1982) A comparison of
      combination chemotherapy and combined modality therapy for
      locally advanced gastric carcinoma. Cancer 9: 1771-1777.

8.   Ansfield F. (1975) A randomized phase III study of four dosage
      regimens of 5-FU. A preliminary report. Proc Am Soc Clin
      Oncol 67: 224.

9.   Mitchell EP, Killen JY, Smith FP, Willis LL, Schein PS and
      Woolley PV. (1981) A phase II trial of 1-(2-Chloroethyl)-3-
      (2,6-dioxo-1-piperidyl)-1-Nitrosourea (PCNU) in colorectal
      carcinoma. Cancer Treat Rep 65: 1129-1130.

10.   Killen JY, Mitchell EP, Hoth DF, Willis LL, Gullo JJ, Smith
      FP, Schein PS. and Woolley PV. (1982) Phase II studies of methyl
      gloyoxal bis-guanyl hydrazone (NSC 32946) in carcinoma of the
      colon and lung. Cancer 50: 1258-1261.

11.   Bonnem EM, Mitchell EP, Woolley PV, Smith FP, Neefe J, Smith L.
      and Schein PS. (1982) A phase II trial of 1,4-Dihydroxy-5,8-bis
      ((2-(Hydroxyethyl)Amino Ethyl))-9-10 anthracenedione dihydro-
      chloride (NSC 301739) in advanced colorectal cancer. Cancer
      Treat Rep   66: 1995-1996.

12.   Haller D, Woolley PV, Macdonald JS and Schein PS. (1978) Phase
      II trial of FAM in advanced colorectal cancer. Canc Treat Rep
      62: 563-565.

13.   Woolley PV, Ayoob MJ, Smith FP, Lokey L. and DeGreen P. (1982)
      A controlled trial of the effect of allopurinol on the toxicity
      of a single bolus dose of 5-fluorouracil. Proc Am Soc Clin Onc
      1: 20.

Fluoropyrimidines in Cancer Therapy
K. Kimura, S. Fujii, M. Ogawa, G.P. Bodey, P. Alberto, eds.

COMBINATION CHEMOTHERAPY REGIMENS CONTAINING FLUOROPYRIMIDINES FOR ADVANCED GASTRIC CANCER

Tatuo Saito, Takao Kanko, Ichiro Nishi, Isao Nakao
Tadashi Yokoyama and Yasuhiko Ohashi

1. INTRODUCTION

The application of combination chemotherapy to the treatment of cancer is becoming increasingly popular, and many methods have been proposed and applied both in Japan and abroad. Combination chemotherapy including fluoropyrimidines is also common, especially for the treatment of gastrointestinal tumors.

This paper described the results obtained to date by combination chemotherapy including fluoropyrimidines on gastrointestinal tumors, mainly stomach cancer in Japan, mainly in the Department of Internal Medicine, Cancer Institute Hospital. Several methods are reported in detail and the results are discussed.

2. CHEMOTHERAPY OF GASTRIC CANCER

Gastric cancer is a major form of gastrointestinal tumor and is still the most common type of cancer in Japan in both men and women. However, good results have not generally been obtained in the chemotherapy of gastric cancer.

Table 1 shows the results obtained from single chemotherapy mainly using mitomycin C (MMC) and

TABLE 1 Chemotherapy of stomach cancer

A) Systemic administration
1) Single

Agent : Route	Dose	Interval		Response rate (%)
5-FU : i.v.	250 mg	daily	drip infusion	8.7-36
dry syrup	300 mg	daily	t.i.d.p.c. Sum.	24-35.6
tablet	300 mg	daily	t.i.d.p.c. Sum.	23.3
Tegafur : i.v.	800 mg	daily	drip infusion	17-31
p.o.	800 mg	daily	q.i.d.	17-32
supp.	1000-2000 mg	daily	d.d. or b.i.d.	17-26.1
UFT : p.o.	600 mg	daily	b.i.d.	19-37.5
MMC : i.v.	6-8 mg	1-2/w	drip infusion	12-38.5

2) Combined

Agent	Dose	Interval	Route	Response rate (%)
MF (I) : MMC	4-12 mg	1-2/w	i.v.	20.1
5-FU	250 mg	daily		
MF (II) : MMC	0.08 mg/kg	2/w	i.v.	28.9
5-FU	10 mg/kg			
MFt : MMC	0.34-0.4 mg/kg	one shot	i.v.	25
Tegafur	800 mg	daily	p.o.	
FU (I) : 5-FU	8-10 mg/kg	daily	i.v.	38-41
BCNU	40 mg/kg			
FU (II) : 5-FU	300 mg/m^2	day 1-5	i.v.	52
Methyl-CCNU	175 mg/m^2	day 1	p.o.	
MFC : MMC	0.08 mg/kg	2/w	i.v.	34-44
5-FU	10 mg/kg	first 2w		
Ara C	0.8 mg/kg	then 1/w		

(continued)

331

2) Combined (continued)

	Agent	Dose	Interval	Route	Response rate (%)
MFU	MMC	0.2 mg/kg	every 2w	i.v.	42.8
	5-FU	5 mg/kg	daily		
	ACNU	2 mg/kg	every 6w		
MFT	MMC	4 mg			
	5-FU	500 mg	2/w	i.v.	22.7
	Toyomycin	1 mg			
FAM	5-FU	600 mg/m2	day 1	i.v.	25-55
	ADM	30 mg/m2	day 1,8,28,35	i.v.	
	MMC	10 mg/m2	day 1,28		
FTP	5-FU	250 mg		i.v.	40
	Toyomycin	0.5 mg	daily		
	Prednisolone	30 mg			
FAC	5-FU	350 mg/m2	day 1-5, 36-40	p.o.	27.6
	ADM	40 mg/m2	day 1,36	i.v.	
	Methyl-CCNU	150 mg/m2	day 1	p.o.	
FAMT	5-FU	500 mg			
	EX	200 mg	1-2/w	i.v.	16-56
	MMC	2 mg			
	Toyomycin	0.5 mg			
MFCT	MMC	0.08 mg/kg	2/w	i.v.	26
	5-FU	10 mg/kg	first 2w		
	Ara C	0.4 mg/kg	then 1/w		
	Toyomycin	0.02 mg/kg			

B) Local administration

intraarterial :	MMC	16 mg	one shot combined
	ADM	30 mg	
	NCS	3000-6000u	
intraperitoneal:	MMC	8-16 mg	
intrapleural :	MMC	8-16 mg	
	ADM	40-60 mg	

ADR: adriamycin, EX: cyclophosphamide, NCS: Neocarzinostatin, MMC: mitomycin C

5-fluorouracil (5-FU) which have shown the highest efficacy, as well as combination chemotherapy based mainly on these two drugs and local administration reported in recent years, especially by the Department of Internal Medicine, Cancer Institute Hospital (1).

In the case of single administration, the response rate ranged from 8.7 to 38.5%, while that for combination chemotherapy was from 16 to 56%. In all cases, there were considerable discrepancies in the results, but the general trend was that combination chemotherapy shows better results than single administration.

TABLE 2 Clinical results of chemotherapy for gastric cancer

	No.	PR	NC	(MR)	PD	Response rate(%)
F	29	4	18	(3)	7	13.8
FTP	6		4		2	0
MF	37	4	21	(4)	12	10.8
MF+IM	13		10		3	0
MFC	11	1	6		4	9.1
MFCT	21	6	13	(4)	2	28.6
MFU	31	10	16	(3)	5	32.3
Total	148	25	88	(14)	35	16.9

F:5-FU: FTP:5-FU, Toyomycin, Prednisolone, MF:MMC, 5-FU.
IM:Immunomodulator, MFC:MMC, 5-FU, Cytosine arabinoside,
MFCT:MMC, 5-FU, Cytosine arabinoside, Toyomycin,
MFU:MMC, 5-FU, ACNU.

The results of combination chemotherapy including 5-FU and MMC on gastric cancer obtained in the 10 years between 1971 and 1981 in the Department of Internal Medicine, Cancer Institute Hospital are shown in Table 2. The best response rate obtained to date was 32.3% for

MFU therapy, i.e. MMC, 5-FU and ACNU. This was followed by 28.6% for MFCT therapy.

3.   MF AND MFU THERAPIES AGAINST GASTRIC CANCER

As mentioned above, MFU combination chemotherapy showed the best response rate against gastric cancer in the author's department. Therefore, a comparative clinical trial was performed using MF therapy which has been widely applied and MFU therapy (2).

3.1   Administration method and subjects

Table 3 shows the administration schedule. In MF therapy, 0.2 mg/kg of MMC was administered once every other week and 5 mg/kg of 5-FU was given daily. In MFU therapy, the schedule was the same as that for MF therapy with 2 mg/kg of ACNU administered once every six weeks.

TABLE 3   Methods of administration

MFU Therapy
MMC	0.2 mg/kg/2 weeks
5-FU	5 mg/kg every day
ACNU	2 mg/kg/6 weeks

MF Therapy
MMC	0.2 mg/kg/2 weeks
5-FU	5 mg/kg every day

The subjects were inoperable or recurrent patients with gastric cancer hospitalized in our department. The selection standards for the subjects were as follows, based on the Cancer Chemotherapy Direct Effect Evaluation Standards.

(1) Patients with histologically confirmed gastric adenocarcinoma

(2) Patients with a measurable cancerous lesion

(3) Patients without active double cancer

(4) Patients whose performance status was from 0 to 3 according to ECOG criteria

(5) Patients without significant impairment of renal, hepatic or hematological functions

(6) Patients without severe complications

(7) Patients without influence from previous therapy within an interval of at least 4 weeks

Randomization was performed by the sealed method using the table of random numbers, and 41 cases have been included to date (Table 4). However, a total of eight cases, including three found not to have gastric cancer during the trial or at autopsy, three cases with PS-4 and two lacking evaluable lesions, were excluded. There were also three cases in which treatment was not performed as specified and two which did not receive adequate clinical observations. Therefore, the final number of cases evaluated was 28, 13 for MF therapy and 15 for MFU therapy, or 70% of the total.

Among the background factors of these evaluable cases (Table 5), there were no major differences in the sex ratio, no marked differences in age which averaged 50.0 for MFU therapy and 46.9 for MF therapy, and no significant differences in the performance status (PS) which was 0 - 1 for four MFU cases and one MF case and 2

335

TABLE 4 Subjects

		MFU	MF
Excluded	Non-gastric cancer	1	2
	PS-4	1	2
	Without measurable lesion	1	1
Withdrew	Did not receive adequate therapy	2	1
Dropped out	Dit not undergo clinical observation	1	1
Evaluable cases		15	13
Total		21	20

TABLE 5 Characteristics of cases

		MFU	MF
Male		6	8
Female		9	5
Age distribution	30	1	5
	40	3	1
	50	7	3
	60	3	2
	70	1	1
	80		1
Performance status	0		
	1	4	1
	2	6	4
	3	5	8
Prior therapy	Yes	6	5
	No	9	8
Primary site	Yes	11	9
	No	4	4
Histology types (inoperable cases)	Undifferentiated	9	7
	Differentiated	2	2

336

- 3 for 11 MFU cases and 12 MF cases. There were also no differences between the two groups concerning previous treatment. The other background factors also showed no intergroup differences.

3.2 Clinical results

Evaluation of clinical results was based on the new efficacy evaluation standards of the Japan Society of Cancer Therapy (equivalent to the WHO Efficacy Evaluation Standards). As shown in Table 6, there were no CR cases in either group. There were four PR cases in the MFU group (27%) and one in the MF group (8%). The response rate tended to be higher in the MFU group, but the difference was not significant.

TABLE 6 Results of evaluation

	CR	PR	NC (MR)	PD	No.	Response (rate)	
						Responder/ evaluable cases	Responder/ total cases
MFU		4	9 (1)	2	15	4/15 (26.7%)	4/18 (22.2%)
M F		1	8 (1)	4	13	1/13 (7.7%)	1/15 (6.7%)

CR: complete response, PR: partial response, NC: no change, MR: minor response, PD: progressive disease

Evaluation of the results in the effusion cases is shown in Table 7. Two out of six cases in the MFU group and two out of seven cases in the MF group were

TABLE 7   Evaluation of effusion cases

	Markedly responsive	Responsive	Not responsive	total	Respons rate
MFU		2	4	6	2/6 (33%)
M F		2	5	7	2/7 (29%)

responsive, and there were no significant differences between the two groups.

Details concerning the five responsive cases are shown in Table 8. Histologically, all of the cases were undifferentiated, four were inoperable and one had a recurrence after surgery. The region occupied by the lesion was the total stomach in three of the four inoperable cases. The PS was one in two cases, two in two cases and three in one case. No prior therapy had been given in four out of five cases. The time until response was 2 - 9 weeks and the duration of response was 4 - 40 weeks.

As shown in Fig. 1, there was no difference in the MFU and MF groups in the 50% survival time, but there were more long-term survival cases in the MFU group. This was mainly due to the longer survival times of PR cases.

338

TABLE 8 Details of responsive cases

Age Sex	Histology	Macro-scopic findings	PS	*	Target organs	Evalu-ation	**	***	Total doses (mg)	Survival time (w)
1 57 F	Poorly differen-tiated	B III A	1	No	Fluoroscopic and endocopic findings	PR	9	20	M 20 F 18,250 U 100	54
2 45 F	Poorly differen-tiated	B IV A	1	Yes	Abdominal tumor	PR	7	16	M 30 F 8,500 U 100	49
3 30 F	Poorly differen-tiated	Recur-rence	2	No	Krukenberg's tumor Ascites	PR	3	16	M 40 F 12,750 U 80	44
4 55 F	Poorly differen-tiated	B IV CMA (E)	2	No		PR	3	40	M 20 F 20,000 U 100	69
5 70 F	Poorly differen-tiated	B IV CMA	3	No	Abdominal tumor	PR	2	4	M 30 F 14,500	34

B: Bormann, M: Mitomycin C, F: 5-FU, U: ACNU
* : Prior therapy, ** : Time to response (w), *** : Duration of response (w)

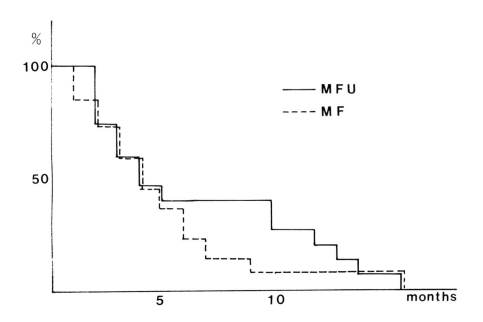

FIGURE 1   Survival time of gastric cancer patients

The side effects are shown in Table 9.   Side effects related to the gastrointestinal tract, i.e., nausea and vomiting, and anorexia, showed a higher frequency in the MFU group than the MF group.   However, the most characteristic side effects were seen in hematological tests.   Leukopenia of $4,000/m^3$ or less was seen in 10 out of 14 cases (71%) and thrombocytopenia of $10,000/m^3$ or less in one out of 14 cases (7%) in the MF group.   In the MFU group, leukopenia was found in 11 out of 16 cases (68%) and thrombocytopenia in eight out of 16 cases (50%).   The frequency of hematological side effects was higher and there were more cases with severe decreases in the MFU group.

TABLE 9   Side effects of MFU and MF therapy

	Grade	MFU	M F
Nausea and vomiting	1 2 3 4	 2 	
Anorexia		1	1
Stomatatis	1 2 3 4	1 	
Skin pigmentation		1	
Hemorrhggic state	1 2 3 4	1 	
Fever	1 2 3 4	 1 	
Leukopenia	1 2 3 4	 3 4 4	3 5 2
Thrombocytopenia	1 2 3 4	1 5 2	 1
None		6	6
Total		16	14

3.3   Summary

These results indicated that MFU therapy tended to be more effective in the treatment of gastric cancer, and the usefulness of a combination with ACNU was suggested. However, MFU therapy causes more severe side effects and this must be taken into consideration when this method is used.

4. ETP AND FAP THERAPIES

The main combination chemotherapies using 5-FU are the MF and MFU methods described above, but many other combinations are now under investigation. These methods are still under development and good results have not always been obtained, but they are introduced briefly here.

4.1 FTP therapy

Excellent results using a combination of three drugs, i.e. 5-FU, chromomycin A_3 (Toyomycin) and prednisolone, were already reported in 1977 (3). As shown in Fig. 2, the administration schedule of FTP therapy consists of daily doses of 250 mg of 5-FU, 0.5 mg of chromomycin A_3 (Toyomycin, CHRM) and 30 mg of prednisolone divided into three administrations in principle.

As indicated in Fig. 2, the authors have revised this method by gradually reducing the dose of prednisolone every week from the second month of administration, and administering only 5-FU and CHRM only from the third month. This method has been attempted on 39 cases, but the results have been extremely poor, i.e. only one PR case as shown in Table 10. These results are probably related to the severity

of the new efficacy evaluation standards, but this
method has still not shown its full effects. Although
the efficacy has been low, the side effects are
comparatively few and the authors hope to improve this
method further in the future.

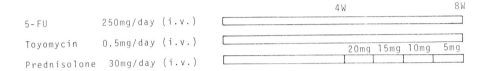

5-FU   250mg/day (i.v.)

Toyomycin   0.5mg/day (i.v.)

Prednisolone 30mg/day (i.v.)

FIGURE 2 Method of administration of 5-FU, toyomycin and
         prednisolone

4.2 FAP therapy

The authors are now investigating the FAP method
which is based on the above-mentioned FTP method. The
main mechanism of action of 5-FU is to inhibit the
synthesis of DNA and the function of RNA. Chromomycin
A_3 is a DNA-dependent RNA synthesis inhibitor, and
prednisolone strengthens the effects of the
carcinostatic agents and decreases the side effects.
Therefore, these three drugs were combined in FTP
therapy. Aclacinomycin A (ACM-A) is an anthracycline
type anticancer agent discovered by Dr. Umezawa, and it
was combined with 5-FU and prednisolone in place of
chromomycin A_3 because it inhibits DNA synthesis at

TABLE 10   Patients treated with 5-FU, Toyomycin and Prednisolone

Name	Sex	Age	Primary	Metastasis	Prior therapy	P.S.	Doses (mg)			Re-sponse		Prog-nosis
							5-FU	CHRM	Pred.	*	**	(month)
1 J.I.	M	48	Stomach	Lung	(-)	3	7750	15.5	930	NC	1-A	4 D
2 K.O.	M	61	Stomach		(-)	2	38500	72.5	4530	NC	0-A	7 D
3 M.Y.	F	51	Stomach	Liver	Tegafur	4	8000	8.5	640	NC	0-0	2 D
4 C.K.	M	78	Stomach		(-)	4	4000	8.0	480	NC	0-0	8 D
5 T.M.	F	70	Stomach	Retroper.	MF	2	14750	24.5	1980	NC	0-0	3 D
6 I.U.	M	80	Stomach		A-145	2	9000	18.0	1080	NC	0-0	12 D
7 T.K.	F	56	Stomach		(-)	4	3750	15.0	375	NC	0-0	1 D
8 S.S.	F	83	Stomach		(-)	4	18500	37.0	1800	NC	0-0	5 D
9 S.K.	F	54	Stomach		MF, Tegafur	4→2	33250	66.5	1640	NC	0-A	25 D
10 T.K.	F	53	Stomach		MFt	3→2	25000	50.0	1550	NC	0-A	6 D
11 E.K.	M	50	Stomach		(-)	2	22250	44.5	1520	NC	0-0	10 D
12 K.F.	F	25	Stomach		MFt	4	7500	15.0	900	PD	0-0	4 D
13 Z.K.	M	66	Stomach		(-)	3	7500	15.0	900	NC	0-0	3 D
14 K.S.	M	63	Stomach	Skin	MF	3	11000	16.5	960	PD	0-0	2 D
15 K.H.	F	40	Stomach	Peritoneum	K-247, M-83	4	2750	5.5	330	NC	0-0	1 D
16 Y.O.	M	53	Stomach	Lung, Bone	MFU	2	15250	17.5	735	NC	0-0	3 D
17 K.N.	M	45	Stomach		(-)	2	4250	8.5	510	NC	0-0	3 D
18 H.I.	M	64	Stomach	Liver, Peri.	(-)	3	5250	9.5	780	NC	0-0	2 D
19 S.M.	M	57	Stomach		MF	2	14250	28.5	1410	NC	0-C	3 D
20 M.G.	F	63	Stomach	Peritoneum	(-)	3	14750	36.0	1100	NC	0-0	3 D

(continued)

TABLE 10 (continued)

Name	Sex	Age	Primary	Metastasis	Prior therapy	P.S.	Doses (mg) 5-FU	CHRM	Pred.	Response *	**	Prognosis (month)	
21 T.N.	F	70	Lung		GANU	3	6250	12.5	750	NC	0-0	2	D
22 G.O.	M	70	Lung		ADM, HCFU	4	7500	15.0	900	NC	0-0	1	D
23 M.K.	M	47	Lung		ADM, VCR, ACNU	3	6250	12.5	750	NC	0-A	6	D
24 J.N.	M	70	Pancreas	Liver	(-)	3	28750	57.5	3850	PR	1-B	5	D
25 S.O.	M	63	Pancreas		(-)	3	6750	13.5	810	PD	0-0	1	D
26 K.T.	M	60	Pancreas		(-)	4	5000	10.0	600	NC	0-0	1	D
27 Y.T.	F	76	Pancreas	Peritoneum	(-)	3	2000	3.5	190	NC	0-0	5	D
28 S.H.	F	69	Colon	Lung, Liver	5-FU, HCFU	4	6000	12.0	720	PD	0-0	6	D
29 K.A.	F	45	Colon	Lung	(-)	3	15500	31.0	1860	NC	0-0	9	D
30 K.O.	F	60	Colon		(-)	3	9000	18.0	(-)	NC	0-0	17	A
31 Y.K.	F	41	Colon	Liver	(-)	3	2000	16.0	(-)	PD	0-0	1	D
32 T.S.	M	60	Colon	Peritoneum	(-)	3	12500	25.0	1050	PD	0-0	3	D
33 H.H.	F	65	Rectum		HCFU, CAM	2	7500	15.0	900	NC	0-0	4	D
34 M.E.	F	60	Uterus	Peritoneum	MFU, Ex, Bleo	4	5750	11.5	670	PD	0-0	1	D
35 H.S.	F	48	Uterus	Bone	(-)	4	1750	3.5	210	PD	0-0	1	D
36 E.M.	F	55	Uterus	Peritoneum	K-247	4	8250	16.5	960	NC	0-0	2	D
37 C.T.	F	42	Ovarium		MFU, NTM	3	15500	31.0	1350	PD	0-0	4	D
38 T.M.	M	61	Prostata	Liver	(-)	3	9250	18.5	(-)	NC	0-0	10	D
39 K.W.	M	70	Unknown	Lung	MF	4→3	18000	28.0	1260	NC	0-0	3	D

MF: MMC & 5-FU, A-145: Ethyl-carbamino-methyl-L-isoleucine, Mft: MMC & tegafur, K-247:
P-aminobenzoic acid-N-xyloside, M-83: Hydoxyphenyl-MMC, MFU: MMC, 5-FU & ACNU, HCFU:
1-Hexylcarbamoyl-5-fluorouracil, VCR: Vincristine, CAM: Etyl-o-[N-(p-carboxyphenil-
carbamoyl]-mycophenolate, Ex: Cylophosphamide, NTM: Neothramycin, Bleo:Bleomycin
D: dead, A: alive
*: JSCT, **: Karnofsky

345

lower doses and shows stronger inhibition of RNA synthesis than chromomycin A_3. This combination is known as FAP therapy.

The details of the FAP regimen are shown in Fig. 3. The dose of ACM-A is currently under investigation. This method has been used on about 8 cases and no good clinical results can be reported as yet, except 2 cases of MR (Table 11).

5. CONCLUSION

In the field of gastrointestinal cancer, there has been active development of carcinostatic agents and treatment regimens using them, but the results obtained so far have not always been good. However, the general trend in all cases has been that combination therapy is better than single administration, and the same trend was seen in our results.

There are many types of fluoropyrimidines used as carcinostatic agents, and new derivatives continue to be developed. There are various reports of combination chemotherapy using these fluoropyrimidines. This has been a report of the results of the authors concerning such combination chemotherapy. In a comparison of MF and MFU therapies, MFU therapy showed a high level of usefulness.

The FTP and FAP therapies have been introduced and, although results cannot always be expected at present,

TABLE 11 Clinical trial of FAP protocol

Name	Sex	Age	Diagnosis	5-FU (mg)	Doses Pred. (mg)	ACM (mg)	Re-sponse	Toxicity	Prognosis
1 T.T.	F	57	Lung ca. Pleuritis	250x16	30x16	40x 8	MR	Nausea Vomiting Diarrhea G-I Bleeding Leukopenia (500) Thrombopenia (0.9×10^4)	2 w dead
2 H.Y.	F	64	Lung ca. Pleuritis	250x15	30x14 20x 6	40x 3 20x13	NC	Diarrhea G-I Bleeding Leukopenia (300) Thrombopenia (0.2×10^4)	3 w dead
3 K.K.	M	82	Stomach ca. Lung meta.	250x17	30x17	20x17	NC	Anorexia Thrombopenia (1.3×10^4)	3 w alive FAP stopped
4 A.T.	F	51	Lung ca.	250x13	30x 9	20x 9	NC	Nausea G-I Bleeding (Gastric ulcer) Leukopenia (2400)	12 w alive FAP stopped

(continued)

347

TABLE 11 (continued)

Name	Sex	Age	Diagnosis	5-FU (mg)	Doses Pred. (mg)	ACM (mg)	Re-sponse	Toxicity	Prognosis
5 S.K.	F	70	Stomach ca. Peritonitis	250x12	30x16	20x15	NC	Nausea, vomiting G-I Bleeding Thrombopenia (1.3x10^4)	4 w dead
6 H.S.	F	40	Stomach ca. Kruckenberg tumor	250x16	30x16	20x15	MR	Nausea Purpura Nasal bleeding Leukopenia (50) Thrombopenia (0.8x10^4)	2 w dead
7 K.I.	F	40	Stomach ca. Kruckenberg tumor	250x37	30x 7 20x 7 15x 7 10x 7	40x 5 20x 2	NC	Hairloss Diarrhea Thrombopenia (5.6x10^4)	11 w dead
8 H.Y.	F	51	Breast ca.	250x75	30x 6 20x30 10x39	20x24	NC	Nausea, vomiting	12 w alive FAP continued

1)	5-FU	250mg/day					
	Prednisolone	30mg/day	20mg	15mg	10mg	5mg.	
	Aclacinomycin	40mg/day					
2)	5-FU	250mg/day					
	Prednisolone	30mg/day	20mg	15mg	10mg	5mg	
	Aclacinomycin	20mg/day					
3)	5-FU	250mg/day					
	Prednisolone	30mg/day	20mg	15mg	10mg	5mg	
	Aclacinomycin						40mg/2/W
4)	5-FU	250mg/day					
	Prednisolone	30mg/day	20mg	15mg	10mg	5mg	
	Aclacinomycin						20mg/2/W

FIGURE 3   Suggested protocols for FAP

investigations are continuing and chemotherapeutic regimens which are more effective against gastric cancer will be developed in the future.

REFERENCES

1. Saito T, Kanko T, Nakao I. and Ohashi Y. (1983) Stomach cancer, Shindan to Chiryo 71: 1608-1611.

2. Nakao I, Kanko T, Yokoyama T, Saito T. and Ishii Y. (1983) A combination chemotherapy of Mitomycin C, 5-FU and ACNU (MFU Therapy) in advanced gastric cancer. Presented at 13th International Congress of Chemotherapy, Vienna.

3. Saito T, Wakui A, Yokoyama M, Himori T, Takahashi H, Kudo T. and Takahashi K. (1977) Combination chemotherapy for solid tumors using 5-Fluorouracil, Chromomycin A_3, and Prednisolone. GANN 68: 375-387.

© 1984 Elsevier Science Publishers B.V.
Fluoropyrimidines in Cancer Therapy
K. Kimura, S. Fujii, M. Ogawa, G.P. Bodey, P. Alberto, eds.

CLINICAL OVERVIEW OF CHEMOTHERAPY FOR GASTROINTESTINAL TUMORS AT MAYO CLINIC

Michael J. O'Connell

1.   INTRODUCTION

This paper will present a brief overview of selected clinical trials involving study of the fluorinated pyrimidines in patients with gastrointestinal carcinomas at the Mayo Clinic. Included will be studies conducted solely within our institution, as well as comparative cooperative group trials based in part on regimens developed at Mayo.

2.   CHEMOTHERAPY STUDIES IN ADVANCED, METASTATIC GASTRO-INTESTINAL CANCER

A. Colorectal carcinoma

A series of controlled prospectively randomized clinical trials in patients with metastatic colorectal cancer has been conducted to examine the therapeutic importance of route of administration and duration of intravenous infusion of 5-FU and FUdR. In addition, the antitumor effect of FUdR and 5-FU were directly compared. The results are summarized in Table 1 (1,2).

TABLE 1   Controlled clinical trials of 5-FU and FUdR in advanced metastatic colorectal carcinoma

Treatment Regimens †	Number of Patients	Objective response rate (%) at 8-10 weeks	
1. 5-FU (rapid I.V.)	74	12	
5-FU (2-hr infusion)	75	12	
2. 5-FU (rapid I.V.)	45	20	N.S.
5-FU (8-hr infusion)	45	11	
3.* 5-FU (rapid I.V.)	53	26	N.S.
5-FU (oral)	47	19	
4. 5-FU (rapid I.V.)	84	12	N.S.
FUdR (rapid I.V.)	84	23	
5. FUdR (rapid I.V.)	63	17	P<.05
FUdR (24-hr infusion)	65	6	

† Treatment given for 5 consecutive days and up to 4 additional doses every other day in studies 1 and 2, with courses repeated at 4-5 week intervals.

* Mean duration of response for I.V. administration (20 weeks) significantly longer than for oral administration (11 weeks). P < 0.02.

It may be concluded that both 5-FU and FUdR can produce objective tumor responses (average duration; 4-6 months) in only 15-20% of patients with advanced colorectal cancer when given as single agents by systemic administration in loading courses. The I.V. route of administration produced more consistent serum levels of 5-FU compared to the oral route, and was associated with longer response durations. There was no significant difference in therapeutic effect between 5-FU and FUdR in these studies, nor was there any advantage to prolonging infusion duration to 2, 8, or 24 hours compared to rapid I.V. administration. Additionally, we have observed objective responses in only 4 of 36 patients (11%) with advanced colorectal cancer treated with tegafur by I.V. loading course technique in a phase II trial (3).

In an attempt to improve on the limited effect of single agent 5-FU, we have conducted a series of controlled trials of 5-FU based combination chemotherapy in patients with advanced colorectal carcinoma. Our initial experience with the combination of 5-FU, MeCCNU, and vincristine yielded an objective response rate of 43% compared to 19% in patients treated with 5-FU alone in a randomized study involving 80 patients (4). However, in a subsequent study (5) we observed objective responses in only 15 of 63 patients (24%) treated with 5-FU, MeCCNU, vincristine. Our overall objective response rate in 150 patients with advanced colon cancer treated with this regimen is 27%, with no improvement in survival compared to randomized controls.

Studies in progress are evaluating biochemical modulation approaches in which PALA and thymidine, given singly or in combination, are administered in conjunction with intravenous 5-FU for the treatment of advanced colorectal cancer patients with disseminated metastases. The prolonged intra-arterial infusion of FUdR with the use of a totally implanted infusion device is being compared to intravenous loading course 5-FU for selected colorectal cancer patients whose clinically apparent metastases are confined to the liver.

B. Gastric carcinoma

Our overall experience with 5-FU given as a single agent in the treatment of advanced gastric cancer has indicated objective tumor responses in 19 of 72 patients (26%), with a median response duration of 4.5 months. A prospective evaluation of 5-FU alone, BCNU alone, or the combination of 5-FU + BCNU in 85 patients with gastric carcinoma demonstrated objective responses in 29%, 17%, and 41%, respectively (6). Furthermore, treatment with 5-FU or combined 5-FU + BCNU afforded a statistically significant survival advantage compared to treatment with single agent BCNU. Subsequently, pilot studies to define tolerable administration schedules were conducted combining loading course 5-FU with adriamycin + mitomycin C (FAMi), and with adriamycin + MeCCNU (FAMe).

These three-drug combinations were then tested against single agent adriamycin, the two-drug combinations of 5-FU + MeCCNU and 5-FU + adriamycin, and three-drug combinations of 5-FU + Ara-C + mitomycin C and 5-FU + MeCCNU + ICRF-159 in a set of three prospectively randomized clinical trials in patients with unresectable gastric cancer conducted by the Gastrointestinal Tumor Study Group (7-9). These GITSG trials have demonstrated a significant survival advantage associated with the FAMe regimen compared to 5-FU + Ara-C + mitomycin C or single agent adriamycin. Furthermore, both FAMe and FAMi were associated with improved survival compared to 5-FU + MeCCNU or 5-FU + MeCCNU + ICRF-159. Finally, the FAMe regimen has shown a significant survival advantage compared to 5-FU + adriamycin. These prospective trials give strong scientific evidence that survival of patients with advanced gastric carcinoma can be prolonged with the FAMe regimen, and provide the basis for ongoing studies of FAMe in combination with radiation therapy or as adjuvant therapy following surgical resection in patients with earlier stage gastric cancer. The limitations of the FAMe regimen in the current management of patients with advanced gastric cancer should be recognized, however, since the median survivals observed in the above-mentioned trials were only 8-9 months with less than 10% of patients surviving beyond two years.

Our current studies in advanced gastric cancer include a randomized assessment of the "FAM" regimen as described by the Georgetown group, 5-FU + adriamycin, versus single agent 5-FU in collaboration with the North Central Cancer Treatment Group. We are also evaluating cis-platinum in combination with 5-FU + adriamycin in a separate phase II trial.

C. Malignant hepatoma

Our experience with single agent 5-FU in treating malignant hepatomas is quite limited: 3 objective respon-

ses among 8 patients receiving I.V. 5-FU and no responses
in 5 patients treated with oral 5-FU. However, 6 of 18
patients (33%) responded to the combination of 5-FU +
BCNU, with 2 of these responses lasting more than 3 years.
The Eastern Cooperative Oncology Group (ECOG) subsequently
studied the 5-FU nitrosourea theme in hepatomas, substituting MeCCNU for BCNU. They subsequently demonstrated
(10) that 5-FU + MeCCNU, 5-FU + streptozotocin, and
adriamycin each showed significant improvement in survival
compared to 5-FU alone. A second generation study (11)
has likewise confirmed a survival advantage for the 5-FU
+ MeCCNU combination. Based in part on these results, our
current research approach to the treatment of malignant
hepatomas involves the use of a single course of intra-
arterial adriamycin as a tumor "de-bulker", followed by
systemic therapy with 5-FU + MeCCNU.

D. Pancreatic islet cell carcinoma

    The nitrosourea streptozotocin is the most active
single agent in treating metastatic pancreatic islet cell
carcinoma, with objective responses reported in 37% of a
collected series from the literature. The addition of
5-FU to streptozotocin resulted in objective responses in
7 of 11 islet cell cancer patients treated at the Mayo
Clinic. This regimen was subsequently compared to streptozotocin alone by the ECOG (12). The combination produced a significant increase in objective response rate (63%

vs 36%), frequency of complete response (33% vs 12%), as well as survival improvement (26 vs 16 months).

3. COMBINED RADIATION THERAPY PLUS 5-FU FOR LOCALLY UN-
    RESECTABLE GASTROINTESTINAL CANCER

A randomized, double-blind trial conducted at the Mayo Clinic (13) demonstrated that the addition of I.V. 5-FU on three consecutive days at the onset of moderate dose radiation therapy (3500 rads in 4 weeks) improved median survival compared to radiation plus placebo in patients with locally unresectable carcinomas of the stomach, pancreas, and rectum. This approach has been studied further by the GITSG in patients with locally un-resectable pancreatic cancer (14). In a randomized trial involving 194 patients it was found that the median surv-ival for patients treated with 5-FU combined with 6000 rads (11.4 months) or 4000 rads (8.5 months) was signific-antly superior to treatment with 6000 rads alone (4.3 months).

We are currently evaluating a new radiation sensitiz-er, hycanthone, in combination with upper abdominal rad-iation compared to 6000 rads + 5-FU as developed by the GITSG for patients with locally unresectable pancreatic cancer. Intraoperative electron beam radiation combined with external beam radiation + 5-FU is also being studied in selected patients with locally unresectable pancreatic cancer.

4. CONCLUSION

The fluorinated pyrimidines 5-FU and FUdR have shown definite, but limited, activity as single agents in advanced gastrointestinal cancer. Combination regimens incorporating other active agents have resulted in improved therapeutic results in gastric cancer, malignant hepatoma, and pancreatic islet cell carcinoma. 5-FU given in conjunction with radiation can prolong survival in selected patients with locally unresectable gastrointestinal carcinoma. However, the long term control of unresectable gastrointestinal carcinomas remains very difficult to achieve with currently available techniques, and therefore further clinical research to develop more effective therapy is clearly needed.

REFERENCES

1. Moertel CG, Reitemeier RJ, Hahn RG. (1969) Slow vs. rapid administration of the fluorinated pyrimidines. IN: Advanced Gastrointestinal Cancer. Clinical Management and Chemotherapy. New York, Harper, pp. 108-118.

2. Hahn RG, Moertel CG, Schutt AJ, et al. (1975) A double-blind comparison of intensive course 5-fluorouracil by oral vs. intravenous route in the treatment of colorectal carcinoma. Cancer 35: 1031-1035.

3. Schutt AJ, Hahn RG, Moertel CG, et al. (1973) Phase II study of ftorafur in previously untreated and treated patients with advanced colorectal cancer. Cancer Treat Rep 67:505-506.

4. Moertel CG, Schutt AJ, Hahn RG, et al. (1975) Therapy of advanced colorectal cancer with a combination of 5-fluorouracil, methyl-1,3-cis (2-chlorethyl)-1-nitrosourea, and vincristine. J Natl Cancer Inst 54: 69-71.

5. Mocrtcl CG, O'Connell JM, Ritts RE Jr, et al. (1978) A controlled evaluation of combined immunotherapy (MER-BCG) and chemotherapy for advanced colorectal cancer. Immunotherapy of Cancer: Present Status of Trials in Man (eds) WD Terry and D Windhorst. New York, Raven Press, pp 573-586.

6. Kovach JS, Moertel CG, Schutt AJ, et al. (1974) A controlled study of combined 1,3-BIS-(2-chloroethyl)-1-nitrosourea and 5-fluorouracil therapy for advanced gastric and pancreatic cancer. Cancer 33: 563-567.

7. The Gastrointestinal Tumor Study Group. (1979) Phase II-III chemotherapy studies in advanced gastric cancer. Cancer Treat Rep 63: 1871-1876.

8. The Gastrointestinal Tumor Study Group. (1982) A comparative clinical assessment of combination chemotherapy in the management of advanced gastric carcinoma. Cancer 49: 1362-1366.

9. O'Connell MJ, Stablein DM. (1982) A prospective clinical trial of 5-fluorouracil/adriamycin based chemotherapy in unresectable gastric cancer. Proceedings ASCO 1: 91 (abstract).

10. Falkson G, Moertel CG, Lavin P, et al. (1978) Chemotherapy studies in primary liver cancer. Cancer 42: 2149-2156.

11. Falkson G, Moertel CG, MacIntyre JM, et al. Primary liver cancer - An ECOG therapeutic trial. (submitted for publication).

12. Moertel CG, Hanley JA, Johnson LA. (1980) Streptozotocin alone compared with streptozotocin plus fluorouracil in the treatment of advanced islet-cell carcinoma. New Engl J Med 303: 1189-1194.

13. Moertel CG, Childs DS, Reitemeier, et al. (1969) Combined 5-fluorouracil and supervoltage radiation therapy of locally unresectable gastrointestinal cancer. Lancet 2: 865-871.

14. The Gastrointestinal Tumor Study Group. (1981) Therapy of locally unresectable pancreatic carcinoma. Cancer 48: 1705-1710.

Fluoropyrimidines in Cancer Therapy
K. Kimura, S. Fujii, M. Ogawa, G.P. Bodey, P. Alberto, eds.

ARTERIAL INFUSION CHEMOTHERAPY FOR GASTROINTESTINAL CANCER

Tetsuo Taguchi, Masahide Fujita, Yosuke Nakano, Masao Usugane
Jun Ohta, Nobuhisa Ueda and Yasuhiko Kimoto

1. INTRODUCTION

Of chemotherapeutic techniques for unresectable or advanced gastrointestinal cancer or its recurrence, intra-arterial infusion chemotherapy is now not a special, but a common technique. Cancer of the liver, in particular, is the most suitable target for intra-arterial infusion chemotherapy, whether it is primary or metastatic, and numerous authors reported the usefulness of this technique in its treatment.[1-5] Meantime, unresectable gastric cancer, colorectal cancer and even carcinomatous peritonitis, for which systemic chemotherapy has so far been the only treatment available, are now being included in the indications for intra-arterial infusion chemotherapy as a result of recent progress in the sub-selective intra-aortic infusion technique, particularly in Japan[6-9].

2. METHOD OF INTRA-ARTERIAL INFUSION CHEMOTHERAPY

Basically speaking, it is desirable to introduce drugs selectively into the artery that supplies tumor. Since the target tumor in many advanced cancers of the digestive system exclusive of hepatic cancer occupies an extensive area below the diaphragm, however, sub-selective infusion by intubation of the aorta is more commonly used in intra-arterial infusion chemotherapy of these cancers.

In sub-selective intra-aortic infusion chemotherapy, the catheter is usually inserted retrograde into a branch of profunda femoris artery until its tip enters aorta. The level of the tip is adjusted according to the location of tumor-supplying artery.

The tip of the catheter is retained in thoracic aorta in gastric cancer, and below renal artery in the upper portion of inferior mesenteric artery in locally advanced sigmoid or rectal cancer [10, 11].

In hepatic cancer or metastasis limited to the liver, selective intra-arterial infusion is preferred. The catheter in this case is inserted retrograde into common hapatic or proper hepatic artery through right gastro-duodenal or right gastroepiploic artery, on which occasion right gastric and gastroduodenal arteries are frequently ligated to prevent influx of excess cancer chemo-therapeutic agents into the gastroduodenal region.

3. DOSE SCHEDULE IN INTRA-ARTERIAL INFUSION CHEMOTHERAPY

There is no established dose schedule for intra-arterial infusion chemotherapy. Of various methods tried at present, those used by us will be presented below.

Roughly speaking, drugs are intra-arterially adminis-tered either by one shot, or daily through a catheter

360

retained in the artery. In the former case, drugs are
infused into tumor-supplying artery during abdominal
surgery, or through a catheter inserted by Seldinger
technique for arteriography, etc. Preferred drugs are
combined 10 - 20 mg mitomycin C (MMC) and 40 - 50 mg
adriamycin (ADR), and combined 10 - 20 mg MMC and 500 -
1000 mg 5-fluorouracil (5-FU). We used 2 - 5 mg esquinone
(CQ) too.

In the latter case, drugs are selectively administered
through a catheter inserted into tumor-supplying artery
during abdominal surgery, or sub-selectively administered
in aorta. Dose schedule usually employed by us consists
of long-term consecutive administrations of 5-FU combined
with intermittent administrations of cytocidal drugs such
as MMC. Actually, we intraarterially administer 250 mg
5-FU and 6000 U urokinase, the basic drug combination,
over 1 - 2 hr once daily, and adjunctively administer 10-
20 mg MMC, or 30 - 40 mg ADR + 3 - 5 mg CQ, or 40 - 100 mg
ACNU, or 20 - 80 mg aclacinomycin (ACM) at certain intervals. Total of 5-FU doses should preferably exceed 10 g
(in 40 or more days), as stated later.

Urokinase is expected to enhance the effect of other
cancer chemotherapeutic agents because of its lysosome
labilizing effect. Its use in intra-arterial infusion
chemotherapy would therefore be beneficial not only in
that it serves to prevent thrombosis within catheter or
peripheral arteries but in that it enhances the antineo-

plastic effect too.

4. TARGET OF INTRA-ARTERIAL INFUSION CHEMOTHERAPY

What advanced cancers of the digestive system can be
the targets of intra-arterial infusion? In 112 cases of
gastric cancer in our series, shown in Table 1, intra-
arterial chemotherapy was aimed at primary lesion in 61
cases (54.5%), hepatic metastasis in 33 cases (29.5%),
carcinomatous peritonitis in 61 cases (54.5%), and others.

TABLE 1   Target of Intra-arterial Chemotherapy in 112
          Cases of Advanced Gastric Cancer

Target	Recurrence (51 cases)	Unresectable (61 cases)	Total
Primary lesion	(cases)	61*(cases)	61 (54.5%)
Hepatic metastasis	20	13	33 (29.5%)
Carcinomatous peritonitis	23	38	61 (54.5%)
Lymph Nodes	7	---	7 (6.3%)
Local recurrence	5	---	5 (4.5%)
Miscellaneous	2	---	2 (1.8%)

* The majority of primary lesions in 61 cases had
  lymph node metastases.

In 37 cases of colorectal cancer, shown in Table 2, it
was aimed at Table 2, primary lesion in 12 cases (32.4%),
hepatic metastasis in 24 cases (64.9%), carcinomatous
peritonitis in 9 cases (24.3%), and others. While hepatic
metastasis and primary lesion are the commonest targets
as stated above, it is characteristic of our practice

362

that carcinomatous peritonitis is also aimed at.

TABLE 2   Target of Intra-arterial Chemotherapy in 37
           Cases of Advanced Colorectal Cancer

Target	Recurrence (25 cases)	Unresectable (12 cases)	Total
Primary lesion	*(cases)	12 (cases)	12 (32.4%)
Hepatic metastasis	16	8	24 (64.9%)
Carcinomatous peritonitis	5	4	9 (24.3%)
Lymph Nodes	1	0	1 (2.7%)
Local recurrence	4	0	4 (10.8%)
Miscellaneous	1	0	1 (2.7%)

  * Pulmonary metastasis was detected in 7 of 25 cases of
    recurrence of colorectal cancer. The pulmonary meta-
    stases were unsuitable as targets.

5.   EFFECT OF INTRA-ARTERIAL INFUSION CHEMOTHERAPY

     We calculated the response rate in intra-arterial
infusion chemotherapy according to the criteria for
evaluation of the direct effect of chemotherapy on solid
cancers by Koyama and Saito [13], defined success in chemotherapy as the survival for at least 1 yr from the day of
exploratory laparotomy in cases of unresectable, advanced
gastrointestinal cancer, and from the day of confirmation
of recurrence in cases of recurrence, and calculated the
rate success.

     The effect was evaluated in 89 of 112 gastric cancer
cases and 31 of 37 colorectal cancer cases, with the
result that PR or higher response was confirmed to be

present in 22 gastric cancer cases and 7 colorectal
cancer cases as shown in Table 3.

TABLE 3   Response Rate and = 1 year-Survival Rate in
           Patients Treated by Intra-arterial Chemotherapy

| Diagno-sis | Popula-tion | No. of evaluated cases | PR or higher | Response rate | | = 1 yr survival rate |
				Popula-tion	No. of evaluated cases	
Gastric cancer	112	89	22	19.6%	24.7%	21 18.8%
Colorectal cancer	37	31	7	18.9%	22.6%	11 29.7%

The response rate was 19.6% in gastric cancer and
18.9% in colorectal cancer in the whole population, and
24.7% in the former and 22.6% in the latter in the evaluated cases. Survival for 1 yr or longer was observed in
21 cases of gastric cancer, 18.8% of whole gastric cancer
population, and in 11 cases of colorectal cancer, 29.7%
of whole colorectal cancer population.

Since cases of carcinomatous peritonitis, that poorly
responds to treatment, are included in the above cases,
the aforesaid response and 1-year survival rates are
considered quite good. It must be added that patients
who survived more than 1 yr have been largely restored
to society, even if temporarily.

6. EFFECTS CLASSIFIED BY THE DRUG

It is of vital importance in intra-arterial infusion
chemotherapy to select suitable drugs.

The efficacy of 5-FU against gastrointestinal cancers has been proved abroad too in arterial infusion chemotherapy [14], and 5-FU is highly valued. According to our dose schedule, 5-FU serves as the base, and cytocidal drugs such as MMC are administered intermittently.

Recent analysis of data from our series disclosed that the higher the total of 5-FU doses, the more markedly the tumor responded to treatment with the resulting prolongation of life span. We tried various methods of intermittent administration of drugs too, to clarify their characteristics.

The results of our efforts are shown in Table 4 on gastric cancer and Table 5 on colorectal cancer.

Though it is difficult to evaluate the relative efficacy of a drug by analysis of data obtained in an uncontrolled study, 5-FU is undoubtedly the most suitable of available drug for the role of basic drug in intra-arterial chemotherapy. The problem is in what dosage and at what intervals the other drugs should be administered. My impression is that MMC and ACNU both produce a good effect when combined with 5-FU, and the effect persists. ADR + CQ has what we call a sharp edge, but recurrence was rapid with this combination.

Our task in future is to clarify the optimal drugs, administration time, and interval between administrations. In the meantime, it is hoped, needless to say, that drugs superior to those currently available will be developed.

TABLE 4   Drugs, Tumor Response and = 1-year Survival
           Cases (Gastric Cancer, Advanced or Recurrence)

Mode of administration	Drugs	No. of cases	Tumor response+	Effect* MR	PR	= 1 yr survival cases**
Shot (26)	MMC	9	1	1		
	ADR	5				
	MMC+5-FU	10	2	1	1	1
	Others	2	1	1		
5-FU -5g (19)	MMC	4				
	ADR+CQ	8	5	4	1	
	ACNU	2				
	ACM	5				
Daily (23) 5-FU 5g-10g	MMC	9	2	1	1	2
	ADR+CQ	5	2	1	1	
	ACNU	7	2	1	1	1
	ACM	2	1	1		
(44) 5-FU 10g-	MMC	10	4	1	3	3
	ADR+CQ	6	3	1	2	3
	ACNU	24	10	1	9	9
	ACM	4	3		3	2
Total		112	36	14	22	21

* Tumor response was evaluated by the criteria for
  evaluation of the clinical effect of cancer chemotherapy by Koyama and Saito.

** Survival period was reckoned from the day of
   confirmation of recurrence in cases of recurrence,
   and from the day of simple laparotomy in unresectable
   cases.

TABLE 5 Drugs, Tumor Response, and 1-year Survival Cases (Colorectal Cancer, Advanced or Recurrence)

Mode of administration		Drugs	No. of cases	Tumor response+	Effect MR	Effect PR	= 1 yr survival cases
Shot (4)		MMC	2				
		ADR+CQ	1				
		MMC+5-FU	1				
(8)	5-FU -5g	MMC	4	2		2	2
		ACNU	1				
		---	2				1
		Others	1				1
Daily (10)	5-FU 5g-10g	MMC	5	1	1		
		ADR+CQ	2				
		ACNU	2	1	1		
		---	1				
(15)	5-FU 10g-	MMC	3	1		1	1
		ADR+CQ	1				1
		ACNU	9	3		3	3
		MMC+ACNU	2	1		1	2
Total			37°	9	2	7	11

° Including 6 cases in which measurement of lesion was not feasible.

7. ADVERSE REACTION TO INTRA-ARTERIAL INFUSION CHEMO-THERAPY

Adverse reactions to intra-arterial chemotherapy are roughly divided into those caused by intubation and those induced by drugs themselves.

The former group of reactions include infections and thrombosis at the site of puncture, and bleeding due to breaking of the catheter. These can be prevented by sterilization, adequate heparinization at the time of insertion of the catheter, adjunctive use of urokinase in intra-arterial infusion, and careful handling of the catheter.

Of the drug toxicities, thrombocytopenia occurred with a high frequency in ACNU-administered cases, and leukopenia in MMC-administered cases. Alopecia was characteristic of ADR. Gastrointestinal disturbance was frequent with 5-FU plus ACNU. As intra-arterial infusion chemotherapy was continued longer, the incidence of skin necrosis at the lateral chest and the back increased. This seemed attributable to the influx of drugs into intercostal arteries.

To prevent adverse reactions to drugs, it is necessary to watch the patient's condition carefully during intra-arterial infusion, perform blood biochemical tests periodically, and confirm the location of the tip of the catheter with X-rays occasionally. The catheter is sometimes located completely wrong, which may induce an unexpected reaction.

8. CONCLUSION

Intra-arterial infusion chemotherapy for gastrointestinal cancers was discussed on the basis chiefly of data obtained by us in gastric and colorectal cases, with references to the methods of drug administration. Table 6 shows indications for intra-arterial infusion sites suitable for intubation.

TABLE 6

Indications for intra-arterial chemotherapy	Arterial site for intubation
Inoperable primary lesion	
primary hepatic cancer	Hepatic artery
gastric cancer	(common or proper)
colorectal cancer	Aorta
cancer of pancreas & biliary tract	
Metastatic hepatic cancer	
(primary lesion resected and recurrence limited chiefly to liver)	Hepatic artery (common or proper)
(primary lesion remains or recurrence outside liver present)	Aorta
Carcinomatous peritonitis Lymph node metastasis (above N_3)	Aorta

For evaluation of the effect, we intend to use tumor measurements as the indicator as far as possible in accordance with the criteria by Koyama and Saito. Recent progresses in scintiscan and ultrasonography and CT scan will allow us to evaluate tumor response in a considerably large proportion of cases if we keep our mind on the evaluation of effect.

Finally, a multidisciplinary approach is necessary in the treatment of advanced gastrointestinal cancers, which

369

alone can provide prolongation of life span and resto

ration, even if it is temporary, to society. Intra-

arterial chemotherapy is one of multidisciplinary treat-

ments, and must be used tractfully so that its characte-

ristics prove most beneficial to individual patients.

REFERENCES

1. Watkins E, et al.(1970) Surgical basis for arterial
    infusion chemotherapy of dissemirated carcinoma of the
    liver. Surg Gynecol Obstet 130: 581-605.

2. Fortuny IE, et al. (1975) Hepatic arterial infusion
    for liver metastases from colon cancer: Comparison of
    Mitomycin C and 5-Fluorouracil. Cancer Chemother
    Rep 59: 401-404.

3. Ansfield RJ, et al. (1975) Further clinical studies
    with intrahepatic arterial infusion with 5-fluorouracil.
    Cancer 36: 2413-2417.

4. Taguchi T. (1977) Surgical chemotherapy for hepatic
    cancer intra-arterial chemotherapy. Jpn J Cancer
    Chemother 4: 61-66.

5. Miura K, et al. (1979) The current state of intra-
    arterial chemotherapy with intubation of hepatic artery
    for hepatic cancer. Shujutsu (Surgery) 33: 1131-1146.

6. Ishida M, et al. (1975) Intra-arterial infusion,
    gastrointestinal cancer. Geka-chiryo (Surgical treat-
    ment) 33: 268-275.

7. Yoshikawa K. (1973) Chemotherapy of gastric cancer -
    with special reference to the evaluation of effect
    produced by continuous intra-aortic infusion -
    Gan no Rinsho (Cancer Clinics) 19: 776.

8. Kamata T, et al. (1976) Problems in intra-arterial
    chemotherapy for gastrointestinal cancer. Jpn J
    Cancer Chemother 3: 515-522.

9. Nakano Y, et al. (1978) Intra-arterial chemotherapy
    for advanced gastrointestinal cancer - a study on the
    evaluation of effect. Jpn J Cancer Chemother 5:
    321-327.

10. Miura K, et al. (1974) Indications for local intra
    arterial infusion and local perfusion techniques and
    their limitations. Chiryo (Therapy) 56: 895-902.

11. Taguchi T, et al. (1979) Intra-arterial chemotherapy
    for advanced gastrointestinal cancer. Shokaki-geka
    (Gastrointestinal Surgery) 2: 1081-1088.

12. Fujita M, et al. (1977) Treatment of Bormann IV gast-
    ric cancer intra-arterial chemotherapy for unresec-
    table cancer. Jpn J Cancer Chemother 4: 1315-1322.

13. Koyama Y, et al. (1980) Criteria for evaluation of
    the clinical effect of cancer chemotherapy. Report
    of study sponsored by Health & Welfare Ministry's
    Cancer Research Fund.

14. Hisao-Sheng, et al. (1980) Intra-Arterial Infusion
    of Anticancer Drugs: Theoretic Aspects of Drug
    Delivery and Review of Responses. Cancer Treat
    Rep 64: 31-40.

© 1984 Elsevier Science Publishers B.V.
Fluoropyrimidines in Cancer Therapy
K. Kimura, S. Fujii, M. Ogawa, G.P. Bodey, P. Alberto, eds.

DISCUSSION

Sadée: I would just like to know whether the hypoxanthine rescue is largely related to reversing the purine-directed effects of methotrexate rather than modulating the 5-FU effects.

Tattersall: No, it isn't due to reversing the methotrexate effects because one can add the hypoxanthine during the regrowth period, and one still sees the same effect.

Ogawa: Your program for locally advanced gastric cancer is of interest because I know you stop treatment at six cycles and there is no maintenance treatment. I would like to know what proportion of the patients are recurrence-free after the discontinuation of your treatment. Secondly, if you get definite recurrence, what kind of treatment do you try?

Woolley: Most of the patients are not disease-free at the end of treatment. There are not many complete responders. Less than 20% of patients are remaining disease-free since the curve does seem to be flattening out. After recurrence, there is no effective treatment. I am encouraged by what I have heard today that some patients who have failed FAM will respond to methotrexate-directed 5-FU. I think that is good because we are not doing well with empiric drug testing. Our approach is to use phase II and phase I drugs. We have used triazinate in some FAM failures. Now we have started using some methotrexate and 5-FU, but really not with a great deal of benefit.

Ogawa: I think radiation plus FAM appears to be a good treatment for locally advanced gastric cancers. But how many patients have local recurrence after the radiation?

Woolley: It looks as if it is about 50% local recurrences and about 50% systemic recurrences - metastases in the liver - so both adequate local treatment and adequate systemic treatment are still a problem.

Woolley: Do you believe that a trial of 5-FU alone versus 5-FU-adriamycin or FAM is ethically defensible? Exactly what do you tell the patients who are randomized to 5-FU alone? According to the literature, no one has demonstrated a response rate or response duration for 5-FU alone in either controlled or uncontrolled trials that approaches those that have been repeatedly demonstrated with FAM combination therapy.

O'Connell: What was the median survival for the patients with gastric cancer treated with the FAM regimen in your report in the *Annals of Internal Medicine?*

Woolley: It was about twelve months for responders, and for all patients treated it was about seven months.

O'Connell: Right, and the median survival of patients treated with the FAMe regimen was 34 weeks. So if we look at the overall survival curves generated in the various studies that I presented, the median survival and the two-year survival, your data would coincide very closely with the various combination regimens and, with 5-FU given alone. What do I tell my patients that I'm approaching for treatment of advanced gastric cancer? In discussing that particular treatment protocol, I tell them that there has never been a controlled trial demonstrating that any combination chemotherapy regimen has improved survival in patients with advanced gastric cancer compared to single-agent 5-FU. I tell them, furthermore, that there have been very interesting results reported from your group that would support the use of combination chemotherapy and invite them to participate in this randomized trial.

Woolley: I would not argue that, it you plot the survival for all patients, it is difficult to show a change in the median survival when the response rate is less than 50%. But considering the subset of patients who actually have responded, there is a difference and those are the patients with whom I am principally concerned. The question is the quality of response.

O'Connell: I have a very hard time interpreting survival data that are presented in that manner. Do patients that respond to chemotherapy live longer because of response to chemotherapy, or is it because the patients who are destined to live longer in the first place (those with better performance status, less aggressive tumors, etc.) are also those more likely to respond to treatment? I am uncertain whether presenting survival of responders versus non-responders is really the best way to present the data. In the present trials, the responders definitely lived longer than the non-responders.

Woolley: I think that improvement of survival in responders, or a difference in survival between responders and non-responders, is a necessary but not sufficient result. But there are randomized studies, and you presented some of them, that indicate a benefit for combination therapy.

Ogawa: Conducting a phase II trial of cisplatinum, I found that the drug is active for advanced gastric cancer. However, the initial study performed at Georgetown discouraged us from performing another pilot study. But the preliminary results are very promising. Could you kindly tell us the doses you employed for the three drugs?

O'Connell: The dose of cisplatinum was 60 mg/m^2 rather than 75 mg/m^2. The 5-FU dose was approximately 300-325 mg/m^2 daily for five days, and the adriamycin dose was 40 mg/m^2 on day 1, with cycles repeated every five weeks.

Ogawa: Do you think it is worthwhile to include cisplatinum in combination chemotherapy for advanced gastric cancer?

O'Connell: Yes. We are planning on studying this particular program further in patients with advanced measurable gastric cancer.

Bodey: The issue that Dr. Woolley raised is somewhat peripheral to the subject under discussion, but I think I must respond to Dr. O'Connell's comment. It has been well demonstrated over the years that the improvement in survival associated with the administration of chemotherapy is related to response. In other words, chemotherapy does not do something magic independent of its effect on the tumor resulting in measurable response. Median survival, to be affected by chemotherapy, means that there must be a response rate in excess of 50% because that is the median. Survival curves cannot be used as a reliable indication of improvement in a chemotherapeutic regimen when the response rates are low. An increase from a 20% to a 40% response rate may represent a significant improvement as a consequence of improved chemotherapy but it would have no effect whatsoever on the median duration of response. The median survival increases only when the response rate increases to greater than 50%. So I don't think that your answer to Dr. Woolley's question was an appropriate answer.

O'Connell: I think the real question when we approach a patient or a population of patients with chemotherapy is how long that entire population of patients will survive from the point that we intervene with the treatment. That includes patients who respond and those who are non-responders - immediate progressions and patients who are stable. In my view, the most accurate and effective way to evaluate the overall impact of a treatment program on a population is to look at the survival of each and every patient who received that treatment, and not to break out a subgroup to compare. I think the most forthright and accurate way to look at treatment efficacy is to look at the overall survival of all patients approached with the therapeutic modality.

Holyoke: Dr. Taguchi, I enjoyed your paper. One of the problems we have - and I wonder if you have given any thought to it - is formalizing some type of staging for recurrent or advanced cancer, because the baseline, for example in liver disease, is unknown. It ranges from a liver filled with tumor to a small lesion, and this makes the results with infusion therapy very difficult to measure.

I wonder if you use any precise staging methods.

Taguchi: In our clinic, those treated with intraarterial infusion chemotherapy are usually stage IV with multiple metastases.

Spears: I have a comment and a question I would like to address to the speakers generally. A recent analysis by Dr. Lokich of Boston of 1300 colorectal carcinoma patients treated with 5-FU alone revealed a very important observation. The patients who responded apparently had longer periods from the time of diagnosis until initial treatment than the non-responders. In other words, possibly patients who responded had a more indolent disease than patients who failed to respond. I find this scientifically very attractive, because if a tumor is growing slowly it might have a very low level of thymidylate synthetase to reflect a low growth fraction. Therefore, it would be easily inhibited by lower levels of activated FdUMP. Tumors that are superficial, such as basal subepitheliomas and actinic keratoses, that are virtually curable with 5-FU, are very slow-growing tumors. The question that I would like to address to the speakers is: have you evaluated in your responders the period before patients are entered on the chemotherapy to see if there is a longer period in responders than for non-responders?

Woolley: We have not done our analysis. Nevertheless, it is my impression that there is not a significant difference between those who respond and those who do not respond in terms of this interval.

O'Connell: We don't have the data analyzed in precisely that fashion either for gastric cancer, but perhaps I could comment on colorectal cancer. We have examined the possible association of responsiveness of colorectal cancer to the fluorinated pyrimidines, particularly 5-FU, related to histology - degree of anaplasia, which is a correlate of rapidity of tumor growth - and have not seen any direct relationship between responsiveness to 5-FU and degree of tumor anaplasia. That was one point of interest in our PALA-5-FU-thymidine program. It seemed to be those with rapidly advancing tumors that were responding best - just the opposite from the hypothesis that Dr. Spears mentioned.

Taguchi: I have no data on the subject.

Majima: I am interested in results with platinum compounds used in stomach cancer. At our institution, platinum caused two serious problems: one was a perforation of the stomach and the other was a large gastric hemorrhage. In both of the cases, the primary lesion was not in the stomach. If we apply platinum to stomach cancer, the possibility of such occurrences must be kept in mind. Should we reduce the amount of this agent, or should we wait for the second generation of platinum compounds like CBDCA or CHIP?

Tattersall: Has anybody evaluated the second generation of platinum compounds in gastric cancer? I was at a meeting recently where they were being evaluated in other tumor types, but I haven't heard of their being tested in gastric cancer.

Woolley: I don't think there are any data at the moment. We are just finishing up the phase I studies with both of those compounds and going into phase II. The emphasis is on other tumors. We based our inclusion of platinum into a 5-FU-adriamycin-platinum compound upon some data from the EORTC indicating single-agent activity of platinum in gastric cancer. Attempts to reproduce those results with platinum as second-line therapy of gastric and pancreatic cancer were not very successful. I am not particularly enthusiastic about any generation of platinum compounds as a therapy for gastric cancer at this point, unless they turn out to be synergistic in some way with other compounds.

Tattersall: Would you make the same comment about second generation anthracyclines other than aclacinomycin?

Woolley: I know of two studies of aclacinomycin, one from the University of Pennsylvania and the other ongoing in the Pan-American Health Organization group. Neither study using full phase II doses has shown any activity with that drug. As far as I know, bisantrene isn't helping too much, and mitoxantrone is not showing any activity. So we're back to adriamycin: I would be very interested to know if any of the Japanese investigators have new compounds with activity.

CHEMOTHERAPY FOR ADVANCED CANCER:
BREAST CANCER

© 1984 Elsevier Science Publishers B.V.
Fluoropyrimidines in Cancer Therapy
K. Kimura, J. Fujii, M. Ogawa, O.P. Bodey, P. Alberto, eds.

COMBINATION CHEMOTHERAPIES CONTAINING TEGAFUR IN ADVANCED BREAST CANCER

Makoto Ogawa, Jiro Inagaki, Noboru Horikoshi and Katsuhiro Inoue

1. INTRODUCTION

Breast cancer is known to be moderately sensitive to various antitumor agents including alkylating agents, vinca alkaloids, antimetabolites, antibiotics and others. Single agent efficacies of L-PAM, cyclophosphamide (CPM), vincristine (VCR), 5-fluorouracil (5-FU), methotrexate (MTX), adriamycin (ADM) and mitomycin C (MMC) can produce response rates exceeding 20% in advanced breast cancer; furthermore, combination regimens containing these agents can increase response rates more than 50% with approximately 10% of complete responses (1,2).

However, it is rare to obtain cure by chemotherapy alone in advanced breast cancer, hence the purpose of chemotherapy in recurrent and advanced disease is to prolong patient's survival duration.

In recurrent breast cancer, the majority of patients have been exposed to adjuvant chemotherapy using L-PAM, CMF (CPM, MTX, 5-FU) and others. Therefore, these patients have possibily gained resistance to various antitumor agents such as L-PAM, CPM, MTX and 5-FU which have

379

been commonly used in adjuvant chemotherapeutic regimens. For the treatment of these patients, ADM is one of the most appropriate drugs to be selected due to both lack of cross resistance to these agents and sufficient anti-tumor efficacy (3).

This paper describes the results obtained from three sequential studies performed in our department in order to establish the standard combination chemotherapy in recurrent advanced breast cancer.

2.   MATERIALS AND METHODS

Table 1 summarizes regimens studied. The first study employing a combination chemotherapy consisting of ADM, CPM and oral tegafur (ACF) was initiated in September 1977 and terminated in February 1979 (4).

The second study was a prospective randomized study comparing two regimens: ACF versus ACFM (ACF plus MTX) which started in March 1979 and completed in April 1983 (5).

The third study on a combination regimen consisting of ACF plus tamoxifen initiated in May 1983 is now ongoing.

These regimens were repeated in 3 week intervals and dose modifications were performed by severity of hematologic toxicities. Eligible conditions for these studies were histological proof of breast cancer, adequate hepatic, renal and bone marrow functions, performance status more than 40% by Karnofsky's scale, and age less than 75 years old. In addition, the second study required clearly measurable lesions.

TABLE 1 Combination regimens in three studies

Ist Study (ACF regimen)

    Adriamycin $40mg/m^2$ iv day 1

    Cyclophosphamide $130mg/m^2$ iv days 1-5 q 3w

    Tegafur* $500mg/m^2$ po daily

IInd Study

                  ACF

    Randomize<

                  ACF + Methotrexatc 10 $15mg/m^2$ iv days 1,5

IIIrd Study

    ACF + Tamoxifen   40mg/d   po daily

---

*Tegafur continued until leukocyte count below 2,000/cm.

    Patients characteristics are summarized in Table 2. Among 67 patients entered in the first study, 18 patients were excluded from evaluation because the regimen was used as adjuvant chemotherapy. Thirty-five patients were premenopausal and 36 patients had received various chemotherapies containing L-PAM, CPM, 5-FU, oral tegafur and others in both adjuvant chemotherapy and prior chemotherapy after recurrence was observed.

    In the prospective randomized study, patients populations entered to both arms were very similar in major prognostic factors including age and performance status. In the latest ongoing study, 11 patients had positive ER receptor, while 14 patients had negative ER receptor, and the receptor was unknown in 23 patients. This study included 32 patients who had not been exposed to any prior chemotherapy after recurrence.

TABLE 2   Patients characteristics

	Ist Study	IInd Study		IIIrd Study
	ACF	ACF vs ACFM		ACFT
Patients entered	67	30	30	48
Evaluable patients	49	28	30	48
Age (range)	52 (32–75)	55 (32–69)	49 (31–68)	48 (30–72)
Performance status (range)	80 (40–100)	80 (40–100)	80 (40–100)	90 (40–100)
Menopausal status				
Premenopausal	35	5	6	29
Postmenopausal	14	23	24	19
Prior chemotherapy				
(–)	13	7	4	32
(+)	36	21	26	16

3.   RESULTS

Clinical results are summarized in Table 3. Among 49 evaluable patients in the first study, there were one complete and 25 partial responses (53%), 16 no changes and 7 progressive diseases. A median duration of responses was 4.4 months ranging from 1 to 28 months.

Thirty-eight patients with better performance status ($\geq$60%) had a 63% response rate comparing to a 18% response rate in 11 patients with poorer performance status and this difference was statistically significant (P=0.01).

In thirteen patients who had not been exposed to prior chemotherapy, a significantly high response rate of 77% was obtained in comparison with the response rate of 44% in 36 patients who had received various chemotherapies (P=0.04).

TABLE 3   Clinical efficacy of three studies

Regimen	Evaluable Patients	Responders		CR+PR (%)	Median Duration of Response (mos)	Median Survival Time (mos)		
		CR	PR			All	Resp.	Non-Resp.
Ist Study								
ACF	49	1	25	53	4.4	9	10	7
IInd Study								
ACF	28	4	14	43	21	21	23	16
ACFM	30	2	16	60	6.9	13	14	10
IIIrd Study								
ACFT	48	7	12	40	8	8	10	7

The response rates analyzed by major metastatic sites were 47% for lung, 60% for liver, 54% in soft tissue and 50% for bone. Menopausal status and numbers of metastatic sites did not influence on response rates. The median survival time of all patients treated was 9 months: 10 months ranging from 2.5 to 29 months for responders and 7 months ranging from 2.3 to 17 months for non-responders.

There were 4 complete and 14 partial responses (43%), 14 no changes and 2 progressive diseases in 28 patients treated by ACF. On the other hand, there were 2 complete and 16 partial responses (60%), 10 no changes and 2 progressive diseases in 30 patients receiving ACFM.

The median durations of responses were 21 months in ACF and 6.9 in ACFM. The median survival time of all patients on ACF arm was 21 months: 23 months for responders and 16 months for non-responders.

On the other hand, the median survival time on ACFM regimen was 13 months: 14 months for responders and 10 months for non-responders. Thus, the response rate was slightly higher with no statistical significance in ACFM regimen, whereas the duration of response and the survival duration were longer in ACF regimen but the difference was statistically not significant.

The metastatic lesion in soft tissues was more responsive comparing to those in bone and lung in both regimens. Hematologic toxicities seen in the first course in both regimens are compared in Table 4. Leukopenia was the dose-limiting toxicity in both regimens and nearly all patients became below 3,000/cmm. Severe leukopenia less than 1,000/cmm occurred approximately twice higher in incidence in ACFM.

TABLE 4   Hematologic toxicity in ACF vs ACFM

		Incidence(%)	
		ACF	ACFM
Leukopenia ($\times 10^3$/cmm)	<3	36	26
	<2	53	47
	<1	11	20
	Total	100	93
Thrombocytopenia($\times 10^3$/cmm)	<100	11*	37*
	<60	3	10
	<30	7	6
	Total	21	53
Hemoglobin (<3 g/dl)		11	23

*P<0.05

Thrombocytopenia less than 10 x 10^3/cmm occurred more frequently in ACFM and the difference was statistically significant.   Anemia was also more frequent in ACFM. The result indicated that ACFM had more profound hematologic toxicities than ACF.

Non-hematologic toxicities are summarized in Table 5. The incidence and grade of gastrointestinal toxicities, alopecia and elevations of hepatic enzymes were nearly identical in both regimens. Palpitation and mild angina attack occurred in one patient each in both regimens but these were reversible.

TABLE 5   Non-hematologic toxicity in ACF vs ACFM

Symptoms	Incidence (%)	
	ACF	ACFM
Nausea	82	90
Vomiting	57	67
Anorexia	75	70
Diarrhea	18	10
Stomatitis	21	13
Pigmentation	21	27
Alopecia	100	100
Hepatotoxicity	11	17
Cardiotoxicity	4	3

Overall, ACFM, adding methotrexate to ACF, demonstrated both slightly enhanced efficacy and increased hematologic toxicity and did not prolong the survival time.

The third study is a pilot study employing a chemo-endocrine therapy consisting of ACF plus tamoxifen which was selected based on the results obtained in the previous studies.

As summarizing in Table 2, seven complete and 12 partial responses (40%), 17 no changes and 12 progressive diseases have been reported until the end of September 1983 in this ongoing study. The median response duration is 8 months and the median survival time of all patients is 8 months: 10 months for responders and

7 months for non-responders.

Hematologic and non-hematologic toxicities were similar to those seen in ACF as shown in Table 5 and there has been no specific toxicity relating to the addition of tamoxifen.

The result observed to date has suggested that this chemoendocrine therapy may be beneficial for patients with positive ER receptor and/or for postmenopausal patients but the conclusion has to wait the final analysis.

4.   DISCUSSION

Carter (1) summarized a 26% of response rate of 5-fluorouracil (5-FU) from 15 literatures and 5-FU has been included in various combinations due to the reasonable activity and mild hematologic toxicity.

Cooper (6) included 5-FU in a five-drug combination, CMFVP (CPM, MTX, 5-FU, VCR, prednisone) and reported a 90% response rate in 60 patients with advanced breast cancer resistant to hormone treatments.

Subsequently, many confirmatory studies have been performed and from these studies, it has been recognized that a three-drug combination CMF (CPM, MTX, 5-FU) can yield an equivalent response rate of approximately 50% which is similar to the results of subsequent confirmatory studies of CMFVP (1).

5-FU has been included in three-drug combinations

named FAC, CAF or AFC, which consist of the same drugs, 5-FU, ADM and CPM (7-10). The response rates reported range from 43% to 82% with median durations of 8-10 months.

We used oral tegafur instead of 5-FU due to several reasons as follows.

Firstly, oral form was first developed in Japan and studied. Secondly, the response rates reported were 39% (11) and 41% (12) and judged as a comparable efficacy to 5-FU. Finally, oral form was thought to be more convenient for out-patient use. Thus, we have included the drug combining with ADM and CPM. The results obtained both in the first and the second study were nearly identical to those reported in the US studies; however, it is noteworthy to mention that majority of our patients had been exposed to prior chemotherapies after recurrence, whereas the US studies were conducted in the first line chemotherapy after recurrence.

There were three studies adding MTX to the three-drug combinations described previously and the response rates reported ranged from 55% to 62% with the median duration of 8.3 - 12 months (9,13,14). These studies including our studies were randomized trials comparing either two-drug or three-drug regimens and indicated that a four-drug combination (ADM, CPM, 5-FU, MTX) showed slightly better response rates than those in two-drug regimens

AC (ADM, CPM) and AF (ADM, 5-FU), or three-drug regimens AFC and ACF but the four-drug combination did not contribute to survival time.

In our previous phase II study of tamoxifen (15), there were one complete and 6 partial responses (20%) in 35 patients with advanced breast cancer and toxicities were extremely mild.

Consequently, we initiated a pilot study using ACF plus tamoxifen. The study is still ongoing and preliminary result suggests that patients with positive ER receptor and/or with postmenopausal status are more responsive than those in patients with premenopausal status. Two randomized studies compared chemotherapy alone and chemotherapy plus tamoxifen suggested that the latter could yield higher response rates than the former but the contribution to survival durations was not significant (16,17). Thus, the combined modality needs further studies in order to establish a clinical role in advanced breast cancer.

5. CONCLUSION

Three sequential studies conducted in our department have provided following results.

Firstly, a three-drug combination consisting of ADM, CPM and oral tegafur (ACF) is an effective regimen for recurrent and advanced breast cancer. Secondly, the addition of MTX to ACF enhanced the response rate, while it increased toxicities with no contribution to survival time. Finally, the current result obtained in an ongoing study employing ACF plus tamoxifen has demonstrated no clinical advantage of this regimen over ACF.

REFERENCES

1. Carter SK. (1976) Chemotherapy of breast cancer: Current status in breast cancer. In: Trends in Research and Treatment (eds) JC Hansen, WH Mathöum and M Rozencweig. Ravan Press, New York, pp. 198-215.

2. Carbone PP, Davis TE. (1978) Medical treatment for advanced breast cancer. Seminors in Oncology 5: 417-427.

3. Carter SK. (1975) Adriamycin-A review. J Natl Cancer Inst 55: 1265-1274.

4. Murosaki SJ, Inagaki J, Horikoshi N, et al. (1981) ACF combination consisting of adriamycin, cyclophosphamide and oral futraful for recurrent advanced breast cancer. J Jpn Soc Cancer Ther 16: 8-14.

5. Inoue K, Ogawa M, Inagaki J, et al. (1983) A randomized trial of adriamycin, cyclophosphamide, ftorafur (ACF) and adriamycin, cyclophosphamide, ftorafur, methotrexate (ACFM) in patients with advanced breast cancer. Cancer Chemother Pharmacol (in press)

6. Cooper R. (1980) Combination chemotherapy in hormone resistant breast cancer. Proc Am Assoc Cancer Res 10: 15.

7. Bull J, Tormey MDC, Li S-H, et al. (1978) A randomized cooperative trial of adriamycin versus methotrexate in combination drug therapy. Cancer 41: 1649-1657.

8. Hortobagyi G, Guttermen JU, Blumenschein GR, et al. (1979) Combination chemoimmunotherapy of metastatic breast cancer with 5-fluorouracil, adriamycin, cyclophosphamide and BCG. Cancer 43: 1225-1233.

9. Traum B, Hoogstraten B, Kennedy A, et al. (1978) Adriamycin in combination for the treatment of breast cancer. Cancer 41: 2078-2083.

10. Smalley RV, Carpenter J, Bartolucci A, et al. (1977) A comparison of cyclophosphamide, adriamycin, 5-fluorouracil (CAF) and cyclophosphamide, methotrexate, 5-fluorouracil, vincristine, prednisolone (CMFVP) in patients with metastatic breast cancer. Cancer 40: 625-632.

11. Konda C. (1975) The effects of oral and rectal administration of N-(2-tetrahydrofuranyl)-5-fluorouracil in the treatment of advanced cancer. Jpn J Cancer Clin 21: 1044-1050.

12. Watanabe H, Naito T, Uchiyama T, et al. (1974) Clinical result of oral ftorafur conducted by a cooperative study group. Jpn J Cancer Chemother 1: 111-121.

13. Kannealey GT, Boston B, Michell MS, et al. (1978) Combination chemotherapy for advanced breast cancer. Cancer 42: 27-33.

14. Creech RH, Catalano RB, Harris DT, et al. (1979) Low dose chemotherapy of metastatic breast cancer with cyclophosphamide, adriamycin, methotrexate, 5-fluorouracil (CAMF) versus sequential cyclophosphamide, methotrexate, 5-fluorouracil (CMF) and adriamycin. Cancer 43: 51-59.

15. Cocconi G, De Lisi V, Boni C, et al. (1982) CFM vs CMF plus tamoxifen in postmenopausal metastatic breast cancer. Proc Am Soc Clin Oncol 1: 75.

16. Akman FR, Jones SE, Davis S. (1983) The effect of initial treatment (Rx) with chemotherapy (C), sequential hormonal-chemotherapy (H C) or combined hormonal-chemotherapy (H+C) on long term survival (S) in metastatic breast cancer. Proc Am Soc Clin Oncol 2: 108.

© 1984 Elsevier Science Publishers B.V.
Fluoropyrimidines in Cancer Therapy
K. Kimura, S. Fujii, M. Ogawa, G.P. Bodey, P. Alberto, eds.

FLUOROPYRIMIDINES IN BREAST CANCER

Gerald P. Bodey, George R. Blumenschein, Gabriel N. Hortobagyi
Aman U. Buzdar and Sewa S. Legha

1. INTRODUCTION

Breast carcinoma is a malignancy which responds to many antitumor agents. The introduction of combination chemotherapy has improved the response rate and duration of response in this disease. In 1973, studies of the combination of 5-fluorouracil (5FU), adriamycin and cyclophosphamdide (FAC) were initiated at our institution. During the past decade, we have attempted to improve upon the results of the original studies by modifying this basic chemotherapeutic regimen. The results of these studies will be reviewed in this presentation.

2. MATERIALS AND METHODS

The dosage schedules of the chemotherapeutic regimens are shown in Table 1. The FAC regimen was administered intravenously at 21 day intervals, providing the patient had recovered from the acute side-effects of the previous course of chemotherapy. Dosages of drugs were increased or decreased during subsequent courses depending upon the toxicity of the preceding course. The total dose of adriamycin was limited to 450-500 mg/M^2 in order to minimize

TABLE 1   Chemotherapeutic regimens for breast carcinoma

I.   FAC-BCG

5-FU	500 mg/M^2, day 1
Adria	50 mg/M^2, day 1
CTX	500 mg/M^2, day 1
BCG	6x10^8 viable units, day 9, 13 and 17

II.   CMF Maintenance

CTX	500 mg/M^2, day 2
MTX	30 mg/M^2, day 1&8
5-FU	500 mg/M^2, day 1&8
BCG	6x10^8 viable units, days 9, 13 & 17

III.   VAC-FUM

A. VCR	1.5 mg/M^2 q wk x 7 wks then d 1 only
Adria	59 mg/M^2, day 2
CTX	750 mg/M^2, day 2
BCG	6x10^8 viable units

B. 5-FU	500 mg/M^2, d 1-5
MTX	30 mg/M^2, d 1,8&15
BCG	6x10^8 viable units, days 9, 16, 23

IV.   ACFTOR

Teg	2 gm/M^2, days 1-5
Adria	50 gm/M^2, day 1
CTX	500 mg/M^2, day 1
BCG	6x10^8 viable units days 9, 13, 17

V.   FAI

5 FU	500 mg/M^2, day 1&8
Adria	50 mg/M^2, day 1
Ifos	800 mg/M^2, day 1-5
BCG	6x10^8 viable units days 9, 13 & 17
Levam	100 mg/M^2, days 9, 10, 13, 14, 17 18

VI.   FAC/L-Asp/Mtx

5-FU	as above
Adria	as above
CTX	as above
L-Asp	10,000 u/M^2, d 1 day 8 & 15
MTX	120 mg/M^2, d 10
CP	2 mg/M^2, d 9&16
PV	0.5 mg/M^2, days 7, 12 & 17

---

the risk of cardiotoxicity.   Thereafter the CMF regimen
was administered orally as maintenance therapy at 21 day

intervals. BCG (Tice, Connaught, or Pasteur strain) immunotherapy was administered by scarification alternating between the upper arms and thighs. The VAC-FUM regimen consisted of 3 courses of VAC, given at 21 day intervals followed by 3 course of FUM given at 28 day intervals. This sequence was repeated. The ACFTOR regimen substituted Tegafur (Ftorafur) for 5FU in the FAC regimen. Tegafur was administered in 100 to 200 ml 5% dextrose solution over a one hour period.

In the FAI study, patients were randomly assigned to receive FAI or FAC. Ifosfamide was given in 500 ml 5% dextrose solution over 2-3 hours. Patients received oral levamisole in addition to BCG as immunotherapy. This immunotherapy regimen was also administered during CMF maintenance. In a subsequent study, L-asparaginase plus methotrexate were added to the FAC regimen along with non-specific immunotherapy, consisting of intravenous C. parvum (CP) or subcutaneous Pseudomonas vaccine (PV). This was a four-arm study in which patients were randomly assigned to FAC, FAC + CP, FAC + L-asp + Mtx or FAC + L-asp + MTX + PV.

Standard criteria were used to evaluate results of treatment. Pretreatment characteristics which affected response were similar in each group of patients in these studies. In the randomized studies, patients were stratified according to known prognostic factors.

394

TABLE 2   Results with FAC ± BCG in metastatic breast
carcinoma

	FAC	FAC + BCG	VAC–FUM + BCG	ACFtor + BCG
Evaluable Pts	44	105	156	91
Complete Rem (%)	14	19	20	20
Partial Rem (%)	59	57	47	46
Stable Dis (%)	27	18	25	29
Progressive Dis (%)	0	6	8	5

3.   RESULTS

A total of 44 evaluable patients were treated with
the FAC regimen (1,2).   Subsequently, 105 evaluable
patients were treated with FAC + BCG. The complete remission rates and response rates were similar with both of
these regimens (Table 2).   Response occurred by 2 months
of treatment in 42% and by 3 months in 71%.   The median
duration of response was 9 months for the FAC regimen and
14 mos. for the FAC + BCG regimen (p=0.04).   The median
duration of stable disease was 8 months for both groups
of patients.   Among responding patients, the median duration of survival was 16 months for the FAC group and 24
months for the FAC + BCG (p=0.004).   Hence, the addition
of BCG immunotherapy did not affect the response rates
but did affect the duration of response, and especially
duration of survival for responding patients.

The VAC-FUM regimen was designed to try to increase the response rate and duration of response in breast carcinoma by cycling two chemotherapeutic regimens early in the treatment program (Table 1). Unfortunately, these objectives were not accomplished with this regimen. The complete remission rate was 20% and the overall response rate was 67% (Table 2). The durations of response and survival with the VAC-FUM regimen did not differ significantly from the FAC regimen. Hence, changing therapy after 3 courses did not improve the results.

The dose-limiting toxicity of the FAC regimen was myelosuppression. Tegafur is an analogue of 5FU which has similar antitimor activity. However, this analogue has less myelosuppressive toxicity. It was anticipated that by substituting ftorafur for 5FU in the FAC regimen, there would be less toxicity, thus permiting the administration of higher doses of chemotherapy. Consequently, a new regimen ACFTOR was designed in which tegafur replaced 5FU (Table 1). The results with this regimen were compared to those obtained with the FAC regimen. All of these patients received BCG immunotherapy.

Ninety-one evaluable patients were entered on this study (3). The complete remission rates were the same for both regimens, although the overall response rate was higher for the FAC regimen (76% vs 66%) (Table 2). The median duration of response was 12 months for patients who received ACFTOR and 14 months for patients who received FAC (p=0.53). The median durations of survival for responding patients were 24 months and 22 months respectively (p=0.19).

TABLE 3 Hematological toxicity of FAC and ACFTOR regimens

| | FAC | | ACFTOR | |
	Median	Range	Median	Range
Lowest WBC	1.1	0.5 - 3.1	2.3	0.1 - 7.0
Lowest P''N	0.8	0.3 - 2.6	1.1	0.0 - 4.4
Lowest Platelets	180	45 - 345	200	10 - 458

Expressed as number per cu mm x 10^3

Myelosuppressive toxicity was more severe with the FAC regimen (Table 3). Although it was anticipated that dosage escalation would be possible with the ACFTOR regimen, this was not accomplished. The frequency of nausea and vomiting was similar for the two regimens but there were important quantitative differences. Severe vomiting occurred five times more often in patients receiving ACFTOR. In 76% of evaluable courses of ACFTOR, weight loss exceeded 5 lbs during the 5 day treatment period whereas this occurred in only 2% of evaluable courses of FAC. Some patients required hospitalization for intravenous fluid and electrolyte replacement. Lethargy, dizziness, fever, chest pain, hypotension, visual and personality changes were observed in some patients receiving ACFTOR, but did not occur in patients receiving FAC. No therapeutic advantage with respect to response rate or duration of response was achieved by the substitution of tegafur for 5FU and it caused some unpleasant side-effects when administered by this schedule.

A second attempt was made to develop a less myelosuppressive regimen in order to be able to administer higher doses of chemotherapy. Ifosfamide was substituted for cyclophosphamide in what was designed to be a prospective randomized comparative trial (Table 1). Randomization could not be maintained due to supply problems with ifosfamide and the FAI arm was eventually discontinued due to the bladder toxicity of ifosfamide. Of the 166 evaluable patients, 117 received FAC and 49 received FAI (4). All of these patients also received BCG and levamisole (Table 4). Both the complete remission rates and response rates were comparable for the 2 treatment

TABLE 4   Results with FAC or FAI in breast carcinoma

	FAC	FAI
Evaluable Patients	117	49
Complete Remission (%)	16	16
Partial Remission (%)	56	50
Stable Disease (%)	23	29
Progressive Disease (%)	4	6

All pts also received BCG and Levamisole immunotherapy

regimens. The median duration of remission was 17 months for the patients receiving FAC and 17.8 months for the patients receiving FAI. The median survival for all patients was similar for both regimens (21.4 mos vs 23.5 mos, p=0.4). The FAI regimen proved to be unsatisfactory because 25% of patients developed hematuria, including 12% who developed gross hematuria. Ifosfamide had to be discontinued in 5 of these patients because of this side-effect. Myelosuppression was comparable with both regimens, although neutropenia was somewhat more severe with the FAI. Consequently, the substitution of ifosamide for cyclophosphamide did not permit the administration of higher doses of chemotherapy, did not increase therapeutic efficacy, and was associated with hematuria.

L-asparaginase (L-asp) protects against the toxicity of methotrexate (MTX) and permits the addition of higher doses in patients with breast carcinoma. L-asp plus MTX was added to the FAC regimen in an attempt to improve the results (5). It was anticipated that, by including L-asp, no additional toxicity would occur. C. parvum (CP) and Pseudomonas vaccine (PV) were also evaluated in this study. Patients were prospectively randomized to receive: FAC alone, FAC plus CP, FAC plus L-asp and MTX, or FAC plus L-asp and MTX plus PV (Table 1). The results of this study are shown in Table 5. Patients who received L-asp plus MTX experienced stomatitis and prolonged myelosuppression requiring omission of doses of 5FU and

TABLE 5   Results of comparative trial of therapeutic regimens in breast carcinoma

	FAC	FAC + CP	FAC + L-asp+MTX	FAC + L-asp + MTX + PV
Evaluable Pts	12	14	10	16
Complete Rem	3 (25%)	1 (7%)	0	3 (19%)
Partial Rem	4 (33%)	6 (43%)	5 (50%)	11 (69%)
Stable Dis	4	6	5	1
Progression	1	1	0	1

CP = C. parvum   PV = Pseudomonas vaccine

MTX and dosage reductions during subsequent courses. Severe infection occurred in only 1 (3%) patient who received FAC, but in 13 (40%) patients who received FAC plus L-asp and MTX. Unacceptable side-effects also were associated with the administration of PV. Because of the excessive toxicity, this study had to be discontinued. Presumably the unexpected toxicity was due to an adverse interaction between L-asp and FU, because L-asp has been given with MTX and adriamycin without difficulty.

Between March 1973 and June 1976, a total of 619 patients with metastatic breast carcinoma were treated with Regimens I-IV listed in Table 1 (6). Of these, 116 (19%) achieved a complete remission. The median time to achieve complete remission was 5 months (range, 1 to 23 months). The time to achieve complete remission was significantly longer for patients with bone metastases (12 months vs 4 months, p <0.01). Chemotherapy was discontinued in 47 patients usually after they had remained in complete remission for at least 2 years.

The median duration of CR was 17 months and all patients were followed for more than 24 months. Eighty-one (70%) of the 116 patients have relapsed from 3 to 44 months after onset of CR. During the first 6 months, 1.8% of the patients relapsed each month, whereas thereafter 5% relapsed each month. The only pretreatment factors which influenced duration of CR were the number of metastatic sites and onset time of chemotherapy following oophorectomy. The median duration of CR was 19 months for patients with 1 or 2 metastatic sites compared to 13 months for patients with 3 or more metastatic sites (p=0.10). The median duration of CR was 33 months for patients who received chemotherapy within 4 weeks after oophorectomy, but only 13 months for patients whose chemotherapy was delayed until disease progression (p <0.01).

Fifty-six (69%) of the 81 patients who relapsed, had their recurrence at a site initially involved by tumor. The remaining 25 patients had recurrence at new sites. In 12 patients, the new site was the central nervous system. Approximately 60% of these patients have survived for 3 years after the onset of chemotherapy. Only a small proportion of patients remain disease-free off chemotherapy and it is likely that most of these will develop recurrent disease. Consequently, curative therapy for patients with metastatic breast cancer remains to be discovered.

Those variables which affected response rate and duration of response were determined from 619 patients (7). Obviously, the degree of response to chemotherapy had a major impact on survival. The median survivals for patients experiencing CR, PR, stable disease and progression were 33, 24, 16 and 3 months, respectively. Important pretreatment variables which significantly ($p<.05$) affected response included extent of disease, weight loss, performance status, platelet count, alkaline phosphatase, extent of prior radiotherapy, response to prior hormonal therapy, prior chemotherapy, disease-free interval, hemoglobin, white blood count, absolute lymphocyte count, lactic dehydrogenase, SGOT, bilirubin, albumin and calcium. The intensity of chemotherapy also influenced response. Patients who received <80% of the standard dose had a response rate of 53%, whereas patients who received 80-99% of the standard dose had a response rate of 66% ($p=0.01$). Patients who received their treatment at 3 week intervals had a response rate of 72%, whereas patients who received their treatment at >4 week intervals had a response rate of 46%. The median survival of these latter two groups of patients was 103 and 76 weeks, respectively. Considering all of these variables it has been possible to develop a logistic regression equation to predict for response and duration of response (8).

There is a steep dose-response when antitumor agents are used for the treatment of experimental animal tumors. The dose-limiting toxicity of most antitumor agents is myelosuppression which is associated with an increased risk of infection. The use of laminar air flow rooms and prophylactic antibiotics (PEPA) reduces the risk of infection during chemotherapy and permits the administration of more intensive chemotherapy. We conducted a prospective randomized trial of the PEPA program in perimenopausal women with breast carcinoma. The major objectives were to determine whether the PEPA program permitted the administration of more intensive chemotherapy and increased the response rate and duration of response. Patients were randomly assigned to receive three courses of remission induction chemotherapy on the PEPA program or as controls. All control patients were hospitalized in a private room to insure comparability of patient care. Details of the PEPA program have been published elsewhere (9). The patients received the FAC regimen and were required to receive dosage escalation during second and third courses if they did not develop major infection during the preceding course, regardless of the degree or duration of myelosuppression (Table 6). 5FU was administered by continuous intravenous infusion to minimize the myelosuppressive toxicity. Patients who developed major infection received a reduction in the dose of subsequent

TABLE 6   PEPA study in premenopausal breast cancer
          patients

	COURSE 1	COURSE 2	COURSE 3
Initial Schedule			
5FU (mg/M^2/d x 5 d)	500	500	500
Adriamycin (mg/M^2, d 1)	50	65	80
Cyclophosphamide (mg/M^2, d 1)	500	750	1000
Subsequent Schedule			
5FU (mg/M^2/d x 5 d)	500	500	500
Adriamycin (mg/M^2, d 1)	60	70	80
Cyclophosphamide (mg/M^2, d 1)	1000	1200	1500

5FU administered as a 24 hr continuous infusion

courses.   Patients   received   conventional   maintenance
therapy thereafter.

Thirty-two evaluable patients were entered on study.
There were no significant differences in complete remission rates or response rates. Thirteen (81%) of the PEPA
patients received maximum dosage escalation compared to 4
(25%) of the control patients. The complete remission
rate was substantially higher for the patients who
received maximum dosage escalation but the overall
response rates were similar (Table 7). The median
duration of response was 14 months (range, 5-30 months)
for the PEPA patients and 16 months (range, 5-55 months)

TABLE 7   PEPA in breast carcinoma, response to therapy

	PEPA	CONTROL	ADRIAMYCIN DOSE (mg/M^2)	
			<185	>185
Evaluable	16	16	11	21
Complete Rem (%)	56	38	36	62
Partial Rem (%)	31	56	45	29
Total Resp (%)	87	94	91	91

for the controls. The median duration of response was 18 months for those patients who received maximum dosage escalation compared to 16 months for the remaining patients (p=0.48). This study demonstrated that the PEPA program permitted the administration of intensive chemotherapy. Unfortunately, intensive chemotherapy failed to have a major impact on degree or duration of response.

4.   CONCLUSION

Combination chemotherapy has had a substantial impact on the natural history of breast carcinoma. 5-Fluorouracil has played an important role in many combination regimens. Overall response rates of about 70% have been achieved with complete remission rates of 20%. Despite numerous modifications of the basic FAC regimen, little improvement has been obtained. Hopefully, the discovery of additional active agents will lead to more effective chemotherapeutic regimens in the future.

REFERENCES

1. Gutterman JU, Cardenas JO, Blumenschein GR, et al. (1976) Chemoimmunotherapy of advanced breast cancer: prolongation of remission and survival with BCG. Brit Med J 2: 1222-1225.

2. Hortobagyi GN, Gutterman JU, Blumenschein GR, et al. (1979) Combination chemoimmunotherapy of metastatic breast cancer with 5-fluorouracil, adriamycin, cyclophosphamide, and BCG. Cancer 43: 1225-1233.

3. Hortobagyi GN, Blumenschein GR, Tashima CK, et al. (1979) Ftorafur, adriamycin, cyclophosphamide and BCG in the treatment of metastatic breast cancer. Cancer 44: 398-405.

4. Buzdar AU, Legha SS, Tashima CK, et al. (1979) Ifosfamide versus cyclophosphamide in combination drug therapy for metastatic breast cancer. Cancer Treat Rep 63:115-119.

5. Hortobagyi GN, Yap H-Y, Wiseman CL, et al. (1980) Chemoimmunotherapy for metastatic breast cancer with 5-fluorouracil, adriamycin, cyclophosphamide, methotrexate, L-asparaginase, Corynebacterium parvum, and Pseudomonas vaccine. Cancer Treat Rep 64:157-159.

6. Legha SS, Buzdar AU, Smith TL, et al. (1979) Complete remissions in metastatic breast cancer treated with combination drug therapy. Ann Intern Med 91:847-852.

7. Swenerton KD, Legha SS, Smith TL, et al. (1979) Prognostic factors in metastatic breast cancer treated with combination chemotherapy. Cancer Res 39:1552-1562.

8. Hortobagyi GN, Smith TL, Legha SS, et al. (1983) Multivariate analysis of prognostic factors in metastatic breast cancer. J Clin Oncol (In press).

9. Bodey GP, Rosenbaum B. (1974) Effect of prophylactic measures on the microbial flora of patients in protected environment units. Medicine 53:209-228.

Fluoropyrimidines in Cancer Therapy
K. Kimura, S. Fujii, M. Ogawa, G.P. Bodey, P. Alberto, eds.

COMBINATION CHEMOTHERAPY IN THE TREATMENT OF WOMEN WITH ADVANCED BREAST CANCER

Baha'Uddin M. Arafah, James S. Marshall and Olof H. Pearson

1. INTRODUCTION

Endocrine and cytotoxic chemotherapy are the main systemic treatments used in women with advanced breast cancer. Endocrine therapy provides effective palliation in about 40% of unselected patients. The introduction of estrogen receptor (ER) measurement in the tumor provided a major advantage in selecting patients likely to respond to endocrine therapies. Whereas the response rate to endocrine treatments is 60 to 70% in women with ER-positive tumors (1), such therapy is virtually ineffective in women with ER-negative tumors. Endocrine treatments can be hormone additive (estrogens, androgen and progestins) or hormone ablative in nature (hypophysectomy, oophorectomy and adrenalectomy).

Cytotoxic chemotherapy can also provide effective palliation in women with advanced breast cancer (2-5). Cooper (2), using a 5-drug combination chemotherapy, reported a high incidence of remissions in women with advanced breast cancer. The agents used in that regimen included: cyclophosphamide, methotrexate, 5-fluorouracil (5FU), vincristine and prednisone. We report here an

407

update of a previous report (6) on our experience in treating 169 patients with this regimen of chemotherapy. We also present our data on the response to Adriamycin used as a single agent following 5-drug chemotherapy. We have evaluated the responses to chemotherapy in patients who responded and those who did not respond to endocrine treatments.

2. PATIENTS AND METHODS

A total of 169 evaluable patients with progressive, stage IV breast cancer were treated with combination chemotherapy. Patients' ages ranged between 29 and 80 years (mean±SEM: 54.1±0.8, median; 52 years). Except for 3 patients, all were postmenopausal at the time of treatments. The disease free interval ranged between 0 and 156 months (mean: 33.3, median: 39 months). ER determination performed on the primary tumor or metastatic lesions was positive (>3 fmol/mg cytosol protein) in 57, negative in 32 and unknown in 80 patients. Sixty-six patients did not receive prior endocrine treatment either because they had an ER negative tumor (n=32) or had advanced liver metastasis (n=34). The remainder of the patients (n=103) were treated with one or more endo-crine therapies prior to the institution of 5-drug chemo-therapy. However, of those treated with endocrine ther-apies (n=103) the responses to such treatment were evaluable in only 79 patients. The dominant sites of disease were visceral in 91 (54%), bone in 69 (41%) and soft tissue in 9 (5%) patients.

The chemotherapy regimen used in our initial experience is described here. Prednisone (0.75 mg/kgm/day) was given orally. The dose was reduced every 10 days until it was stopped after 1 month. Cyclophosphamide was given orally at a daily dose of 2 mg/kgm. 5-Fluorouracil (5FU, 12 mg/kgm) and methotrexate (0.6 mg/kgm) were given intravenously every week for the first 3 months, every other week for the next 3 months and every 3 weeks thereafter. Vincristine (35 µg/kgm) was given intravenously with 5FU and methotrexate during the first 6 treatments and every 6 weeks thereafter. Some patients were hospitalized during the first 2 weeks of treatments and thereafter chemotherapy was administered in the ambulatory service. However, following our initial experience with this regimen and because of severe myelosuppression seen in many patients, the doses of cytotoxic agents were reduced to tolerable levels: cyclophosphamide 100 mg daily, methotrexate 20 to 30 mg and 5FU 500-650 mg given according to the schedule described above. The doses of drugs were adjusted according to blood counts. Vincristine was withheld whenever neurotoxicity occurred. This regimen of chemotherapy (except prednisone) was continued until disease progression was noted. One hundred patients who relapsed or failed this combination chemotherapy were treated with Adriamycin as a single agent (50-60 mg IV every 3 weeks). The total dose of Adriamycin was less than 500 mg/m^2 in all patients.

Remission is defined as complete or partial (>50%) regression of measurable lesions, or recalcification of osteolytic lesions with no new lesions appearing for 3 months or more. Failure is defined as >25% progression of measurable lesions and/or the appearance of new lesions after an adequate trial of at least 6 weeks. Stable disease is defined as <50% regression and <25% progression of measurable lesions with no new lesions appearing for a period of at least 6 months.

ER assays on the primary or metastatic tumors were performed using the dextran-coated charcoal technique (7). Statistical analysis of the results was done using the chi-square or the unpaired Student-t-test.

TABLE 1   Results of 5-drug chemotherapy in 169 patients with advanced breast cancer

	Patients		Dominant disease % of patients			D.F.I.†
	No.	%	Visceral	Bone	Soft tissue	(months)
Remissions	110*	65	52%	43%	5%	35.4±4.8
Failure	59	34	58%	38%	4%	28.7±5.5
Total	169	100	-	-	-	

* Includes 6 patients with stable disease.
† Disease free interval.

410

3. RESULTS

3.1   Overall response to 5-drug chemotherapy

Table 1 summarizes the overall results of 5-drug chemotherapy in all patients. Sixty-five percent of our patients treated with 5-drug chemotherapy obtained an objective remission lasting for 3 to 54+ months (mean ± SEM: 12.2±2, median: 10 months). There was no significant difference between those who responded and those that did not with respect to age, menopausal status or dominant disease. The disease free interval was slightly but not significantly longer in patients who responded to chemotherapy. Nine of the 110 patients who responded to chemotherapy are still in remission. In general patients tolerated the treatments well. The predominant side effects were nausea, fatigue and myelosuppression. These were controlled with antiemetics and appropriate reduction in the doses of drugs.

TABLE 2.   Response to 5-drug chemotherapy in relation to ER level in the tumor

	Positive	Negative	Unknown
Total no.	57	32	80
Remissions	34	18	58
%	60%	56%	72%
Duration (months) mean±SEM median	11.91±1.9 10	11.1±1.5 9	13.2±2.6 10.5

3.2 Response to chemotherapy in relation to endocrine
    therapy

Table 2 summarizes the data on all patients in relation to ER level on the primary or metastatic tumors.
There was no significant difference in the response rate
to chemotherapy between patients with positive, negative
or unknown ER. We then evaluated the response to chemotherapy in patients with unknown or positive ER who were
treated with 2 or more endocrine therapies (tamoxifen,
hypophysectomy, oophorectomy, androgens, progestins and
estrogens). Table 3 summarizes the data in these
patients.

TABLE 3.   Response to 5-drug chemotherapy in relation to
           previous response to endocrine therapy

	Patients who responded to ≥ 1 endocrine Rx	Patients not responding to ≥ 2 endocrine Rx	P value
Total	46	25	-
Remissions	33*	14	0.08
%	72%	56%	
Duration of remission mean	12.3±2.1	10.1±1.5	NS
median	11.5	9.5	-

* There are 4 additional patients with no change, thus
  making the response rate 37/56 or 80%.

412

Of 46 patients who responded previously to at least one endocrine treatment, 33 or 72% obtained objective remissions with 5-drug chemotherapy. In addition 4 patients had stabilization of disease. Thus the response rate in this group was 37/56 or 80%. In contrast, of 25 who did not respond to >2 endocrine treatments 14 patients or 56% responded to 5-drug chemotherapy. The difference between the 2 groups was of borderline significance. The duration of remission was slightly but not significantly longer in patients who responded to endocrine therapy. Thus 5-drug chemotherapy was effective in patients with hormone responsive as well as hormone non-responsive tumors. However, a major difference in the 2 groups is the significant increase in survival (see below) in patients responding to various endocrine treatments.

3.3 Response to Adriamycin after 5-drug chemotherapy

One hundred patients were treated with Adriamycin as a single agent. Of those, 57 patients responded initially and then relapsed on 5-drug chemotherapy while 43 failed to benefit from that treatment after an adequate trial was given. Of 100 patients treated, 26 obtained an objective remission, 10 had stable disease and 64 patients failed to benefit from Adriamycin (table 4). There was no significant difference in response rate to Adriamycin between patients who responded or those who

TABLE 4.   Response to Adriamycin after 5 drug chemo-
           therapy in 100 patients

Response	Patients No. and %	Duration of response (months) Mean±SEM	Median
Remission	26	6.5±0.8	5.5
Stable disease	10	7.8±0.6	7
Progression	64	-	-

failed to benefit from 5-drug chemotherapy.

3.4 Survival

Survival from the onset of metastasis in all patients
ranged between 9 and 148+ months (median 36 months,
mean±SEM: 40.2±4.2). There was no significant difference
in survival between patients who responded to or failed
5-drug chemotherapy (43±4 vs 35±6 months respectively).
However, when the data are analyzed according to response
to endocrine therapy one can appreciate a significant
prolongation of survival in patients responding to these
treatments (table 5). In this current series of patients
treated with 5-drug chemotherapy, patients who responded
to tamoxifen survived significantly longer (p = 0.03)
than those who did not irrespective of response to subsequent treatment. We have recently published (8) a
detailed summary of long term follow up of the initial
113 patients treated with tamoxifen and subsequently with

TABLE 5. Survival in women with breast cancer in
          relation to response to endocrine therapy

	Responders*	Failures†	ER negative
Total number	46	25	32
Survival (months) mean±SEM median	51.9±4.1 50	29.1±2.9 24	24.1±3.1 22
p value††		0.006	0.0046

*   Patients who responded to ≥one endocrine therapy.
†   Patients who did not respond to ≥2 endocrine treat-
    ments.
†† As compared to responders.

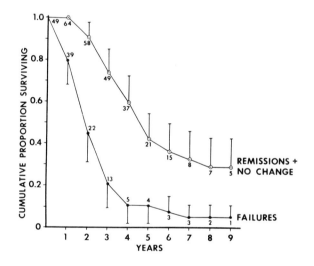

FIGURE 1   Life table plots of survival from the onset of

metastasis for patients who benefited from and those who

failed to respond to tamoxifen.   p<0.001 (generalized

Wilcoxon test).   Bars indicate 2SE.   Reproduced from

Breast Cancer Research and Treatment (1981) 1: 97-103,

with permission.

other endocrine treatments or chemotherapy. Figure 1 summarizes the survival data on those patients. It is apparent that patients who obtained palliation from anti-estrogen therapy lived significantly longer than those who failed to benefit from that treatment.

4. DISCUSSION

Our data show that the modified Cooper regimen utilized here provided excellent palliation to women with advanced breast carcinoma. The regimen was well tolerated by patients and the side effects were easily controlled with antiemetics and appropriate reduction in the doses of drugs administered. Reports on several clinical trials utilizing different combinations of cytotoxic drugs (3-5) have shown a response in one half to two-thirds of patients. Our data compare favorably with those reported in the literature. We have utilized Adriamycin as a single agent after 5-drug chemotherapy and as our data show, we were able to obtain significant palliation in approximately one-third of the patients regardless of their previous response to 5-drug chemotherapy. Some clinical studies (5,9) have indicated that regimens using Adriamycin in combination may be superior to those utilizing various combinations of cyclophosphamide, methotrexate, 5FU and vincristine. However, it remains to be established whether it is more advantageous to use Adriamycin initially in combination

416

with other drugs or as a follow-up treatment after the
5-drug combination regimen.

Of particular interest in our study was the relationship between response to chemotherapy and previous endocrine therapy. Our data show that the combination chemotherapy was effective in patients who responded to and
those who failed endocrine treatments. This is in agreement with other series in the literature (10,11). The
value of ER level in the tumor in predicting response to
hormone therapy is well established. In contrast, the
value of ER in predicting response to chemotherapy
remains controversial. Whereas Lippman et al. (12)
found a significantly lower response rate to chemotherapy
in patients with ER-positive tumors, Kiang et al. (11)
reported data to support a completely opposite conclu-
sion--that is, patients with ER rich tumors had a higher
response rate to chemotherapy than those who had receptor
poor tumors. The reason for this discrepancy is not
apparent at the present time. In our experience the
response rate to chemotherapy was similar in patients
with ER positive or negative tumors.

One group of patients in our series, namely those
with hormone responsive tumors, deserves a special comment. This represents a favorable group of patients who
responded to several endocrine treatments before being
treated with combination chemotherapy. With the sequential use of optimal treatments (endocrine and chemo-

therapy) these patients obtained significantly longer remissions and survival. It is remarkable that in this group of patients and with the sequential use of treatments the median survival after the onset of metastasis was greater than 4 years. Our approach in treating patients with metastatic breast cancer is to try to obtain maximal benefit from sequential endocrine therapies before introducing cytotoxic chemotherapy unless the patient has an ER-negative tumor or advanced liver metastasis. Endocrine treatments are more readily acceptable and well tolerated by the patients. The question that may arise is whether it would be more beneficial to use chemotherapy in conjunction with endocrine therapy rather than sequentially. The answer is not available at the present time, but can be approached through a large prospective, randomized study.

ACKNOWLEDGEMENT

The authors wish to thank all referring physicians. The help and support of the staff of the Oncology Center is greatly appreciated.

REFERENCES

1. Manni A, Trujillo JE, Marshall JS, et al. (1979) Antihormone treatment of stage IV breast cancer. Cancer 43: 444-450.

2. Cooper RG (1969) Combination chemotherapy in hormone resistant breast cancer. Proc Am Assoc Cancer Res 10:15.

3. Canellos GP, DeVita VT, Gold LG, et al. (1976) Combination chemotherapy for advanced breast cancer: response and effect on survival. Ann Intern Med 84: 389-392.

4. Kennealey GT, Boston B, Mitchell MS, et al. (1978) Combination chemotherapy for advanced breast cancer. Two regimens containing Adriamycin. Cancer 42: 27-33.

5. Smalley RV, Carpenter J, Bartolucci A, et al. (1977) A comparison of cyclophosphamide, Adriamycin, 5-fluorouracil (CAF) and cyclophosphamide, methotrexate, 5-fluorouracil, vincristine, prednisone (CMFVP) in patients with metastatic breast cancer. A Southeastern Cancer Study Group Project. Cancer 40: 625-632.

6. Manni A, Trujillo JE, Pearson OH (1980) Sequential use of endocrine therapy and chemotherapy for metastatic breast cancer; effects on survival. Cancer Treat Rep 64: 111-116.

7. McGuire WL, DeLaGarza M (1973) Improved sensitivity in the measurement of estrogen receptor in human breast cancer. J. Clin Endocrinol Metab 37: 986-989.

8. Manni A, Pearson OH, Marshall JS, Arafah BM (1981) Sequential endocrine therapy and chemotherapy in metastatic breast cancer: effects on survival. Breast Cancer Res Treat 1: 97-103.

9. Muss HB, White DR, Richards F II, et al. (1978) Adriamycin versus methotrexate in five-drug combination chemotherapy for advanced breast cancer. A randomized trial. Cancer 42: 2141-2148.

10. Henderson MD, Buroker TR, Samson MK, et al. (1975) Responses of patients with carcinoma of the breast to hormonal therapy and combination chemotherapy. Surg Gynecol Obstet 141: 232-234.

11. Kiang DT, Frenning DH, Goldman AI, et al. (1978) Estrogen receptors and responses to chemotherapy and hormonal therapy in advanced breast cancer. N Engl J Med 299: 1330-1334.

12. Lippman ME, Allegra JC, Thompson EB, et al. (1978) The relation between estrogen receptors and response rate to cytotoxic chemotherapy in metastatic breast cancer. N Engl J Med 298: 1223-1228.

Fluoropyrimidines in Cancer Therapy
K. Kimura, S. Fujii, M. Ogawa, G.P. Bodey, P. Alberto, eds.

A COMBINATION OF TEGAFUR AND TAMOXIFEN FOR ADVANCED BREAST CANCER

Hiroki Koyama and Tomio Wada

1. INTRODUCTION

    Chemo-endocrine therapy has been attracting much attention recently as a new modality for advanced breast cancer (7,9). Most trials, however, deal with combinations of tamoxifen and massive multiple drug chemotherapy. Patients with metastatic breast cancer are usually obliged to receive the treatment for a long period. To improve quality of life in these patients, effective treatment on an outpatient basis is urgently required. In an attempt to establish a standard chemo-endocrine regimen for ambulatory patients, we combined tamoxifen and tegafur, both of which are characterized by moderate response rates and mild toxicities.

    This article presents the results of a sequential study comparing the effects of tamoxifen alone and tamoxifen plus tegafur in advanced breast cancer.

2. MATERIALS AND METHODS

    A total of 123 patients with primary advanced or recurrent breast cancer were entered in this study during the 7 year period between 1976 ~ 1982. All had objectively evaluable lesions and were judged able to tolerate the treatment on an outpatient basis from their acceptable performance status (Ps 0 ~ 3). The trial was designed as a sequential study. During the first $2^1/_2$ years 45 consecutive patients were treated with tamoxifen alone (TAM). During the second $4^1/_2$ years 70 consecutive patinets received tamoxifen and tegatur simultaneously (TAM + TF). Tamoxifen was given in a daily oral dose of 20mg (10mg bid) and tegafur in a daily oral dose of 600mg (200mg tid). The treatments were continued for at least 12 weeks.

Routine laboratory tests and chest radiography, if necessary, were done every 4 weeks. Lesions were evaluated every 2 ~ 4 weeks during the visits of the patients to our clinic. Eight patients were excluded from the study because of protocol violation or for socioeconomic reasons, leaving 115 patients that were eligible for further analysis. Background factors of these patients are shown in Table 1.

TABLE 1   Background factors in patients studied

Regimen	TAM	TAM + TF
No. of patients	45	70
Age (mean)	36 ~ 67 (57.4)	36 ~ 75 (55.6)
Menstruation		
Premenopausal	21	23
Postmenopausal	24	47
Dominant site of lesion		
Soft tissue	23	32
Bone	12	20
Viscera	10	18
Estrogen receptor		
Positive	14	19
Negative	16	16
Unknown	15	35
Prior therapy		
Not given	18	22
Given	27	48

3.   RESULTS

The overall response rate (CR + RR) was 28.9% for TAM and 38.6% for TAM + TF as shown in Table 2.   TAM + TF was characterized by the higher CR rate of 12.8%.

TABLE 2 Overall response rate

Regimen		TAM	TAM + TF
No. of patients		45	70
Responder	CR	2 (4.4) ⌝	9 (12.8) ⌝
		(28.8)	(38.6)
	PR	11 (24.4) ⌟	18 (25.7) ⌟
Non-responder	NC	14 (31.1) ⌝	24 (34.2) ⌝
		(71.1)	(61.4)
	PD	18 (40.0) ⌟	19 (27.1) ⌟

( ): %

Table 3 illustrates the response rate according to dominant site of lesions. The response rate in soft tissue and bone did not show much difference between the two groups. But in visceral lesions, the majority of which were pulmonary metastases, there was no responder in 10 patients receiving TAM while 7 out of 18 patients responded to TAM + TF, including 5 patients with CR.

TABLE 3   Response rate by dominant site of lesion

Regimen	TAM	TAM + TF
Soft tissue	10/23 (43.5)	16/32 (50.0)
Bone	3/12 (25.0)	4/20 (20.0)
Viscera	0/10 (0)	7/18 (38.9)

( ): %

Table 4 shows the response rate according to meno-pausal status and estrogen receptor (ER) status. In post-menopausal patients, TAM + TF produced a response rate of 44.7%, significantly higher than that with TAM alone (20.0%). In premenopausal patients, however, no improve-ment in favor of TAM + TF was observed.

As is generally accepted, TAM was highly effective in ER-positive patients but much less effective in ER-negative patients. TAM + TF was also more effective in ER-positive patients (63.2%) than in ER-negative (6.3%). Both the groups included a considerable number of ER-unknown patients. These ER-unknown patients showed a relatively high response rate of 40.0% with TAM + TF, which roughly corresponded with the overall response rate of 38.6%.

TABLE 4   Response rate by menopausal status and estrogen
          receptor status

Regimen	TAM	TAM + TF
Premenopausal	8/21 (38.1)	6/23 (26.1)
Postmenopausal	5/24 (20.8)	21/47 (44.7)
Estrogen receptor		
Positive	9/14 (64.3)	12/19 (63.2)
Negative	1/16 (6.3)	1/16 (6.3)
Unknown	3/15 (20.0)	14/35 (40.0)

As to prior therapy given to the patients, TAM + TF
was equally effective regardless of whether they had previously received any anticancer therapy (36.4% response
rate in prior therapy group and 39.5% in no prior therapy
group).

The median interval between the start of treatment
and the onset of PR was 8 weeks for both regimens, as
shown in Table 5.   The duration of response was 10 to 57
weeks with a median of 37 weeks with TAM and 8 to 145 +
weeks with a median of 34 weeks with TAM + TF.   Some patients are still responding to the latter regimen.

TABLE 5   Interval from start of treatment to onset of
          response and duration of response

Regimen	TAM	TAM + TF
Interval to onset of response (median)	4 - 17 (8) weeks	4 - 48 (8) weeks
Duration of response (median)	10 - 57 (37) weeks	8 - 145 + (34) weeks

Survival of the patients was calculated as the period from start of treatment to death, disregarding treatments, if any, subsequent to the present protocol. As shown in Table 6, the median survival with TAM + TF was 48 + months for responders, 24 months for non-responders and 32 months overall. The overall value for TAM + TF was longer than that for TAM (24 months).

TABLE 6   Median survival after start of treatment

Regimen	TAM	TAM + TF
Responder	32 months	48 + months
Non-responder	12 months	24 months
Overall	24 months	32 months

426

Table 7 illustrates the incidence of side effects in the two groups. Some patients receiving TAM alone developed mild gastro-intestinal disorders, but the incidence was very low. No patients on TAM had leukopenia below 3,000 in WBC. With TAM + TF, gastro-intestinal disorders occurred in 20.0% and leukopenia in only 5.7%. Liver dysfunction, defined as elevation to 100 or higher of either GOT or GPT, occurred in only 5.7%. No patient on either regimen had to discontinue taking the drugs due to their toxicities.

TABLE 7 Side effects

Regimen	TAM	TAM + TF
Nausea, vomiting	5 (11.1)	14 (20.0)
Leukopenia ($\leq$3,000)	0	4 (5.7)
Liver dysfunction (GOT, GPT $\geq$100)	0	4 (5.7)
Hot flushes	0	1 (1.4)

( ): %

4. DISCUSSION

Breast cancer involves several types of cancer cells. As to the estrogen receptor (ER) status for example, ER-positive tumors contain a certain number of ER-negative

cancer cells, and vice versa (2,4). These findings provide a theoretical basis for combining drugs with different modes of action and for chemo-endocrine therapy. In
clinical studies, however, it still remains controversial
as to whether there is any practical advantage in chemo-
endocrine therapy over chemotherapy alone or over endocrine therapy alone. Tormey et al. (6) reported that the
combination of tamoxifen, adriamycin (ADR) and dibromodulcitol showed a higher response rate and longer duration
of response than did only adriamycin plus dibromodulcitol.
Glick et al. (1) showed that CMF combined with tamoxifen
was more effective than CMF alone. On the other hand,
Link et al. (3) claimed that no definite evidence was
available as to the benefit of chemo-endocrine therapy.

The most characteristic feature of our chemo-
endocrine regimen was that two drugs of mild toxicity,
tamoxifen and tegafur, were combined to treat patients on
an outpatient basis. Tegafur has a response rate of approximately 20% in advanced breast cancer, according to
several publications (8). Side effects of this drug included mild gastro-intestinal disorders and leukopenia.
But bone marrow depression was encountered only rarely
and the safety of this drug for prolonged ambulatory use
had already been established. Tamoxifen used alone was
effective in 20 ~ 30% patients (5,10) and presented only
mild side effects, including gastro-intestinal disorders.

428

In our sequential study, tamoxifen combined with tegafur had a higher overall response rate, a higher CR incidence, and better response in visceral lesions than did tamoxifen alone. The response rate of this regimen was also higher than that of tegafur alone.

The effect of tamoxifen was extremely poor in ER-negative tumors, which are found in about one-half of patients with metastatic breast cancer. We had expected that the addition of tegafur to tamoxifen might improve the response rate in the ER-negative tumors. The results obtained, however, failed to clearly demonstrate such improvement. Since the ER status was unknown in one-half our patients, this problem required further analysis.

The incidence of toxicities in the combined regimen was slightly higher than with tamoxifen or tegafur alone, but was still much lower in comparison to other conventional multiple drug chemotherapies, such as CMF and CAF, which were usually given to inpatients. Therefore, the present regimen proved to be safe and acceptable when given to ambulatory patients for a prolonged period, and it is expected to play an important role as a basic chemo-endocrine regimen in the treatment of breast cancer.

REFERENCES

1. Glick J, Creech RH, Torri S et al. (1980) Tamoxifen plus sequential CMF chemotherapy versus tamoxifen alone in postmenopausal patients with advanced breast cancer: A randomized trial. Cancer 45: 735-741.

2. Leclercq G, Heuson JC, Deboel MC et al. (1975) Oestrogen receptors in breast cancer: A changing concept. Brit Med J 1: 185-189.

3. Link H, Rückle H, Waller HD et al. (1981) Kombinierte Chemo-Antiöstrogen Therapie beim metastasierten Mammakarzinom. Dtsch Med Wsch 106: 1260-1262.

4. Mercer WD, Carlson CA, Wahl TM et al. (1978) Identification of estrogen receptors in mammary cancer cells by immunofluorescence. Am J Clin Path 70: 330.

5. Mouridsen H, et al. (1978) Tamoxifen in advanced breast cancer. Cancer Treat Rev 5: 131-141.

6. Tormey DC, Falkson H, Falkson G et al. (1978) Evaluation of chemotherapy+tamoxifen in breast cancer (abstr). Proc AACR and ASCO 19: 34.

7. Wada T, Koyama H and Terasawa T. (1981) Tamoxifen alone versus tamoxifen plus 1-(2-tetrahydrofuryl)-5-fluorouracil in the treatment of advanced breast cancer: A sequential trial. Breast Cancer Res Treat 1: 53-58.

8. Wada T, Koyama H and Terasawa T. (1981) Recent advances in chemotherapy for advanced breast cancer. Recent Result Cancer Res 76: 315-324.

9. Wada T, Koyama H, Nishizawa Y et al. (1982) A combined chemo-endocrine therapy with tamoxifen, tegafur and cyclophosphamide in a treatment of advanced breast cancer. J Jpn Soc Cancer Ther 17: 2093-2100.

10. Yoshida M, Miura S, Murai H et al. (1980) Clinical evaluation of tamoxifen in advanced breast cancer (primary & recurrent) — Double blind study —. Clin Eval 8: 321-352.

© 1984 Elsevier Science Publishers B.V.
Fluoropyrimidines in Cancer Therapy
K. Kimura, S. Fujii, M. Ogawa, G.P. Bodey, P. Alberto, eds.

A RANDOMIZED COMPARISON OF THREE CHEMOTHERAPY REGIMENS INCLUDING ORAL OR I.V. 5-FLUOROURACIL WITH AND WITHOUT HORMONE TREATMENT IN BREAST CANCER PATIENTS

Pierre Alberto, Kurt W. Brunner, Bernadette Mermillod and Francesco Cavalli

The chemotherapeutic agents most frequently used in the treatment of breast cancer are cyclophosphamide (or another alkylator), methotrexate, 5-fluorouracil (5-FU), adriamycin and vincristine. Various combinations of these agents have been investigated in concurrent or sequential administration schedules. Also, combination chemotherapy has been supplemented with hormonal treatments consisting in prednisone or another glucocorticoid, estrogens, progestins and hormone antagonists. Marginal differences in terms of activity or tolerance have been reported but no treatment emerged as significantly better.

High dose multidrug treatments may achieve a higher rate of early tumor response, when compared with low dose treatments. However, the influence of higher response rates upon remission duration and patient survival has not been clearly defined. Also the feasibility of a high dose multidrug chemotherapy combined with an hormonal treatment for the whole duration of remission deserve further investigation.

The objective of this study was to compare a concurrent and a sequential combination of chemotherapy and hormonotherapy in breast cancer patients, and to compare chemotherapy programs of different intensities. Results have been, in part, already published elswhere (1,2,3).

MATERIALS AND METHODS

Four hundred and sixty-four patients with measurable
advanced breast cancer were entered. No patient had a
previous chemotherapy or hormonal treatment. Patients with
brain metastases, serum creatinine of 1.5 mg/ dl or more
and serum bilirubin of 3 mg/dl or more were excluded.
Osteoblastic bone metastases and malignant effusions were
not accepted as measurable lesions. Before randomization,
patients were stratified according to menopausal status
and prognostic factors. All patients were randomized to
receive either chemotherapy and hormonal treatment concurrently (group A) or hormonal treatment alone, followed
by chemotherapy after 6 to 8 weeks in case of no response
(group B). In this latter group, the same chemotherapy was
administered in case of tumor relapse following a response
to the hormonal treatment. In treatment groups A and B,
patients were also randomized to receive one of three
chemotherapy schedules shown in table 1. Regimen I was a
mild treatment with oral 5-FU, methotrexate, chlorambucil
and prednisone during 2 weeks with 2-week rest periods.
Regimen II was a cyclic 4-week treatment with intravenous
5-FU and vincristine alternating with oral chlorambucil
and methotrexate. In regimen II prednison was given un-
interrupted orally, starting with 30 mg/sq.m. daily,
progressively reduced to 7.5 mg/sq.m. daily. Regimen III
was an alternating treatment of two 2-week cycles with
oral chlorambucil and predison and intravenous 5-FU and
methotrexate in one cycle and adriamycin alone in the
other cycle. In case the treatment was to be given for
longer than 6 months, a 4-week rest period was introduced
between each cycle after the sixth month. Adriamycin was
discontinued when the total dose reached 450 mg/sq.m.
Patients older than 65 years or with extensive bone metastases had reduced dosages for adriamycin (40 mg/sq.m.),

5-FU (400 mg/sq.m.) and methotrexate (30 mg/sq.m.) in regimen III. Dose reduction or suppression was provided in case of toxicity, particularly leukopenia below 2'500 or 4'000 and thrombopenia below 75'000 and 100'000/mm3. Hormonal treatment consisted in surgical ovariectomy in premenopausal patients and tamoxifen, 20 mg daily orally, in postmenopausal patients.

TABLE 1   Chemotherapy regimens

I	CLB	5	mg/m2/D	D	1-14	p.o.	
	MTX	10	mg/m2/W	D	1+8	p.o.	Q 4 WKS
	5-FU	500	mg/m2/W	D	1+8	p.o.	
	PDN*	30	mg/m2/D	D	1-14	p.o.	
II	CLB	5	mg/m2/D	D	1-14	p.o.	
	MTX	15	mg/m2/W	D	1-3, 8-10	p.o.	
	PDN*	30	mg/m2/D	D	1-28	p.o.	Q 4 WKS
	5-FU	500	mg/m2/W	D	15+22	i.v.	
	VCR	1.2	mg/m2/w	D	15+22	i.v.	
III	CLB	5	mg/m2/D	D	1-14	p.o.	
	MTX	40	mg/m2/W	D	1+8	i.v.	
	5-FU	600	mg/m2/W	D	1+8	i.v.	Q 8 WKS
	PDN*	30	mg/m2/D	D	1-14	p.o.	
	ADM	60	mg/m2	D	28	i.v.	

* Dose of prednison progressively reduced to 7.5 mg/m2/D in subsequent cycles.

The tumor response was defined at the time of maximum tumor regression. Responses were classified in 5 categories. Progression, stabilisation, partial and complete

response correspond to the WHO tumor response criteria
(4). Minor responses were measurable responses of less
than 50% but more than 25%. Survival and time to progression were calculated from the first day of treatment.
Actuarial survival curves were computed according to
Kaplan and Meyer. The statistical significance of comparisons of actuarial curves was performed with the "logrank
test", the Mantel-Cox test and the generalized Wilcoxon
test. The least significant result was selected. The
median observation time from onset of treatment was longer
than 5 years.

RESULTS

Four hundred and fifteen patients were accepted for
evaluation. Fourty-nine patients were rejected : 7 were
not eligible, and 42 were unevaluable because of insufficient documentation, major protocol violation or early
death. Concerning hormonal treatment alone, 12 of 54
premenopausal patients had a partial tumor response within
6 to 8 weeks, and 8 further patients showed a minor response. In 145 postmenopausal patients receiving tamoxifen
alone 25, or 17% were considered as partial responders in
the first 6 to 8 weeks and 21 (14%) as minor responders.
All other evaluable patients were changed to the randomized chemotherapy program after this first phase of treatment. Seventeen patients showed a second remission among
40 patients with primary response to the hormonal treatment. From the 109 patients having received chemotherapy
after primary failure of ovariectomiy or tamoxifen, 57
(52%) had either a partial or a minor response. The median
overall survival was significantly influenced by the
initial response to the hormonal treatment. The median
survival was 43.4 months for partial responders, 36.1
months for stable disease and 16.1 months for initial

disease progression (p = 0.0001).

A comparison of treatment groups A and B in terms of response rate and survival shows no statistically significant differences. The overall response rate was 46% in group A and 43% in group B for premenopausal patients, 40% in group A and 33% in group B for postmenopausal patients. The median survival time was in premenopausal patients 25.3 months in group A and 21.0 months in group B, in postmenopausal patients 23.7 in group A and 27.5 in group B. A significant difference was observed in postmenopausal low-risk patients between group B (40 months) and group A (21.8 months) with a p value of 0.003.

A direct comparison of the 3 chemotherapy regimens is available in treatment group A where the patients had no previous therapy. Of the 216 evaluable patients, 74 were allocated to regimen I, 70 to regimen II and 72 to regimen III. In premenopausal patients, ovariectomy was performed within 10 days prior to the onset of chemotherapy. In postmenopausal patients, tamoxifen was initiated concurrently with the drug combination. Table 2 shows the characteristics of the evaluable patients. The tumor responses are shown in table 3. The response rate was 32% only with the low dose oral regimen, 52% and 54% with the two alternating regimens in groups II and III. The difference between regimen I and regimens II and III together is highly significant (p = 0.0001). Considering complete responses the difference is still significant, with 10% for regimen I and 20% respectively 21% for regimens II and III. Concerning the influence of prognostic factors upon response rate for regimen I and regimens II + III, a significantly higher response rate was observed with regimens II + III in postmenopausal patients, patient with high risk disease, poor performance status and

TABLE 2   Characteristics of the 216 evaluable patients
with concurrent hormono- and chemotherapy

	treatment group		
	I	II	III
Median age (years)	57.9	57.2	57.6
Median free interval (months)	28	21	29
N. premenopausal pts	20	18	20
N. postmenopausal pts	54	52	52
N. high-risk pts	21	17	17
N. low-risk pts	53	53	55
N. of metastatic lesions :			
1	20	21	24
2	31	27	24
3 or more	23	22	24
Performance status :			
0 - 1	51	47	48
2 - 4	23	23	24
Site of metastases			
- local	4	7	4
- skeletal	13	10	13
- local + pleural	3	2	1
- local + skeletal	12	10	11
- visceral + local	11	8	8
- visceral + skeletal	21	27	26
- visceral only	10	6	9

visceral metastases. The superiority in postmenopausal
patients is related to the higher response rate in patients 60 or more years old. Regimens II + III was also
significantly superior for patients with 2 tumor sites,

TABLE 3   Tumor response according to treatment group

TREATMENT	CR	PR	MR	NC	PD
			in %		
I	10	22	13	24	31
II	20	32	22	16	10
III	21	33	19	19	8

Distribution of results among the 3 treatments: p = 0.005
Distribution of results II vs III: p = n.s.
Distribution of results I vs (II+III): p < 0.001

and a free interval of 12 to 60 months. The median time to disease progression was 19.6 months for all patients with a complete or partial response. This result was similar in the three regimens : 20.5 months for I, 18.5 for II and 19.5 for III. The median survival time was 23.5 months for regimen I, 27 months and 30 months for regimens II and III (p = 0.003). Comparing pre and postmenopausal patients the values were 26 and 25.5months. In the postmenopausal group, where the number of observations is sufficient for statistical comparison there is also a significant difference between regimen I and regimens II + III. Table 4 summarizes the influence of pronostic factors upon survival for regimens I and II + III. A statistically significant advantage for the more intensive regimens was observed for postmenopausal patients, and again particularly those of 60 or more years, patients with poor performance status, visceral lesions, particularly in the liver, 2 tumor sites or a free interval of 12 months or longer. The survival is shorter with regimen I in both risk-groups, although this difference is significant at the level of 0.005 in the low-risk group only.

TABLE 4   Influence of prognostic factors upon median
           survival (in months) in patients treated with
           different regimens

	I	II+III	p.value
Premenopausal	26	25	n.s.
Postmenopausal	17	28.5	0.018
Low-risk	26	31	0.043
High-risk	19.5	27	n.s.
N. of sites: 1	28.5	33	n.s.
2	13.5	25	0.02
$\geqslant$ 3	15	26	n.s.
Performance status: 0-1	27.5	33.5	n.s.
2-4	13	22.5	0.002
Age (years): $\leqslant$ 50	25	26	n.s.
50-60	18	19	n.s.
$\geqslant$ 60	19	33	0.03
Free interval (months): 0-12	16.5	19	n.s.
12-60	25	33.5	0.05
$\geqslant$ 60	17.5	32.5.	0.04
Site of metastases:			
osseous only	28	31	n.s.
osseous + local	26.5	30.5	n.s.
visceral + local	8	21.5	0.05
osseous + visceral	12	22	n.s.
liver (dominant)	7	20.5	0.004
lung (dominant)	16	32.5	0.03

The median survival was 51.5 months for patients with complete response, 38 months for partial response, 17 and 18 months for stable disease and minor response and less than 8 months for progressive disease. The longest median survival was observed in patients older than 60 years and the shortest in those 50 to 60 years. This difference is also significant (p = 0.05).

The overall tolerance was good in the three chemotherapy treatment groups. Non-hematological toxicity was mild and never dose limiting. Alopecia was negligible, neurological toxicity rare and mild and cardiac toxicity absent. Table 5 summarizes the myelosuppression elicited by the three regimens I, II and III in treatment goup A. As expected, regimen I was significantly less myelotoxic than II and III.

TABLE 5   Hematologic toxicity according to chemotherapy

Chemotherapy	grade of hematologic toxicity*		
	0	1	2
Regimen I	29 %	51 %	20 %
Regimen II	13 %	48 %	39 %
Regimen III	8 %	47 %	45 %
	I vs (II+III) $p < 0.001$		

* grade 0 : Leukocytes $> 4000/mm3$, Platelets $> 100'000/mm3$
  grade 1 : Leukocytes $2500-4000/mm3$,
           Platelets $75'000-100'000/mm3$
  grade 2 : Leukocytes $< 2500/mm3$, Platelets $< 75'000/mm3$

DISCUSSION

This study compared tumor response, survival and tolerance in patients with advanced breast cancer treated
with a concurrent or sequential combination of a hormonal
manipulation and chemotherapy regimens of different intensities. The difference of intensity of chemotherapy was
achieved by differences in dose and route for 5-FU and
methotrexate, and by the adjunction of vincristine and
adriamycin in the alternating schedules. For 5-FU, an oral
weekly dose of 500 mg/sq.m. is particularly low. This
suggests that the superior activity observed with the more
intensive regimens is not completely explained by the
adjunction of adriamycin or vincristine but also, at least
partially, by a difference in the dose of 5-FU.

Significant differences in the results of different
treatments have been observed for different patients subgroups. Those patients in postmenopausal age and low-risk
category obtain a longer survival if they are treated with
tamoxifen alone until hormonal failure, and then with
chemotherapy. For the low-risk patients the more intensive
chemotherapy regimens does not produce superior response
rates, although this absence of visible difference may be
due to the relatively low number of observations.

Patients with an isolated recurrent tumor site, a good
performance status, an age between 50 and 60 years and
either a very short or very long free interval do not draw
a significant benefit from a more intensive, and more
toxic chemotherapy. This is also true for patients with
bone metastases only, corresponding in general to a disease category of slow progression. On the contrary, patients with high-risk disease, visceral lesions, poor performance status and an intermediate disease free interval
should be treated with an intensive treatment, even if the
toxicity will eventually be more severe.

These findings emphasize the importance of major pronostic factors (menopausal status, performance status, age, free interval, site of metastatic disease and tumor load including number and volume of tumor localisations) in the definition of the best treatment to be applied. Our results also show that the overall value of combined hormono- and chemotherapy is still limited in the treatment of breast cancer, with a response rate just superior to 50%, and only 20% of complete response. In terms of survival time however, the differences between patient with responsive or non-responsive tumor is more encouraging. The results of our study strongly emphasize the need for more active agents in the treatment of breast cancer.

REFERENCES

1. Cavalli F, Beer M, Martz G, et al. (1982) Gleich-
    zeitige oder sequentielle Hormono/Chemotherapie
    sowie Vergleich verschiedener Polychemotherapien
    in der Behandlung des metastasierenden Mammakar-
    zinoms. Schweiz med Wschr 112: 774-783.

2. Cavalli F, Beer M, Martz G, et al. (1983) Concur-
    rent or sequential use of cytotoxic chemotherapy
    and hormone treatment in advanced breast cancer:
    report of the Swiss Group for Clinical Cancer
    Research. Brit Med J 286: 5-8.

3. Cavalli F, Pedrazzini A, Martz G, et al. (1983)
    Randomized trial of 3 different regimens of combi-
    nation chemotherapy in patients receiving simulta-
    neously a hormonal treatment for advanced breast
    cancer. To be published.

4. WHO (1979) WHO handbook for reporting results of
    cancer treatment. World Health Organization,
    WHO, Geneva.

Fluoropyrimidines in Cancer Therapy
K. Kimura, S. Fujii, M. Ogawa, G.P. Bodey, P. Alberto, eds.

PREOPERATIVE CHEMOTHERAPY WITH TEGAFUR FOR INFLAMMATORY BREAST CANCER

Nadezhda G. Blokhina

It is a well-known fact that the inflammatory form of breast cancer takes a special place among other forms of cancer of this site.

There are very few literary data on special clinical trials concerning treatment of this form of breast cancer in spite of a great number of publications reflecting the problem of treatment of breast cancer in general.

Poor prognosis is a typical peculiarity of the inflammatory form of breast cancer that is determined by the extensive local diffusion of the tumor, by the lesion of the lymphatic system both of the gland and beyond its limits, by different lymphatic collectors' metastatic spreading from the unilateral side and to contralateral areas. Therefore, treatment of this patients' contingent is a complicated problem and it requires multicomponent therapy, separate stages of which are carried out in different sequence and considerably differs from common standard methods of treatment. The choice of treatment methods, sequence of application for all available agents are accomplished as a rule with individual approach to evaluation and assessment of the local and general patient status. The refusal from surgical treatment at the first stage is a general trend in these patient treatment. However, there is an opinion that the patients with the inflammatory form of breast cancer must be treated by conservative methods only, including irradiation, drug and hormonal therapy.

There are data in literature showing the effect of conservative treatment with 5-year survival rate, which makes 30% in application of X-ray and drug therapy, using cyclophosphamide, adriamycin and 5-fluorouracil. This result of treatment can be achieved only in patients older than 50 years (1). Hormonotherapy application, based on the study of hormonal receptors, had slightly improved the result of treatment.

X-ray therapy only allows to achieve partial or complete tumor regression but then relapse appears rapidly and the average duration of life does not exceed 18 months (2). Drug therapy in combination with hormonotherapy allows to achieve a therapeutic effect in 38% of patients with the average life duration, 24-36 months. Drug therapy with subsequent surgical treatment increases life duration to 45-49 months (3). The resection of the remained tumor after effective preoperative treatment should be considered appropriate based on presented material. Thus literature testifies the fact of the absence of a general point of view concerning the treatment of patients with the inflammatory form of breast cancer. The necessity of application of treatment measures in complex is doubtless and from our point of view this complex must include surgical treatment.

X-ray or drug therapy can be used as preoperative treatment. Each of these two types of treatment has its positive and negative sides.

Preoperative X-ray therapy gives good therapeutic effect directly only on tumor lesion and thus does not influence distant metastases, which often have the stage when they are cannot be differentiated with the help of the existing diagnostic methods. Besides, after the full course of X-ray therapy it is necessary to wait for 3-4 weeks for the surgical stage of treatment to be carried out. X-ray therapy causes serious complications one of which is pneumosclerosis. Distant metastases can appear in interval before an operation. Healing of operative wound is often complicated in postoperative period that is also connected with X-ray skin damage.

Preoperative drug therapy possesses general resorptive effect and effect on visible tumor lesions; therefore, the application of antitumor agents as the first stage of treatment is presented more appropriate.

The use of polychemotherapy is most popular in nowadays. Cooper scheme is one of the combinations of drug agents. The scheme of agents including adriamycin is widely used lately. As it is known Cooper scheme has side effect that delays surgical stage of treatment in some of cases. Meanwhile the application of a single effective drug gives the same antitumor effect without serious complications. Tegafur refers to such kinds of drugs. All Union Cancer Research Center, AMS, USSR has an experience in application of tegafur for conducting of the first stage of treatment in complex therapy of the inflammatory form of breast cancer but this type of treatment was not the subject of a special clinical trial and was carried out without randomization.

At the same time the patients with the above-mentioned form of breast cancer received X-ray therapy on the first stage and part of patients received drug therapy according to Cooper scheme. In present report we tried to analyze the result of treatment in 2 groups of patients, who received tegafur or irradiation on the first stage of treatment. Treatment of patients according to Cooper scheme was carried out on special protocol, therefore, this group of patients is not included in this report. Thus, we discuss 17 patients operated on at the second stage of combination treatment and who received tegafur or irradiation at the first stage.

Age range of patients was within 22-68 years. The average age of the patients was 54-55 years. All 17 patients did not have complicated anamnesis - the absence of breast cancer in near relatives. Two patients had no pregnancy and labors. The rest patients had 1 or 2 children. They gave suck from 3 to 12 months. Duration of the disease to the first consultation of a doctor was 2-6 months. The overwhelming number of patients revealed small breast induration themselves firstly, limited area of hyperemia in the zone of induration and small edema. Because of lack of pain they did not consult a doctor at once. They consulted a doctor with growing of mentioned disorders.

Metastases into lymphatic nodes of the axillary region from the unilateral side were revealed in all 17 patients by the moment of their consulting in All Union Cancer Research Center, AMS, USSR. Two patients out of 17 also had metastases in supraclavicular region on the side of the primary lesion and one patient had crossed metastasis into lymph nodes of axillary region.

Metastatic formations of supraclavicular region and crossed metastasis of axillary region were verified by the data of cytologic trial of punctate.

Eight patients out of the whole number (17 persons) received preoperative X-ray therapy including 2 patients with metastases in supraclavicular region.

Nine patients received preoperative therapy with tegafur including a patient who had crossed metastasis in axillary region.

Evaluation of therapeutic effect (decreasing of

visible tumor lesions by 50% and more) was carried out after cessation of the first stage of treatment and then the second stage of treatment - mastectomy with axillary and infrascapular lymphoadenectomy was accomplished. After histological examination of the tumor and determination of hormonal receptors the treatment was supplemented with ovariectomy and subsequent chemohormonotherapy.

Preoperative treatment as irradiation was carried out with several zones on the first lesion (on mammary region-4500 Grey) of lymph drainage zone in 3-3500 Grey. Single dose - 2 Gr. Such doses of irradiation can give therapeutic effect without serious postradial complications.

The next stage of treatment - mastectomy was carried out 3 weeks later.

Preoperative chemotherapy with tegafur was carried out according to the following methods - single dose 1.2 mg (in 2 or 30 mg/kg - 1,6-2,4 to 3 gr). The drug was given intravenously. Daily dose was divided in 2 parts and was given with an interval in 12 hours. The total dose was 26-40 gr. The treatment was stopped due to the appearance of insignificant side effects, e.g., diarrhea stools 2-3 times a day, or with the achievement of high therapeutic effect. The interval after the cessation of preoperative chemotherapy and between surgical interference was at an average of 3-4 days. Only one

patient was operated on 2 weeks later because of
moderate leukopenia (to 3500 in 1 mm^3) which was
accompanied with catarrhal symptoms in the upper
respiratory tract. Preoperative chemotherapy was
carried out without serious complications in 8 patients
of this group; therefore, surgical treatment was carried
out without delay.

TABLE 1   Number of patients and method of treatment

Methods	Number of patients
Preoperative X-ray therapy	8
Preoperative chemotherapy	9
Mastectomy	17
Ovariectomy	5*
CMF chemotherapy postoperatively	17
CMF chemohormonotherapy**	17**
Tamoxifen	

*   2 patients received preoperative irradiation out of 5
    patients who received ovariectomy because of the
    presence of positive receptors of steroid hormones
    and 3 patients - chemotherapy with tegafur.
** 5 patients out of the whole general number of
    patients received treatment with tamoxifen in
    addition to chemotherapy.

The estimation of direct effect was carried out
after the cessation of preoperative treatment.

Immediate results according to methods of treatment
are presented in Table 2.

As it is seen from the table immediate results of
treatment is practically the same in both methods of
treatment. One patient treated with tegafur achieved
complete tumor regression.

TABLE 2 Immediate results according to methods of treatment

Method of treatment	Complete regression 50%	Partial regression 50%	Partial regression
Preoperative irradiation	-	3	5
Preoperative chemotherapy	1	5	3
Total	1	8	8

Taking into account that severe irradiation of mammary gland results into radiation damage the evaluation of treatment effect is much more difficult than that one of chemotherapy treatment, therefore, this estimation is of rather relative character. It should be pointed out that therapy effect was evaluated in both the primary lesion and metastases..

TABLE 3 Number of metastatic lymph nodes and method of preoperative treatment

Method of treatment	Metastases to lymph nodes of axillary region					Metastases to lymph nodes of subscapular region				
Number of metastatic lymph nodes	2	3	4	5	>5	2	3	4	5	>5
Preoperative irradiation	3	2	-	3	-	1	-	-	-	-
Preoperative chemotherapy	-	3	-	4	2	1	-	-	-	-

The final estimation of treatment effect was carried out according to the survival and relapse-free time.

Morphologic analysis of preparation was carried out after surgical treatment. The data are presented in Table 4.

TABLE 4

Method of treatment	Morphological type of tumor		
	Solid and solid-gland-dular	Medular	Skirrous
Preoperative irradiation	2	4	2
Preoperative chemotherapy	2	4	3

In postoperative period all patients received chemotherapy as CMF combination in which 5-fluorouracil was substituted for tegafur. The treatment included 6 repeated cycles.

Unlike the clinical CMF scheme tegafur was given daily in a single dose 20 mg/kg for 2 weeks.

Five patients in addition received tamoxifen 30 mg per day.

As it was mentioned above the assessment of follow-up results of treatment was carried out according to 2 indexes - survival and relapse-free time.

Therapeutic effect was evaluated according to the method of preoperative treatment after 6 cycles of postoperative chemotherapy.

TABLE 5 The results of combined treatment after accomplishment of the whole complex of therapy (the first year of treatment)

Method of treatment	Results of treatment	
	Complete remission	Partial remission
Preoperative irradiation (8 patients)	5	3
Preoperative chemotherapy (9 patients)	5	4

As can be seen from data represented in Table 5, complete disappearance of all visible tumor lesions was not achieved in all patients; moreover, the results were practically identical and did not depend on character of preoperative therapy. Seven patients out of general number had metastases into lymph nodes, liver and bones, part of which had not been discovered by the beginning of treatment. However, one can suppose that by the beginning of treatment they had already been but could not have been determined with all accessible diagnostic methods. The methods of treatment of all the 7 patients were substituted for the other methods - polychemo-therapy and irradiation.

The survival of patients according to the method of preoperative treatment varied. Better results were achieved in the group of patients receiving preoperative therapy with tegafur. It was found impossible to establish statistical significance of these distinctions because of a limited number of observations.

Comparing the long-term therapeutic results of the inflammatory form of breast cancer using Cooper's scheme in the preoperative period, it appeared that the result was almost the same: 12 out of 21 patients survived for 3 years, 7 of them (33.3%) without signs of relapse and metastases. According to our data 4/9 of patients survived for 3 years and 2/9 (44%) for 4 years.

Summing up the results obtained it should be mentioned that a tendency to an increase of the patient life duration with the inflammatory form of breast cancer was observed with drug therapy at the first stage of treatment. Drug therapy especially in the form of monochemotherapy with tegafur produces a therapeutic effect which is similar to that of polychemotherapy and is devoid of severe side effects.

The use of monochemotherapy as preoperative treatment provides more reserves for subsequent treatment of patients with the inflammatory form of breast cancer.

REFERENCES

1. Victor Lira-Puerto, et al. (1980) Improved survival of inflammatory breast carcinoma with combination chemotherapy and radiotherapy. Proc ASCO (c-351).

2. Krutchik AN, et al (1979) Combined chemoimmuno therapy and radiation therapy of inflammatory breast carcinoma. J Surg Oncol 11: 325-332.

3. Wiseman, et al. (1982) Inflammatory breast cancer treated with surgery, chemotherapy and BCG immuno-therapy. Cancer 49: 1266-1271.

DISCUSSION

Bertino: Dr. Bodey, you discount the high complete response rates in your last study comparing normal and high-intensity chemotherapy. The only variable that I can see there is the five-day infusion of 5-FU. Why don't you think that that change in the way you gave FAC resulted in the higher complete response rate, or do you think that?

Bodey: I think the improvement in the complete remission rate had to do primarily with the more intensive administration of adriamycin-cyclophosphamide. The patients, when they got up to their third course, were getting almost a full dose of each of those drugs. Whether continuous infusion 5-FU contributed or not, I don't really think we can determine from the design of that particular study. What was disappointing was the fact that even though we had a higher complete remission rate, the overall duration of response was no different. That was very discouraging because when we first analyzed these data and saw a better complete remission rate we were quite excited with it. But it didn't really turn out to represent a substantial improvement. One of the problems with that regimen was that it was very difficult to administer maintenance therapy because the patients' bone marrow was compromised by the intensive induction therapy. That probably had contributed to the failure to demonstrate an improvement in the duration of response.

Yan Sun: Why didn't you mention anything about ER negative and positive patients? Did the ER positive patients show better results than ER negative patients?

Bodey: When these studies were done, estrogen receptors were not analyzed regularly.

H. Koyama: You mentioned that being a non-Caucasian was an unfavorable factor for response. Do you have any data showing that non-Caucasians are less responsive to chemotherapy? I raise this question because your FAC regimen response rate would be unexpectedly high in our country. We use FAC according to your regimen, but our obtained response rate was 50% at the most. Therefore, I think there may be racial differences in the responsiveness to chemotherapy.

Bodey: This is a question which is raised not infrequently. As I mentioned when I presented this, I cannot comment on the difference in response between Caucasians and Orientals because the Oriental population in our community is not very large. What we are really looking at is a difference in response rate between Blacks and Caucasians. One of the problems is that as a general rule the Black population is of a lower socio-economic group, and they frequently consult physicians much later on in the course of their disease, and this may be a major factor in their poor response rate. So I am not sure whether this is a genetic difference or whether it reflects the stage of disease at the time of presentation.

Abe: This is quite an enigma, because hormone responsiveness is the same in the United States and Japan, yet the chemotherapy responsiveness is quite different.

Kubo (National Nagoya Hospital, Nagoya): I would like to comment on the discussion between Drs. Bodey and H. Koyama. The difference in the response rate between the two groups - Japanese and American - is, I believe, just because of background factors. The majority of the patients didn't receive any previous systemic treatment, but one-third of Dr. Koyama's patients received previous systemic treatment. That may be the reason. I don't think that genetic factors have much influence on the results of chemotherapy based on my experience in the United States and in Japan.

H. Koyama: In this series we gave a mild chemotherapy and endocrine therapy, so the response rate was naturally low. My previous question concerned another series.

Ogawa: I feel that chemo-endocrine therapy appears to be well established for those patients who are postmenopausal or ER positive. However, for the premenopausal patient, we don't have any appropriate modality of treatment. Therefore, I would like to ask Dr. Alberto about the oophorectomies he performed for hormonal manipulation followed by chemotherapy. I would like to know more details of the results.

Alberto: You must consider that this is a relatively old study, and we stopped doing this in 1975. I am not sure that if we were to start such a study now and we would do it in exactly the same way. I agree with you that the main message from this complicated study with more than 400 patients is that certainly there is no standard treatment for all patients with breast cancer. One has to seriously consider prognostic factors and to select those patients who benefit from a simple hormonal treatment before being engaged in chemotherapy and those patients with poor-risk disease who should be treated from the very beginning with a combination of intensive chemotherapy and hormonal treatment.

H. Koyama: I would like to ask Dr. Blokhina a question. The treatment of breast cancer is a very hard task, not only in Caucasian patients, but also in Japanese patients. I entirely agree with your opinion that preoperative treatment is indispensable for the inflammatory form of breast cancer. Why did you select tegafur as the preoperative chemotherapy? Does it have any advantage over other multiple chemotherapies such as CMF?

Blokhina: We have different kinds of experience in our center. We have tried CMF therapy, Cooper's scheme, and others. We decided to investigate a single drug treatment with tegafur. Before that, we tried 5-FU and in some cases we had good, immediate results. But now we have tried tegafur and we are satisfied with our results, because if the patient develops metastases later on, we have the possibility of using another drug in another combination.

H. Koyama: I am also doing preoperative treatment. I make it a rule to conduct intraarterial chemotherapy, and by this method I obtain 45 months median survival.

Blokhina: We have a similar experience. We tried intravenous and intraarterial infusions. It was a long time ago. We also had good results, but they were only local responses.

Bertino: Dr. Bodey, I was intrigued by your comments about the L-asparaginase and 5-FU. Would you go over again when you gave those two drugs and in what relationship they were given?

Bodey: The L-asparaginase-5-FU relationship? They were given on the same day.

Bertino: I suppose it could have conceivably been that you were intensifying the inhibitory effect on RNA synthesis and maybe protein synthesis. Did you note more L-asparaginase toxicity as well in terms of clotting factor abnormalities?

Bodey: No. There is some disagreement amongst the various people involved in this study as to what was responsible for the excessive toxicity, but my opinion is that it was an interaction between 5-FU and L-asparaginase, because the toxicities were those that are generally seen with 5-FU. We have had experience with other combinations where this toxicity did not occur. There have been some studies where L-asparaginase has aggravated the toxicity of vincristine in childhood leukemia.

Majima: I have just a short comment. There have been a few papers presented in this session about the combination of tamoxifen and fluorinated pyrimidines. Basic studies in vitro have indicated that when we treat with both drugs in cell lines that are ER positive, the accumulation of fluorinated pyrimidines is increased in high molecular weight RNA. So there is the possibility of this combination not only for chemo-endocrine therapy but also intensive chemotherapy cannot be ruled out.

456

Alberto: As with many others, I also have a small series of thirty-five patients with inflammatory breast cancer and initial chemotherapy using a regimen that is definitely less heavy than the one I presented. In this small series, we had 75% response, including 50% complete response measured on the primary tumor. So I completely agree that the selection of patients according to duration of disease and location of tumor site may be responsible for differences in response rate.

Bodey: I think another factor is the intensity of chemotherapy. As you showed in your study and in our review of our large experience we demonstrated that the patients who received less than full-dose chemotherapy or at longer intervals than prescribed did have lower response rates and shorter duration of response. So I think that there is an optimum dosage schedule for each regimen and if that is not utilized then it is likely that the results won't be quite as good. Some of the papers presented here used the doses of adriamycin that were somewhat lower than the doses that we have used. This might possibly account for some of the differences in response rates.

Kubo: I would like to add a comment to the previous comment. I got almost identical response rates with your FAC plus BCG regimen, and I got a 70% response rate with CAMF, which is cyclophosphamide-adriamycin-methotrexate-5-FU. The two series were almost identical in terms of site of disease, age of patient, etc. These results suggest that there is no genetic difference responsible for different responses in Japanese and Caucasian patients.

SURGICAL ADJUVANT CHEMOTHERAPY

© 1984 Elsevier Science Publishers B.V.
Fluoropyrimidines in Cancer Therapy
K. Kimura, S. Fujii, M. Ogawa, G.P. Bodey, P. Alberto, eds.

SURGICAL ADJUVANT CHEMOTHERAPY FOR BREAST CANCER BASED ON EXPERIMENTAL AND CLINICAL STUDIES

Osahiko Abe, Kohji Enomoto, Tetsuro Kubota, Tadashi Ikeda
and Junichi Koh

INTRODUCTION

As an adjuvant therapy for breast cancer, the following condition should be satisfied:

1) To supress the metastasis with minimal side-effect, especially, in early stage, and the fact that breast cancer shows a better prognosis as compared to the other site-specific carcinoma, should be taken into consideration.

2) Adequate effect to prevent metastasis should be expected regardless the stage.

3) Breast cancer is thought to be a generalized disease, that is, metastasis can occur in patients with negative lymph node.

To compromise all these factors, the tentative schedule for adjuvant therapy might be combination of antitumor agent and hormone.

EXPERIMENTAL STUDY

MCF-7 cell line was established by Soul et al. in 1973, which cell was originally obtained from pleural effusion of a premenopausal woman with breast cancer and has been proved to have both estrogen and progesterone receptors. The in vitro doubling time of the tumor cell was 37 hours. Fetal calf serum used in the experiment was treated twice with dextran coated charcoal in order to remove endogenous steroid hormones.

Using MCF-7 cells in culture, the influence of drugs on cell growth was investigated. By using cell count method, it was shown that 40% inhibitory concentration (IC 40) of 5-FU upon cell growth was 0.28 μg/ml, and the concentration of tamoxifen (TAM) was 1.8×10^{-5}M. respectively.

When 5-FU and tamoxifen were used simultaneously, the IC 40 values for 5-FU and tamoxifen were either concentration of 0.01 μg/ml and 4.5×10^{-6}M, or 0.05 μg/ml and 1×10^{-6}M, or 0.1 μg/ml and 1.3×10^{-7}M, respectively.

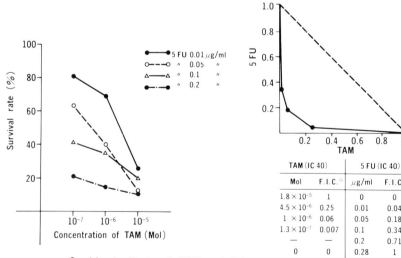

TAM (IC 40)		5 FU (IC 40)	
Mol	F.I.C.*	μg/ml	F.I.C.*
1.8×10^{-5}	1	0	0
4.5×10^{-6}	0.25	0.01	0.04
1×10^{-6}	0.06	0.05	0.18
1.3×10^{-7}	0.007	0.1	0.34
—	—	0.2	0.71
0	0	0.28	1

*F.I.C. = Fractional Inhibitory Concentration

FIGURE 1   Combined effects of TAM and 5FU on the growth of MCF-7 cells

A 40% response isobologram demonstrates graphically the fractional inhibitory concentrations of the two drugs in combination which have resultated in a 40% decrease in cell count. The results indicate a synergistic effect of the two drugs, when analyzed by 40% response on isobologram.

In 1981 in our institution MCF-7 was successfully transplanted into nude mouse which was treated with estradiol dipropionate and progesterone caproate. Since then, it was serially transferred to female nude mice. The experimental model was used for the evaluation of antitumor effects of mitomycin C or tamoxifen alone and their combination. The latter had an effect against MCF-7 in terms of T/C ratio. The administration of mitomycin C alone did not result in a decrease in cytosol estrogen receptor which is required by the additional tamoxifen treatment.

CLINICAL STUDY

The experimental results lead us to design a prospective randomized clinical trial for adjuvant chemoendocrine therapy in patients with primary breast cancer recruited from 25 institutions affiliated with Department of Surgery, School of Medicine, Keio University. All women submitted to mastectomy for primary breast cancer with stage II or III were enrolled in this study during 12 months starting in January 1982.

TABLE 1.   PROTOCOL OF SURGICAL ADJUVANT CHEMO-ENDOCRINE
THERAPY FOR BREAST CANCER

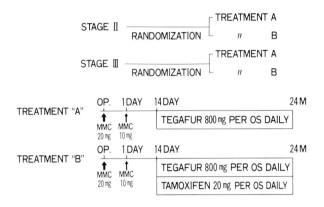

After the patients were stratified according to the
stage of the disease (Stage II or III), they were randomized into two arms either A or B.

A patient assigned to the treatment A is to receive
mitomycin C 20mg per body during operation with addition
of mitomycin C 10mg on the first postoperative day. This
is followed by oral administration of tegafur 800mg per
body daily for a period of two years starting from the
14th day of mastctomy.

In treatment B, the same schedule is taken and is supplemented with tamoxifen in a daily dose of 20mg per body
orally in addition to treatment A.

Two hundred and twenty eight patients were enrolled
in the study, however, thirty eight patients (16.6%) were
excluded due to the violation of protocol of 14 cases
(6.1%) and twenty four ineligible patients (10.5%). The

TABLE 2.   CHARACTERISTICS OF PATIENTS

CHARACTERISTICS	GROUP II-A	GROUP II-B	GROUP III-A	GROUP III-B
Median Age (Range)	47 (26-65)	48 (27-73)	51 (33-76)	53 (27-74)
		(N.S.)		(N.S.)
Menstrual Status				
Pre-menopausal	37	36	16	15
Menopausal	2	2	4	2
Post-menopausal	25	28	10	13
		(N.S.)		(N.S.)
Operation				
Standard	46	50	14	16
Extended	16	12	15	14
Modified	2	4	1	0
		(N.S.)		(N.S.)
Nodal Status				
0	40	37	12	10
1∿3	16	15	8	6
≧ 4	8	14	10	14
		(N.S.)		(N.S.)
Histological Pattern				
Papillotublar	11	9	3	3
Medulary tublar	36	41	21	22
Scirrhous	13	13	5	5
Special type	4	3	1	0
		(N.S.)		(N.S.)
Hormonal Receptor				
ER(+) PgR(+)	14	18	6	7
ER(+) PgR(-)	8	11	4	3
ER(-) PgR(+)	3	0	0	0
ER(-) PgR(-)	12	11	11	9
ER(+)	22	29	10	10
ER(-)	15	11	11	9

figure indicate number of cases

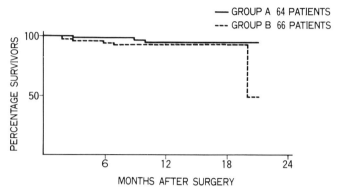

FIGURE 2   SURGICAL ADJUVANT CHEMO-ENDOCRINE THERAPY FOR
BREAST CANCER

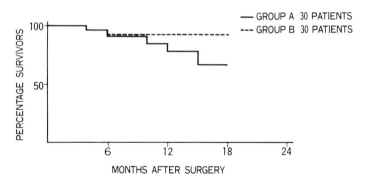

FIGURE 3   SURGICAL ADJUVANT CHEMO-ENDOCRINE THERAPY FOR
BREAST CANCER

190 evaluable patients were assorted into four subgroups:
64 cases in group II-A, 66 in group II-B, 30 in group
III-A and 30 cases in group III-B.

Characteristics of the evaluable patients in the two

treatment arms of stage II and III was shown in table 2. No significant differences were observed in each factor enlisted on the table.

Analysis of disease free survival rate in stage II breast cancer showed no significant differences between group A and B for 20 months after surgery (Figure 2).

Disease free survival rate in stage III revealed no significant difference between Group A and B for a period of 18 months after mastectomy as analized by two tailed generalized Wilcoxan test (Figure 3).

The incidence of 15 recurrent cases were assessed in term of mode of operation (Table 3 and Table 4). Recurrence was observed in ten patients who underwent standard

TABLE 3. SURGICAL ADJUVANT CHEMO-ENDOCRINE THERAPY FOR BREAST CANCER

- LIST OF PATIENTS WITH RECURRENCE OF BREAST CANCER IN THIS STUDY -

CASE	GROUP	AGE	MENOPAUSAL	SURGERY	NODE	ER	PgR	DFI	SITE
C.K	II-A	56	post	extended	0/37	+	-	10	liver
K.T	II-A	55	post	standard	10/11	-	-	9	supraclv
S.S	II-A	46	pre	extended	25/25	-	-	3	bone
M.I	II-B	45	pre	standard	6/9	unknown		20	supraclv
K.S	II-B	47	pre	standard	26/37	-	-	3	local
O.U	II-B	53	post	standard	3/7	+	-	6	bone
Y.S	II-B	55	post	standard	24/26	-	-	2	supraclv
K.H	II-B	65	post	standard	1/9	-	-	7	bone
O.Y	III-A	55	post	extended	7/22	unknown		10	liver
K.S	III-A	43	pre	standard	1/17	+	+	12	breast
N.M	III-A	71	post	extended	69/69	-	-	4	local
K.N	III-A	50	meno	standard	3/6	+	+	15	breast
Y.M	III-A	50	pre	extended	47/47	-	-	6	bone
W.M	III-B	61	post	standard	24/24	unknown		4	supraclv
S.C	III-B	53	post	standard	0/4	-	-	6	colon

Number of DFI (Disease Free Interval) indicates months

TABLE 1. RATE OF RECURRENCE AND BACKGROUND FACTORS

BACKGROUND FACTORS	GROUP II-A	GROUP II-B	GROUP III-A	GROUP III-B
Menstrual Status				
Pre-menopausal	1(2.7)	2(5.6)	2(12.5)	0
Menopausal	0	0	1(25.0)	0
Post-menopausal	2(8.0)	3(10.7)	2(20.0)	2(15.4)
Mode of Operation				
Standard	1(2.1)	5(10.0)	2(14.3)	2(12.5)
Extended	2(12.5)	0	3(20.0)	0
Modifed	0	0	0	0
Nodal Status				
0	1(2.5)	0	0	1(10.0)
1∿3	0	2(13.3)	2(25.0)	0
≧ 4	2(25.0)	3(21.4)	3(30.0)	1(7.1)
Histological Pattern				
Papillo-tubular	2(18.2)	0	0	0
Medullary tubular	1(2.8)	3(7.3)	5(23.8)	1(4.5)
Scirrhous	0	2(15.4)	0	1(20.0)
Special type	0	0	0	0
Hormonal Receptor				
ER(+) PgR(+)	0	0	2(33.3)	0
ER(+) PgR(−)	1(12.5)	1(9.1)	0	0
ER(−) PgR(+)	0	0	0	0
ER(−) PgR(−)	2(16.7)	3(27.3)	2(18.2)	1(11.1)

figure indicate number of cases
( ) indicate per centage

radical mastectomy and five patients with extended radical mastectomy. No recurrence was encountered in group II-B and III-B after extended mastectomy. However no significant difference was found between the two comparable groups. A and B, despite of the stage.

Of the 15 recurrent patients, 13 were positive for lymph node metastasis. With an increase in the number of involved lymph nodes, recurrence tended to be more frequently observed. However, no significant differences were found between the two comparable groups, A and B, regardless of the stage (Table 4).

Surgical adjuvant chemoendocrine therapy is tabulated in terms of recurrence and hormone receptors as shown in the table 4. In group II and III respective overall positivity for estrogen receptor was 66% and 50%. Because of the small number avilable for statistical analysis, no significance can be inferred.

Assessment of relationship between recurrence and histological pattern or recurrence and menopausal status is under way.

In summary, experimental study using MCF-7 which is positive for both estrogen and progesterne receptors showed that the combination of 5-FU and tamoxifen exerted a synergistic action in vitro and that combination of mitomycin C and tamoxifen revealed an additive antitumor action in vivo. The clinical trial using the combination of mitomycin C and tegafur with or without tamoxifen as surgical adjuvant therapy was started.

The fifteen recurrent patients out of 190 cases were found in 18 months follow up without death cases. Although no difference in the rate of recurrence between A and B was found in either stage II and III, it was observed that no recurrence developped in group II-B and group III-B in patients with extended radical mastectomy. Further observation remains to be made to assess the correlation between recurrence and hormonal receptors or menopausal status.

REFERENCE

1. Soule HD, Vazquez JJ, Long A, Albert S and Brennen M. (1983) A human cell line from a pleural effusion derived from a breast carcinoma. Jpn N Cancer Inst 51: 1409-1416.

2. Von S Loewe. (1969) Randbemerkungen zur quantitativen Pharmakologie der Kombinationen. Arzneimittel Forshung 8: 449-456.

3. Kaplan EL and Meier P. (1958) Non-parametric estimation for incomplete observations. J Am Stat Assoc 53: 475-481.

4. Gehan EA. (1965) A generalized Wilcoxan test for comparing arbitrally single censored samples. Biometrika 52: 203-223.

© 1984 Elsevier Science Publishers B.V.
Fluoropyrimidines in Cancer Therapy
K. Kimura, S. Fujii, M. Ogawa, G.P. Bodey, P. Alberto, eds.

ADJUVANT THERAPY IN WOMEN WITH STAGE II BREAST CANCER

Baha'Uddin M. Arafah, Charles A. Hubay, Nahida H. Gordon
Olof H. Pearson, James S. Marshall, William L. McGuire and
Collaborating Investigators

1. INTRODUCTION

Over the past 9 years, we have been conducting a prospective, randomized clinical trial of adjuvant therapy
of stage II breast cancer. The study involved 312 women
with breast cancer who underwent a modified radical mastectomy and who were subsequently stratified according to
the estrogen receptor (ER) status (positive vs negative)
and the number of axillary nodes involved with carcinoma
(1-3 vs $\geq$4 nodes). Following stratification the patients
were randomized to receive one of 3 treatment regimens:
3-drug chemotherapy, chemotherapy plus antiestrogen
(tamoxifen), or chemotherapy plus tamoxifen plus immunotherapy using BCG vaccination. Preliminary data published thus far have shown that the addition of tamoxifen to
chemotherapy significantly prolongs the disease-free
survival of patients with ER-positive tumors (1-3).
Furthermore, the data showed that patients with ER positive tumors survived significantly longer than those with
ER negative tumors regardless of the treatment given.

Supported by NIH Contract CB-23922 (formerly CA-43990).

This report updates the results of this study to 6 years of actuarial analysis. The results confirm the value of ER as an important prognostic factor and the beneficial effect of tamoxifen in patients with ER-positive tumors. In addition, among patients with ER-positive tumors, the study identifies subgroups who are more likely to benefit from antiestrogen therapy. Since the study lacked a control-untreated group, the benefit from chemotherapy could not be assessed adequately.

2. MATERIALS AND METHODS

The details on patient selection, stratification, treatment regimens and follow up have been previously reported (1-3) and will be reviewed briefly here. All patients in this study underwent radical or modified radical mastectomy for primary breast cancer and had histologic evidence of axillary node involvement. ER analyses were performed on all tumors in a single laboratory using the dextran-coated charcoal technique (4). Tumors were considered to be ER-positive if the level was >3 fmol/mg cytosol protein. Seventy-four percent of the tumors were ER positive.

After stratification for ER (positive vs negative) and the number of axillary nodes involved (1-3 vs $\geq$4 nodes) patients were randomized to receive one of 3 modalities of treatment: 1. CMF - chemotherapy, 2. CMF plus tamoxifen, 3. CMF plus tamoxifen and BCG vaccina-

tion. CMF chemotherapy was given in the following regimen: cytoxan (60 mg/m^2) was given orally from day 1
through 14 for each of 12 monthly cycles. Methotrexate
(25 mg/m^2) and 5-fluorouracil, 5FU (400 mg/m^2) were
given intravenously on days 1 and 8 of each cycle. No
chemotherapy was given during the latter two weeks of the
monthly cycle. Tamoxifen was given orally at a dose of
20 mg twice daily for a total of one year. Vaccination
with BCG was given during the second year after completion of one year of chemotherapy and antiestrogen treatment.

Approximately 100 patients were entered into each of
the arms of the study between September 1974 and June
1979. No major differences in the three treatment groups

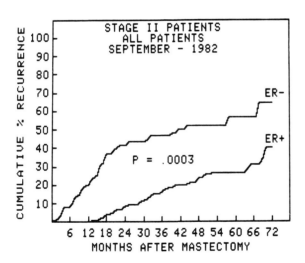

FIGURE 1. Cumulative recurrences for all patients
divided according to ER. ER+, n=234 patients; ER-, n=78
patients.

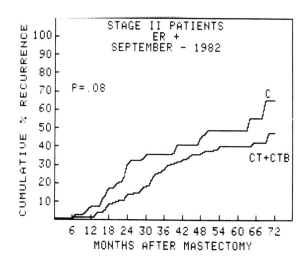

FIGURE 2. Cumulative recurrences in patients with ER-positive tumors divided according to treatments. C: chemotherapy, n=76, T: Tamoxifen, B: BCG vaccination. CT+CTB, n=158.

were observed with respect to patients' age, number of positive nodes, tumor size, ER value and menopausal status. The end point of the study was the time of local recurrence or distant metastasis.

Statistical analysis was performed using a generalization of the Kruskal-Wallis test (5,6) and the generalized Wilcoxon test (7). Furthermore, delay in recurrence was assessed on the basis of quartile analysis (8). Delay in onset of metastasis was obtained whenever at least 25% (first quartile) and possibly 50% (second quartile) of the patients had recurrences in each of the two groups being compared.

TABLE 1.   First and second quartile (in months) of the
            recurrence cumulative distribution function
            of the CMF and CMFT treatment regimens. Delay
            is defined as the difference between the
            quartiles of these two regimens

Group	Quartile	CMF (mos)	CMFT (mos)	Delay (mos)	P* Value
ER+	1	25.2	35.5	10.2	0.024
	2	65.2	>72	>6.8	-
ER+					
1-3 pos. nodes	1	70.0	66.2	-3.8	0.99
4+ pos. nodes	1	21.2	30.3	9.1	0.0034
	2	40.1	49.6	9.4	0.023
ER+					
tumor diameter	1	21.1	30.8	9.7	0.00023
>3cm	2	40.8	>72	>31.2	-
ER+					
premenopausal	1	30.5	39.1	8.6	0.0095
postmenopausal	1	24.2	35.3	11.1	0.0086
	2	50.7	71.4	20.7	<0.000001

* Computed for a one tail test.

3.   RESULTS

The value of ER as an important prognostic factor
was clearly evident (figure 1). Patients with ER negative tumors recurred at a more rapid rate than those with
ER-positive tumors. A similar finding was seen among
the patients treated only with chemotherapy (CMF). There
was no significant difference in recurrence rate between
patients given CMF plus tamoxifen (CMFT) and those given
CMFT plus BCG. Thus the data on these 2 groups have been
pooled and compared with patients treated with CMF alone.
When all patients were included in the analysis, tamoxi-
fen-treated patients tended to recur less rapidly than
those treated with CMF alone, but the difference did not

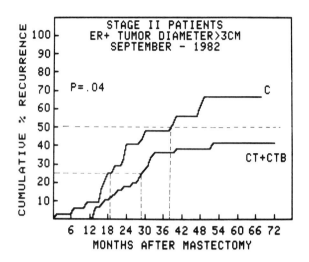

FIGURE 3.   Cumulative recurrences in patients with ER-positive tumors larger than 3 cm divided according to treatments.   C, n=34;   CT+CTB, n=66.

achieve statistical significance (p=0.11).   The beneficial effect of tamoxifen was more apparent when patients with ER positive tumors were evaluated (Figure 2).   When the data were analyzed according to the quartile system, tamoxifen treatment provided a statistically significant increase in disease free survival (table 1).   In contrast tamoxifen treatment did not influence the recurrence rate in patients with ER-negative tumors (p=0.74).   Further analysis of the data revealed that among the ER-positive patients tamoxifen treatment resulted in a significant decrease in recurrence rate in women with large tumors (>3 cm) and those with $\geq$ 4 involved axillary nodes (table 1, figures 3 and 4).   Among women with ER-positive tumors tamoxifen treatment did not influence the recurrence rate

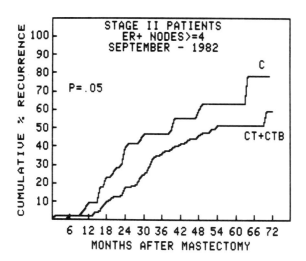

FIGURE 4. Cumulative recurrences in patients with ER-positive tumors who also had >4 involved nodes divided according to treatment. C, n=40; CT+CTB, n=81.

in those who had 1 to 3 nodes involved (table 1). The data were also analyzed according to the menopausal status of the patients. Table 1 clearly shows that both pre- and postmenopausal women with ER positive tumors benefited from tamoxifen treatment. However, when the same data were analyzed according to life table plot analysis, tamoxifen treatment did not result in a significant change in the recurrence rate in premenopausal women (Figure 5) and was of borderline significance (p=0.08) in improving the recurrence rate in postmenopausal women (Figure 6). It is possible that this finding may be due to the fact that a larger number of women were postmenopausal.

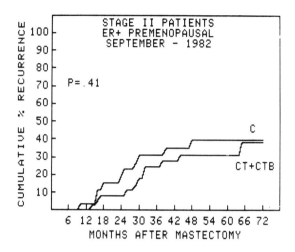

FIGURE 5. Cumulative recurrences in premenopausal women with ER-positive tumors divided according to treatment. C, n=27; CT+CTB, n=37.

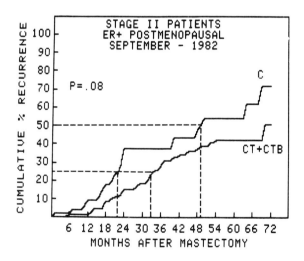

FUGURE 6. Cumulative recurrences in postmenopausal women with ER-positive tumors divided according to treatment. C, n=49; CT+CTB, n=121.

4. DISCUSSION

In 1974, at the outset of this clinical trial of adjuvant therapy, we had hoped to compare patients treated with chemotherapy and/or antiestrogen after surgery to those who did not receive any treatment (i.e., control group) after surgery. However, after the initial promising report by Bonadonna et al. (9) showing the value of CMF adjuvant therapy, we decided to treat all patients with CMF. This left us with no control group to evaluate the value of CMF in our patients. This was early in the study and few patients were affected. The recurrence rate at 5 years was 30% for patients with 1-3 positive nodes and about 65% in those with greater than 4 positive axillary nodes. These recurrence rates are less than what would have been expected if they had received no adjuvant treatment. This suggests that CMF adjuvant therapy had some effect on the disease free interval in our patients.

In long-term studies of patients receiving cytotoxic chemotherapy, there is always a concern for the development of secondary malignancies. Of 312 patients who received adjuvant therapy as outlined here, 12 developed second malignancies 13 to 80 months after mastectomy. Of those 12 malignancies, 4 were new contralateral breast carcinomas, 3 were myeloproliferative disorders, two were colonic cancer and one each of the endometrium, cervix and lung. The spectrum did not seem to be related to treatments or ER status. However, all patients are under surveillance with frequent evaluation to monitor for possible future problems.

Endocrine treatments have also been used as an adjuvant form of therapy in patients with breast cancer (10-13). Surgical or radiation-induced castration has been noted to result in delay in the onset of recurrence in premenopausal women with breast cancer (10-12). In one study (13), the addition of prednisone to radiation-induced castration resulted in a significant increase in disease-free survival and also total survival. With the introduction of antiestrogen drugs such as tamoxifen, new adjuvant trials using tamoxifen were undertaken to evaluate its value as adjuvant therapy in women with operable breast cancer (14-16). Several preliminary reports have shown that tamoxifen can improve disease-free survival in some patients with breast cancer. The 6 year results of our study indicate that a regimen of tamoxifen plus CMF chemotherapy increases the disease-free survival in women with ER positive tumors as compared to CMF chemotherapy alone. However, among the patients with ER positive tumors the ones who benefited the most from tamoxifen were those who had large tumors or those who had 4 or more involved axillary nodes. Thus it appears that patients with a more advanced stage of disease exhibited the most benefit from tamoxifen. Recently, Fisher et al. (14) have confirmed the benefi-

cial effect of tamoxifen added to 2 drug chemotherapy.
Although they indicated that the beneficial effect of
tamoxifen was independent of the number of nodes involved,
close analysis of the data showed that the beneficial
effect of tamoxifen was more significant in women with 4
or more involved axillary nodes. In our study, patients
with 1 to 3 positive nodes treated with tamoxifen had
fewer recurrences than those treated with CMF alone
during the first 2.5 years. It was only after 2.5 years
that the curves crossed over. Since the data reported
by Fisher et al. (14) were at 2 years, it will be of
interest to see their results after a longer period of
follow up. Thus, the duration of treatment with tamoxifen may be important in evaluating its benefit as an adjuvant therapy. In our current adjuvant therapy protocol
we are randomizing patients with ER-positive tumors to
either tamoxifen alone (for 3 years) or tamoxifen (3
years) plus 5-drug chemotherapy for one year. No data
are available at the present time on that study. We
hope that with prolonging therapy with tamoxifen to 3
years, its benefit would be enhanced.

Our data show that ER measurement in the primary
tumor provides important prognostic information. We
have also measured the progesterone receptor (PgR) in a
subset of the patients in this clinical trial, and Clark
et al. (17) have recently reported an analysis of the
data. The PgR level was found to provide significant

prognostic information in these patients independent of the treatment used. Multivariant analysis of prognostic factors showed that PgR and the number of positive nodes remained significant in predicting disease free survival whereas ER was no longer significant. This apparent superiority of PgR over ER needs further confirmation, but clearly suggests that both receptors should be evaluated in future clinical trials.

REFERENCES

1. Hubay CA, Pearson OH, Marshall JS, et al. (1980) Antiestrogen, cytotoxic chemotherapy and bacillus Calmette-Guerin vaccination in stage II breast cancer: a preliminary report. Surgery 87: 494-501.

2. Hubay CA, Pearson OH, Marshall JS, et al. (1980) Adjuvant chemotherapy, antiestrogen therapy and immunotherapy for stage II breast cancer: 45-month follow-up of a prospective, randomized clinical trial. Cancer 46: 2805-2808.

3. Hubay CA, Pearson OH, Marshall JS, et al. (1981) Adjuvant therapy of stage II breast cancer: 48-month follow-up of a prpspective randomized clinical trial. Breast Cancer Res Treat 1: 77-82.

4. McGuire WL, DeLaGarza M (1973) Improved sensitivity in the measurement of estrogen receptor in human breast cancer. J Clin Endocrinol Metab 37: 986-989.

5. Breslow N (1970) A generalized Kruskal-Wallis test for comparing K samples subject to unequal patterns of censorship. Biometrika 57: 579-594.

6. Thomas DG, Breslow N, Gart JJ (1977) Trend and homogeneity analyses of proportions and life table data. Comput Biomed Res 10: 373-381.

7. Gehan EA (1965) A generalized Wilcoxon test for comparing arbitrarily singly-censored samples. Biometrika 52: 203-233.

8. Gross AJ, Clark VA (1975) Survival disturbances: reliability applications. In: Biomedical Sciences,

New York, Wiley.

9. Bonadonna G, Brusamolino E, Valagussa P, et al.
    (1976) Combination chemotherapy as an adjuvant treat-
    ment in operable breast cancer. N Engl J Med 294:
    405-410.

10. Cole MP (1975) A clinical trial of an artificial
    menopause in carcinoma of the breast. INSERM:
    Hormones and breast cancer, vol. 55. May 1975.
    (Les Editions de l'Institut National de la Santé et
    de la Recherche Médicale), pp. 143-150.

11. Nissen-Meyer R (1975) Ovarian suppression and its
    supplement by additive hormonal treatment. INSERM:
    Hormones and breast cancer, vol. 55, May 1975, pp.
    151-158.

12. Bryant AJS, Wein JA (1981) Prophylactic oophorectomy
    in operable instances of carcinoma of the breast.
    Surg Gynecol Obstet 153: 660-664.

13. Meakin JW, Allt WEC, Beale FA, et al. (1977) Ovarian
    irradiation and prednisone following surgery for
    carcinoma of the breast. In Adjuvant Therapy of
    Cancer. Salmon SE (ed), New York North-Holland
    Publishing Co., pp. 95-99.

14. Fisher B, Redmond C, Brown A, et al. (1981) Treatment
    of primary breast cancer with chemotherapy and
    tamoxifen. N Engl J Med 305: 1-6.

15. Baum M, Brinkley DM, Dossett JA, et al. (1983)
    Controlled trial of tamoxifen as adjuvant agent in
    management of early breast cancer. Lancet 1: 257-
    261.

16. Ribeiro G, Palmer MK (1983) Adjuvant tamoxifen for
    operable carcinoma of the breast: report of clinical
    trial by the Christie Hospital and Holt Radium Insti-
    tute. Br Med J 286: 827-830.

17. Clark GM, McGuire WL, Hubay CA, et al. (1982) Com-
    parison of progesterone receptor with estrogen
    receptor in predicting disease free interval in stage
    II breast cancer patients. (Abstr). Clin Res 30:
    532A.

© 1984 Elsevier Science Publishers B.V.
Fluoropyrimidines in Cancer Therapy
K. Kimura, S. Fujii, M. Ogawa, G.P. Bodey, P. Alberto, eds.

COMPARISON OF 5-FLUOROURACIL AND TEGAFUR IN ADJUVANT CHEMOTHERAPIES WITH COMBINED INDUCTIVE AND MAINTENANCE THERAPIES FOR GASTRIC CANCER

Toshifusa Nakajima, Kunio Takagi, Keijiro Kuno and
Tamaki Kajitani

1. INTRODUCTION

Since 1961, seven different trials of adjuvant chemotherapy for gastric cancer have been undertaken in Cancer
Institute Hospital, Tokyo. When a combination of MMC,
5-FU and Ara-C (MFC therapy) was completed in 1974 (the
fourth trial), a new combination chemotherapy, MF'C therapy where 5-FU in MFC is substituted by tegafur, a
derivative of 5-FU, was reportedly effective on tumor
reduction. Either of these therapies reported at that
time was relatively short term regimen. Since 1973, 5-FU
and tegafur have been available for oral use which
allows patients to receive chemotherapy at home for a
long time after surgery. A long term chemotherapy seemed
to meet a clinical need to control the highest hazard of
cancer death at 1 or 1.5 years after surgery. These
circumstances inspired us to initiate a new trial in
1974 to compare the effect of 5-FU and tegafur in the
combination of inductive multidrug therapy and long term
oral maintenance therapy for patients with gastric cancer

after curative surgery. Almost all patients have been
observed more than 5 years at the end of 1982, the
present study therefore deals with the late results of
this trial, showing some encouraging data.

2. PATIENTS AND METHODS

A series of 243 patients with gastric cancer who were
undergone curative gastrectomy was subjected to this trial. On the seventh or tenth day after surgery, patients
were randomized to the following three treatment regimens
by the envelop method.

Patients allocated to Group A (Regimen A) received
one shot i.v. injection of 1.3 mg/m^2 of MMC, 167 mg/m^2 of
5-FU and 13 mg/m^2 of Ara-C twice a week for consecutive
5 weeks (MFC therapy). After four week intermission,
oral administration of 5-FU dry syrup followed the MFC
(i.v.) therapy with a dose of 133 mg/m^2/day for 4 weeks
with 8 week intermission. This oral 5-FU was repeatedly
given 7 times for 2 years after surgery. This treatment
course was designated as MFC + 5-FU. In the Group B,
5-FU in MFC therapy was substituted by tegafur with a
dose of 267 mg/m^2 for i.v. injection and 670 mg/m^2/day
for oral intake on the same schedule as Group A (referred
to as MF'C + tegafur). Patients subjected to Group C
were treated by surgery alone and served as the control.

Among 243 cases, 81 was allocated to Group A, 83 to

Group B, and 79 to Group C. Twenty cases were excluded later from the study due to incomplete requirement for the protocol regimens (11 cases with early cancer, 8 with non-curative surgery which were revealed later by the histological report and one case suffered from uterine cancer). Finally the prognosis of 223 cases was analyzed for the evaluation of adjuvant chemotherapy. There was no significant difference in the composition of prognostic factors among three groups. Postoperative survivals were analyzed according to several prognostic factors such as the extent of lymphatic spread, serosal involvement and clinical stage defined by the General Rule of the Surgical and Pathological Study of the Gastric Cancer issued by the Japanese Research Society for the Gastric Cancer (Jpn Res. Soc. Gastric Cancer, 1981). Postoperative survival was calculated by Kaplan-Meier's method (Kaplan and Meier, 1958) and was examined by χ^2 or logrank test (Peto et al., 1977) for the statistical significance.

3. RESULTS

Postoperative survivals of whole cases

Postoperative survival probabilities of whole cases subjected to the trial indicate that approximately a half of the control group (49.6%) survived more than 5 years with a constant decrease in survival rate thereafter. In contrast, the survival probabilities in adjuvant chemotherapy Group A and B reached almost constant 3 years after surgery. The rates of living more than 5 years was 68.8% in Group A and 63.2% in Group B. Logrank test however did not show a statistical significance (P=0.0934) in the survival difference between Group A and C because of insufficient accumulation of the cases.

Survivals according to the prognostic factors

The following analyses of survivals were done in several subsets according to the prognostic factors.

As to the lymph node metastasis, no significant difference in the survival rate was observed in any subset.

As to the serosal involvement of cancer, survivals of subset S_1 plus S_2 are demonstrated in Fig.1. There was approximately 20% difference in the 5-year survivals between Group A and C. This was statistically significant by logrank test (P<0.005). There was no deviation of background factor between Group A and C. In the subset S_0 where the serosa is not involved by cancer, there was apparently big difference in the survivals among three groups, e.g. 5-year survival rates were 93.3% for Group A, 87.5% for Group B, and 66.2% for Group C.

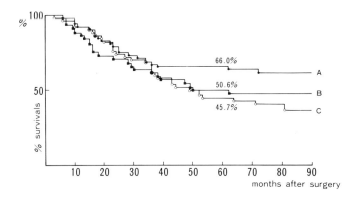

FIGURE 1 Postoperative Survivals According to the
Serosal Status (Subset S_1 + S_2). Statistical significance
between Groups A and C (P<0.005).

However, these difference were not statistically significant and seemed to be biased by an uneven composition of
nodal state among three groups.

Analyzing the survival possibilities according to the
clinical stages which are defined by nodal and serosal
states in curative cases, big differences in survival
between the treatment regimens were observed in the
subsets Stage II (Fig.2). 5-year survival rates in Stage
II were 100%, 87.5%, and 72.4% for Group A, B and C,
respectively. These differences among three groups did
not reach the statistical significance in both tests. In
the subset Stage II + III, on the contrary, Group A was
significantly superior to Group C in relation to the
survivals.

488

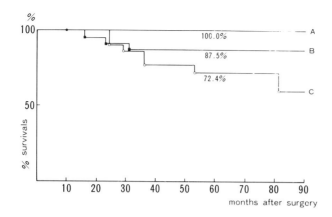

FIGURE 2   Postoperative Survivals According to the
Clinical Stages (Stage II). Statistical significance
between Groups A and C (P<0.025).

Types of recurrence according to the treatment modalities

Analysis of the causes of death in these groups is
necessary for elucidating the mechanism of life-prolonga-
tion with the adjuvant chemotherapy.

Incidences of deaths occurred during whole
observation period are listed in Table 1. Death due to
recurrence was observed in 28.7% of Group A, 36.9% of
Group B, and 47.4% of Group C. When the type of
recurrence was classified into the following three
categories, e.g. peritoneal dissemination, hematogenous
metastasis and local recurrence, a slight decrease in
the incidence of peritoneal dissemination and local
recurrence was found in Group A, and hematogenous
metastasis was slightly reduced in Group B compared with
the control. Death resulted from diseases other than
recurrence was observed in three groups with almost same

TABLE 1 TYPES AND TIMING OF CANCER RECURRENCE

Type of recurrence	Treatment regimens							
	A		B		C		Total	
	3 postoperative year							
	before	after	before	after	before	after	before	after
Peritoneal dissemi-nation	8 (11.0)	6 (8.2)*	8 (10.5)	10 (13.2)	6 (8.1)	15 (20.3)	22 (9.9)	31 (13.9)
Hematogen-ous metas-tasis	2 (2.7)	3 (4.1)	2 (2.6)	2 (2.6)	5 (6.8)	3 (4.1)	9 (4.0)	8 (3.6)
Local re-currence	2 (2.7)	0 (0)	5 (6.6)	1 (1.3)	3 (4.1)	4 (5.4)	10 (4.5)	5 (2.2)
Total	12 (16.4)	9 (12.3)	15 (19.7)	13 (17.1)	14 (19.0)	22 (29.8)	41 (18.4)	44 (19.7)
	21(28.7)*		28(36.8)		36(48.8)		85(38.1)	

Figures in parentheses indicate % incidence.
* P<0.05 (A : C).

incidence. Four percent of all cases died in unknown
circumstances. When the causes of death were compared
among three groups within 3 years and thereafter since
surgery, a remarkable decrease in the peritoneal
dissemination was observed in Group A later than 3 years
after surgery. The difference between Group A and C was
statistically significant, though not significant
between Group B and C. Within 3 years after surgery,
there was no remarkable difference in the incidence of
cancer death among 3 groups.

4. DISCUSSION

When a chemotherapeutic effect is evaluated between two drugs, comparison between an equivalent dose of each drug must be an essential prerequisite for the study. Based on the experimental and clinical results of tumor reduction, or those of acute toxicities with 5-FU or tegafur, we employed 5-FU to tegafur ratio of 1:1.6 for i.v. injection, and 1:5 for oral administration. As the result of this dose-setting, our preliminary report (Nakajima and Kajitani, 1980) showed that bone marrow suppression was observed at almost the same rate in both groups (13.9% and 10.5%, respectively), although dysfunction of G.I. tract was observed more frequently in Group B than in Group A (52.6% and 40.3%, respectively). These findings suggest that our dose-setting is not deviated far from the biologically equivalent dose.

Differences in the postoperative survivals among whole cases of three groups did not reach the statistical significance by logrank test (P=0.0934). However, these differences could be attributed to the suppressive effect of adjuvant chemotherapy on the recurrence of cancer by the following facts that over-all incidences of recurrence in the treated groups were significantly reduced as compared with the control group. Thus, the non-significant differences in the survivals between the treated and the control groups could be attributed to the small scale of the study and to non-cancer death which were excluded from the calculation of survival rates.

Analysis of various subsets categorized by prognostic factors revealed that Regimen A is effective for patients with moderately locally advanced diseases, especially in the subset of involved serosa ($S_1 + S_2$). This is consistent with the reduced incidence of peritoneal dissemination (P<0.005) and local recurrence in Group A. Free cancer cells in the peritoneal cavity exfoliated from the gastric serosa were reportedly found in 16% of patients with "curative" gastrectomy (Nakajima et al., 1978). Regimen A seems to inhibit such a latent peritoneal dissemination. Regimen B yielded better survivals than the control, but the difference in survivals between Group B and C did not reach a statistical significance in any subset.

At present, it might be allowed to state that the combination chemotherapy including 5-FU (MFC + 5-FU) is effective in the limited groups of patients with moderately advanced disease. Difficulty in improving the prognosis of Stage IV patients may explain one of the reasons why many previous studies have provided negative data on the effectiveness of adjuvant chemothrapy for gastric cancer. As for Stage IV cancer, more intensive modalities of therapy, for instance, a combination of local and general administration of anti-cancer drugs, or a combined radio-chemotherapy, should be considered. Prognosis of patients with Stage I disease are very good, requiring no farther adjuvant therapy after surgery.

These method of assessing treatment difference in the stratified subsets are referred to as exploratory data analysis by Fleming (Fleming, 1982), lacking the confidence of estimation. However, informations from these analysis may be helpful for the proper selection of patients in future studies. Statisticians (Simons, 1982; Starmer and Lee, 1982) claim it inevitable to conduct an independent study for confirming the suggestive results. From these point of view, our present trial could serve as a pilot study. Since 1987, in our hospital, patients with Stage II and III diseases have been exclusively subjected to the ordinary type of adjuvant chemotherapy.

It is an another interest for clinicians to confirm whether the oral maintenance therapy with 5-FU or tegafur has any additive effect to the preceding induction therapy, though the present study is, regretfully, not designed for this purpose. It is not reasonable to make a direct comparison of the survival rates between the present and previous protocols (Nakajima et al., 1980), it could be allowed to compare among the subsets where the survival rate of control group (surgery alone) is identical in both regimens. In the subset S_{1-3}, 5-year survival rates were 64.9% for MFC + 5-FU, and 61.9% for MFC. This minimum difference in the survival between both regimens indicates that the validity of long term oral maintenance therapy is not yet established in the present trial. On the other hand, Taguchi (1981) reported that intravenous MMC combined with oral tegafur was superior to MMC alone in regard to the postoperative survival of the patients with gastric cancer. Additive effect of oral maintenance therapy may possibly depend on the induction therapy, e.g. a powerful induction therapy may overweigh the additive effect of consecutive maintenance therapy. Another possibility may be that there is a slight difference in the method of maintenance therapy between Taguchi's and ours; the former employed continuous administration of relatively low dose of tegafur (600 mg) and the latter, intermittent administration of high dose 5-FU (200mg) or tegafur (1,000 mg).

As our previous report indicates, chemotherapeutic effect in Group A has become manifest 3 years after surgery. Long-term maintenance therapy did not alter the mode of occurrence of cancer relapse. One possible explanation for this phenomenon is that whether cancer relapses or not is destined in relatively short period by surgery and inductive chemotherapy, but it takes more than 3 years for the remaining minimum cancer to be manifest clinically.

5. CONCLUSION

A prospective randomized trial of adjuvant chemotherapy for gastric cancer was undertaken in Cancer Institute Hospital, Tokyo, from 1974 to 1977. After curative sur-

gery, 243 cases were randomized to three treatment regimens. Patients allocated to Regimen A (MFC + 5-FU) received one shot i.v. injection of 1.3 mg/m^2 of mitomycin
C (MMC), 167 mg/m^2 of 5-fluorouracil (5-FU) and 13 mg/m^2
of cytosine arabinoside (Ara-C) twice a week for consecutive 5 weeks. After 4 week intermission, oral administration of 5-FU with a dose of 133 mg/m^2/day for 4 weeks
with 8 week intermission followed MFC (i.v.) therapy.
Oral administration was repeated 7 times for 2 years. In
the Regimen B (MF'C + tegafur), 5-FU in Regimen A was
substituted by tegafur with a dose of 267 mg/m^2 for i.v.
injection, and 670 mg/m^2/day for oral intake on the same
schedule as Regimen A. Patients subjected to Regimen C
were treated by surgery alone and served as the control.
Regimen A was proved effective on the suppression of
relapse in the limited groups of moderately locally
advanced cancer; 5-year survival rates of the subset of
Stage II and III were 70.6% for Group A (treated with
Regimen A) and 49.9% for the control (Group C). Group B
(allocated to Regimen B) was always superior to the
control in regard to the survivals, but there was no
statistical significant difference in any subset. Improvement in the prognosis of Group A seemed to be
caused by the suppression of peritoneal dissemination.
Validity of the oral maintenance therapy still remained
to be elucidated. These results favor 5-FU in the
adjuvant chemotherapy for gastric cancer. Analysis of

effectiveness according to the prognostic factors
indicates the importance of proper selection of patients
for successful adjuvant chemotherapy.

REFERENCES

1. Fleming TR. (1982) Historical controls, data banks
    and randomized trials in clinical research: a review.
    Cancer Treat Rep 66: 1101-1105.

2. Japanese Research Society for Gastric Cancer (1981)
    The general rules for the gastric cancer study in
    surgery and pathology. Jpn J Surg   11: 127-139.

3. Kaplan EL and Meier P. (1958) Nonparametric estimation
    from incomplete observations. J Am   Stat Assoc 53:
    457-481.

4. Nakajima T, Harashima S, Hirata M, et al. (1978)
    Prognostic and therapeutic values of peritoneal cytolo-
    gy in gastric cancer. Acta Cytolog 22: 225-229.

5. Nakajima T, Fukami A, Takagi K, et al. (1980) Adjuvant
    chemotherapy with mitomycin C, and with a multi-drug
    combination of mitomycin C, 5-fluorouracil and cytosine
    arabinoside after curative resection of gastric cancer.
    Jpn J Clin Oncol 10: 187-194.

6. Nakajima T and Kajitani T. (1980) Adjuvant chemothera-
    py with inductive multi-drug combination and long-term
    oral maintenance therapies for gastric cancer. J Jpn
    Soc Cancer Ther 15: 980-988.

7. Peto R, Pike MC, Armitage P, et al. (1977) Design and
    analysis of randomized clinical trials requiring
    prolonged observation of each patients, II analysis
    and examples. Br J Cancer 35: 1-39.

8. Simon R. (1982) Randomized clinical trials and research
    strategy. Cancer Treat Rep 66: 1083-1087.

9. Starmer CF and Lee KL. (1982) A data-based approach to
    assessing clinical interventions in the setting of
    chronic disease. Cancer Treat Rep 66: 1077-1082.

10. Taguchi T, Hattori T, Kondo T. et al. (1981) Post-
    operative adjuvant chemotherapy with mitomycin C plus
    futraful for gastric cancer. In: Adjuvant Chemotherapy
    III (eds) SE Salmon and SE Jones. Grune & Stratton,
    New York, pp. 511-518.

Fluoropyrimidines in Cancer Therapy
K. Kimura, S. Fujii, M. Ogawa, G.P. Bodey, P. Alberto, eds.

ADJUVANT THERAPY OF GASTRIC CANCER

E. Douglas Holyoke and Harold O. Douglass, Jr.

In spite of a real but unexplained decrease in gastric cancer in the United States over the last 25 years, gastric cancer remains the sixth leading cause of death in America. Of the more than 24,000 patients expected to present with gastric cancer during 1983, between 80-90% will have died after five years. Until we in the United States are able with our lower incidence rates to develop a detection success approaching that seen in Japan, we are not likely to see a significant change. In North America, the majority of patients continue to present themselves at a stage where long term survival is not possible. Because of the high failure rate of surgery per se, gastric cancer has been the subject of study using combined modality therapy for some years.

Comis in 1973 reviewed nearly 7,000 patients with gastric cancer (1). At diagnosis in his series, 18% were inoperable, 26% were unresectable, and 19% underwent palliative resection leaving only one-third for potentially curative procedures. This is still estimated to be the percentage undergoing surgery for cure. The number of patients cured is reduced still further by a severe, although lessening mortality of between 10 and 20% for a proximal or total gastrectomy and a lesser but finite mortality of 3-5% for distal subtotal resection.

Attempts at widening the surgical field revealed the limits of this approach some years ago. Removal of lymph node areas increases survival, but following detailed studies in Japan and elsewhere, the gastric lymphatic drainage areas have been well delineated and the extension of surgery beyond clearly defined borders is not useful (2).

No current treatise concerning one of the solid tumors and adjuvant treatment is complete without a statement concerning staging and stratification. Factors affecting resection and/or survival are listed in Table 1. All of these may apply and must be accounted for in evaluating reported results.

TABLE 1   FACTORS AFFECTING SURVIVAL IN PATIENTS WITH
          GASTRIC CANCER

TUMOR LOCATION	HISTOLOGIC TYPE
SIZE	"INTESTINAL" OR "DIFFUSE" TYPE OF GROWTH
DEPTH OF PENETRATION	BORRMANN'S CLASSIFICATION
SEROSAL PERFORATION	PATIENT ACTIVITY STATUS
LYMPH NODE INVOLVEMENT	PATIENT NUTRITIONAL STATUS
LOCATION AND NUMBER	SURGERY PERFORMED
	DISTANT METASTASES

Comis and Carter published a review of gastric chemotherapy in 1974 in Cancer which was designed to awaken
interest in this area and especially as a means of at-
tracting interest to the possibilities for adjuvant
study (3).

Chemotherapeutic agents discussed included 5-Fluor-
ouracil (5-FU), Fluorodeoxyribose (FUdR), Methotrexate,
and Mitomycin C (MMC). The problems in determing true
response rate for some of these agents are well known and
best illustrated in Dr. Moertel's recitation for 5-Fluor-
ouracil with approximately a ten-fold variation in response rate reported in various series (4). In 1974 and
even today, various approaches to dosage are being tried.
The original Ansfield regime was quite toxic and many
investigators employ the Mayo Clinic 5 week - 5 day
course. In non-protocol care of patients in the United
States, the weekly intravenous maintenance course has become widespread allowing outpatient treatment. 5-Fluor-
ouracil has also been given orally with some demonstrable
result. Currently there is a push for continuous infusion of 5-FU supported by data from Lokich and others.
Other antimetabolites include FUdR with a response rate
similar to 5-FU and Methotrexate which has not proven
effective. The generally accepted response rate for
patients with gastric cancer treated by 5-Fluorouracil is
about 25% with a 4-5 months duration.

Mitomycin C has been reported as having an overall

response rate of 30% but there are problems with
toxicity and cumulative toxicity has been a problem. The
response time is somewhat shorter for Mitomycin C than
for 5-FU, and as the latter is a safe agent, we believe
no advantage is to be seen in using Mitomycin C per se.

In 1974 Kovach et al. reported on a comparison between 5-FU and BCNU singly and in combination in patients
with cancer of the stomach and pancreas. This report
cited 14 of 34 evaluable patients with carcinoma of the
stomach as responding to this combination (41%) as
against (29%) responding to 5-FU alone (5). Subsequently,
the Eastern Cooperative Oncology Group reported a better
than 40% response rate for patients with advanced cancer
for 5-FU combined with another nitroso compound, 1-(2-
chloroethyl)-3-4-methyl-cyclohexyl-1-nitrosourea or Methyl
CCNN (MeCCNU). This information led to several studies of
chemotherapy for gastric cancer based on 5-FU and nitrosourea.

There have been many other gastric adjuvant studies
around the world in addition to those we will discuss in
detail.

It is clear that in most instances for whatever
reasons, results have been negative although Mitomycin C
apparently had some effect in these earlier Japanese
studies. More recent Japanese findings are to be presented in this symposium.

TABLE 2   STUDIES OF ADJUVANT* CHEMOTHERAPY: A PARTIAL
           LIST

Year	Author	Trial	Result
1976	Hattori	(1)	-
1977	Goto	(1)	-
1977	Serlin	(3)	-
1978	Koyama	(6)	+
1978	Nakakma	(1)	-
1979	Dent	(1)	-
1980	Huguier	(1)	-
1980	Blake	(1)	-

* Exclusive of those discussed in detail

In 1976 Higgins summarized the status of a number of adjuvant chemotherapy studies for gastric cancer in progress around the world (6). This included studies of surgery alone versus 5-FU and MeCCNU as an adjuvant to surgery by the Eastern Cooperative Oncology Group (ECOG), the Veterans Administration Surgical Adjuvant Group (VASAG), and the Gastrointestinal Tumor Study Group (GITSG). The Eastern Cooperative Oncology Group Study 3275 has been completed and results have been updated at the 1983 ASCO Meetings (7). There were 180 evaluable patients entered on ECOG Protocol 3275 between September 1975 and June 1980. Stratification was for depth of invasion, lymph node status and tumor site. Patients were randomized within seven weeks of surgery to a non-treatment control or to a ten-week cycle of 5-FU, 325 mgm/m^2 I.V. daily days 1-5, with Methyl CCNU 150 mgm/m^2 P.O. day one. As of the Spring 1983 report, 47/89 surgery only patients and 49/91 chemotherapy treated patients have recurred. Forty-seven control and 51 adjuvant therapy patients have died. At two years, the disease-free rates

were 49% and 59% for the surgery versus the surgery and
chemotherapy arms, P ∿ 0.87, so that, this study indicated no significant effect of chemotherapy with 5-FU and
Methyl CCNU as adjuvant.

The Veterans Administration Surgical Adjuvant Group
report was published in Cancer in September of 1983 (8).
This study was begun in August 1974 and continued through
May of 1980. All patients were male in this series.
Therapy was begun postoperatively less than 45 days following surgery. Stratification was into three groups:
(A) no proven residual disease - this group does include
patients with residual disease suspected on clinical
grounds, (B) proven palliative resection - this group does
define a patient with microscopic tumor at the edge of the
removed operative specimen as undergoing a palliative
operation, (C) no resection carried out. As in the ECOG
and GITSG studies, the protocols were for prospective
randomization into a combined modality versus surgery
alone arm. In this study Group A represents the adjuvant
patients.

Recurrence rates in Group A ran 15% in the surgery
and adjuvant arm after one year, 14% and 16% in the
second year, and 9% (2 patients) and 0% in the third
year (P=0.77) for Group A survival results are seen
in Table 3.

There was no significant difference demonstrated in
survival in the adjuvant group of patients between the

502

surgery alone and combined modality arms. While the combined arm did trend towards a more favorable survival during the first year, this was not apparent by two years
and did not approach statistical significance in any event.

TABLE 3   GASTRIC ADJUVANT (VASAG) RELATIVE FAILURE RISK
          ADJUVANT VERSUS SURGERY ONLY

Without Adjustment

Patients	Relative Risk	95% Limits
Adjuvant	0.93	0.57 - 1.52
High Risk	0.94	0.57 - 1.56
Low Risk	0.91	0.26 - 4.09

With Adjustment

Patients	Relative Risk	95% Limits
Adjuvant	0.92	0.55 - 1.54

After Higgins et al., Sept. 1983

When the high risk subset of these patients was examined,
it did appear that the small advantage which appeared was
contained in this group as one might postulate, but this
finding still did not approach significance. As can be
seen in Table 3, adjustment for lymph node involvement or
serosal penetration, etc., made no difference.

It is also of interest that the residual disease
group failed to show any advantage to therapy. As in all
of this type of study it is necessary for a chairman or
committee to review all deaths or recurrences. In this
study, the study site chairman reviewed 214 of 238
deceased patients by manuscript submission time. The
necessity for this evaluation has become apparent over the
last decade. Of 32 deaths in the combined modality arm

24 were attributed to cancer. Similarly for the surgery only, 27 of 35 deaths were attributed to cancer. But of these, 9 of each were labeled "presumable" and 7 and 14 respectively "probable". When the problems associated with stratification are reviewed, it is apparent that 65-70 patients per treatment arm even with a greater than 50% mortality at five years is not a large number.

The first report of the findings from the GITSG Protocol for adjuvant chemotherapy following curative resection for gastric cancer (GITSG 8174) appeared in 1982 (9). This study was underway from January 1975 to September 1980, and was, as were the two studies just reported, a comparison of a surgery only arm with a treatment arm using 5-FU and MeCCNU. Patients were entered with a detailed stratification; type of resection, site - cardia versus all others, extent of tumor invasion - confined to the gastric wall or invading beyond, lymph node involvement and tumor histology - limitis plastica versus other.

The adjuvant treatment arm received 5-FU 325 mgm/m^2 I.V. days 1-5, and 375 mgm/m^2 I.V. on days 36-40 plus MeCCNU on day 1 given as 150 mgm/m^2 P.O. Treatment was to begin 3-6 weeks post surgery.

As of 1982 there were 69 deaths. Of these, 40 were in the surgery only arm, and 29 in the surgery chemo-therapy arm. Figure 1 illustrates the overall survival for the two groups. For the carefully staged control group, median survival was 33 months which is quite satisfactory and was at the time of submission greater than 56 months for the combined modality arm. Disease-free survival similarly shows an advantage for the combined modality arm.

FIGURE I **ADJUVANT TREATMENT OF GASTRIC CANCER**

GITSG STUDY 8174

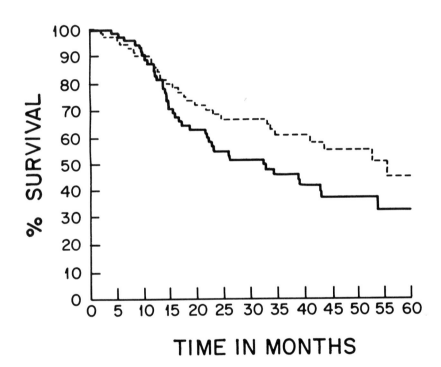

The apparent survival advantage for combined therapy noted above was seen in all subgroups of patients who were analyzed. Although the patients are still being followed subsequent analysis do not show any important change.

It should also be remembered that these treatment programs are not without their price in toxicity. Of the 71 patients randomized in the GITSG study to receive chemotherapy, eight experienced an episode of life threatening toxicity, and 45% experienced at least one GITSG severe or worse episode of toxicity. There was one possible treatment death in this group. An additional problem has been the occurrence in some patients of leukemia following treatment with MeCCNU. This is apparently a rare but finite event which must be figured into an equation when a decision for using this adjuvant approach is made. A considered report and discussion of this problem is to be published in the New England Journal. There are other indications that the indicated response rate of 40-50% for advanced disease entertained when these studies began was somewhat optimistic (10).

One study concerning 5-FU and BCNU has been reported (11). All patients received a potentially curative operation and were Stage II or III (UICC). Chemotherapy courses of 5 days were given 8 times at 6-8 week intervals. 5-FU was at 10 mgm/kg/day and BCNU at 40 mgm/kg/day. Reported in 1980, the study showed 21 recurrences in 54 controls, and 14 in 44 combined modality patients. Both survival and disease-free interval were not affected in this study, and the authors felt there was no benefit from the therapy program.

More recently a second generation of adjuvant
studies has been fathered by a regime brought up from the
ranks of advanced study protocols. MacDonald et al. reported on 36 patients with advanced measurable gastric
cancer treated with 5-Fluorouracil, Adriamycin, and Mitomycin C (12). These authors reported a 50% objective
partial response. Of importance was the reported duration
of that remission of over nine months. This treatment
program has now become known as the FAM regime. As reported by the Georgetown group, FAM is administered in
eight week cycles. 5-Fluorouracil is given at 600 mgm/m^2
on days 1, 8, 29, and 36. Adriamycin was given, also
intravenously, at a dose of 30 mgm/m^2 on days 1 and 29,
Mitomycin C at 10 mgm/m^2 administered on day 1 of each
cycle only. In addition to a rather impressive reported
response rate, this dosage schedule was found to avoid the
gastrointestinal toxicity often associated with the nitrosoureas. Further, the use of Mitomycin C in an intermittent schedule avoided the problem of cumulative bone
marrow depression. Adriamycin given at 60 mgm/m^2 a cycle
or 360 mgm/m^2 per year obviates any problem from cardiac
toxicity.

The Southwest Oncology Group (SWOG) has a study
Phase III Adjuvant Chemotherapy with FAM vs. Surgery Alone
for Locally Advanced Gastric Adenocarcinoma. Stratification is by TNM Stage/Group IB vs. IC vs. II vs. III.
Chemotherapy begins 4-8 weeks after surgery. 5-FU is

given at 600 mgm/m^2 I.V. on days 1,8,29, and 36. Adriamycin and Mitomycin C are according to the Georgetown program. This study is apparently accruing well. A similar study was begun by the Cancer and Leukemia Group B. This was slow to get underway and was closed in March 1982.

Other related ongoing protocols include that of the Mayo Clinic, Adjuvant Chemotherapy with 5-FU and Adriamycin following curative surgery for adenocarcinoma of the stomach. The treatment program consists of 5-FU 350 mgm/m^2 I.V. on days 1-5 and Adriamycin 40 mgm/m^2 on day 1. Courses are repeated at 5 week intervals for 3 courses. One hundred and twenty-six patients were originally planned for entry and as of February 1982, 42 were entered.

The GI Tumor Study Group has followed a related line of investigation. A study in advanced gastric cancer both measurable and non-measurable chaired by Dr. O'Connell is scheduled to appear in January in Cancer. 5-FU and Adriamycin alone was compared to FAM and 5-FU, Adriamycin, Methyl CCNU or FAMe. The result indicates that FAMe is not less effective than FAM, and there may be a slight advantage. Based on this study and the previous GITSG adjuvant protocol building on the previous best arm, Protocol 8180 was activated in November 1980. This called for 5-FU and MeCCNU versus 5-FU, Adriamycin, and MeCCNU to be analyzed in the adjuvant setting. At last analysis 80 patients had been entered in this study.

Other studies include, in addition to ongoing Japanese protocols, a study headed by Dr. Araujo in Argentina studying 5-FU, Adriamycin and Cis-Platinum (FAP). The Sydney Cooperative Oncology Group in Australia is looking at 5-FU, Adriamycin, and BCNU. A number of other agents are being developed from Phase I and II studies in advanced disease.

This symposium will review a number of Japanese studies. Our own experience indicates to us that 5-FU and MeCCNU and probably FAM has or should show a small effect. This effect is not marked and perhaps on reflection does not exceed what could have been anticipated, especially if in the human adjuvant situation the location or accessibility and amount of tumor is such that a significant augmentation in drug effect is not seen over that encountered in advanced disease. For gastric cancer for the relatively low risk patients, the risk to benefit ratio of these programs is not very favorable. And finally, the specter of divergence between results in multiple prospective similar randomized trials deserves thought.

REFERENCES

1. Comis RL. (1973) The chemotherapy of adenocarcinoma
    of the stomach, a brief review. Cancer Therapy
    Evaluation Branch, National Cancer Institute.

2. Lawrence W Jr. and McNeer G. (1960) An analysis of
    the role of surgery for gastric cancer. SG&O 3:
    691-696.

3. Comis RL, Carter SK. (1974) A review of chemotherapy
    in gastric cancer. Cancer 43:1576-1586.

4. Moertel CG. (1969) Clinical management of advanced
    gastrointestinal cancer. Harper and Row, New York.

5. Kovach JS, Moertel CG, Schutt AF. (1974) A controll-
    ed study of combined 1,3-bis(2 chloro-ethyl)-1-nitro-
    sourea and 5-Fluorouracil therapy for advanced gas-
    tric and pancreatic cancer. Cancer 33:563-569.

6. Higgins GA. (1976) Adjuvant studies in gastric can-
    cer in the United States. Rec Results in Cancer
    Research 76:244-248.

7. Engstrom P, Lavin P, for the Eastern Cooperative
    Oncology Group. (1983) Postoperative adjuvant
    therapy for gastric cancer patients. Proc ASCO 114.

8. Higgins GA, Amadeo JH, Smith DE. (1983) Efficacy of
    prolonged intermittent therapy with combined 5-FU and
    Methyl-CCNU following resection for gastric cancer.
    Cancer 52:1105-1112.

9. The Gastrointestinal Tumor Study Group. (1982) Con-
    trolled trial of adjuvant chemotherapy following
    curative resection for gastric cancer. Cancer 49:
    1116-1122.

10. Moertel CG, Lavin PT. (1979) Phase II-III chemo-
    therapy studies in advanced gastric cancer. Cancer
    Treat Rep. 63:1863-1869.

11. Herfarth CH, Schlag P. (1979) A controlled prospec-
    tive study of adjuvant 5-Fluorouracil and BCNU
    therapy in stomach carcinoma. Springer-Verlag,
    pp 357-360, Berlin.

12. MacDonald JS, Schein, PS, Woolley PV, et al. (1980)
    5-Fluorouracil, Doxorubicin, and Mitomycin C (FAM)
    combination chemotherapy for advanced gastric cancer.
    Am Int Med 93:533-536.

510

© 1984 Elsevier Science Publishers B.V.
Fluoropyrimidines in Cancer Therapy
K. Kimura, S. Fujii, M. Ogawa, G.P. Bodey, P. Alberto, eds.

ADJUVANT CHEMOTHERAPY AFTER SURGERY FOR GASTRIC CANCER IN JAPAN

Takao Hattori, Tetsuo Taguchi, Osahiko Abe, Kiyoshi Inokuchi
and Nobuya Ogawa

1. INTRODUCTION

To improve the therapeutic results of gastric cancer, chemotherapy is now considered to be indispensable adjuvant therapy. In Japan, various forms of induction chemotherapy using mitomycin-C (MMC) for patients undergoing gastrectomy in gastric cancer have been prescribed (1,2,3), based on over ten years of clinical experience. Since 1975, the focus has been on detection of long-term maintenance chemotherapy as an adjunct to surgery. For such a study the chemotherapy should be performed on an out-patient basis. Therefore, a drug showing sufficient anticancer activity and low toxicity on the one hand and convenient usage for out-patients on the other had to be selected. Fortunately former trials with oral administration of tegafur provided a very compatible administration for a long time and a considerably good response rate in recurrent or inoperable gastric cancer in Japan. Thus, a study of postoperative long-term adjuvant chemotherapy with MMC and tegafur was planned. To promote the multihospital trial, the Cooperative Study Group of Surgical Adjuvant Chemotherapy for Gastric Cancer

involving 297 major hospitals throughout Japan
(Conductor: Prof. K. Inokuchi) was organized in 1975.
in this paper, two studies of this Cooperative Group are
presented.

2. THE FIRST STUDY OF THE COOPERATIVE STUDY GROUP

The first study was performed from May 1975 to July
1976 and the results were repeatedly reported (4,5,6).
For this study two protocols were planned as shown in
Fig. 1. Each hospital chose one of them. After
gastrectomy patients were assigned at random to either
Group A or B. In protocol I, patients received MMC
intermittently in a single dose of 0.08 mg/kg twice a
week for a total of 8-10 times, starting from the first
postoperative week. In protocol II, they received
large-dose MMC, 20 mg (0.4 mg/kg) on the day of

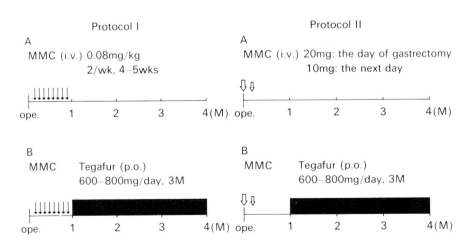

FIGURE 1 Treatment schedule of the first study by the
Cooperative Study Group of Surgical Adjuvant
Chemotherapy for Gastric Cancer in Japan (1975-1976).

gastrectomy and an additional 10 mg (0.2 mg/kg) on the next day. In Group A of each protocol no further treatment was added and in Group B tegafur in a daily dose of 600-800 mg was administered orally for three months starting one month after gastrectomy.

A total of 2834 patients were registered and the details of the clinical backgrounds are indicated in Table 1.

TABLE 1   Clinical backgrounds of the cases entered (the first study)

	Protocol I				Protocol II			
	A		B		A		B	
Entered	912	%	832	%	550	%	540	%
Excluded	258	(28)	330	(39)	164	(29)	171	(31)
Analyzed	654		502		386		369	
Curability		%		%		%		%
curative	468	(72)	351	(70)	301	(78)	289	(78)
noncurative	186	(28)	151	(30)	85	(22)	80	(22)
Stage								
I	119	(18)	94	(19)	94	(24)	79	(22)
II	216	(33)	146	(29)	111	(29)	90	(24)
III	151	(23)	117	(23)	117	(29)	126	(34)
IV	168	(26)	145	(29)	70	(18)	74	(20)
n, ps*								
n(-)ps(-)	132	(20)	98	(20)	98	(25)	89	(24)
n(+)ps(-)	158	(24)	125	(25)	72	(19)	67	(18)
n(-)ps(+)	75	(12)	53	(10)	49	(13)	44	(12)
n(+)ps(+)	289	(44)	226	(45)	167	(43)	169	(46)

*n: histological lymphnode metastasis
ps: histological serosal invasion

Further known prognostic factors as shown in Table 2 were compared between Groups A and B by statistical analysis using Chi square test, and no differences were observed.

TABLE 2   Prognostic   factors   tested   by   statistical
          analysis
───
Tumor
     Location
     Size
     Serosal invasion
     Penetration in the stomach wall
     Peritoneal dissemination
     Liver metastases
     Lymphnode metastases
     Borrmann's classification
     Histological classification
Host
     Sex
     Age
     Classification of gastrectomy based on lymphnode
     removal
     Reconstructive procedure
     Histological examination of the specimen
          cut edge of the oral margin
          cut edge of the anal margin
     Curative or noncurative resection
Agent
     Total dose of MMC
     Total dose of tegafur
───

In general, the actuarial survival rate of Group B was superior to Group A in both protocols. Significant differences were observed in stage III of protocol II at 5 years and in stage II of protocol I and stage III of protocol II at 7 years (Table 3). As for n-factor (histological lymphnode metastasis) and ps-factor (histological serosal invasion), significant increase of survival rate of Group B was observed in n(+)ps(+) group of protocol II at 5 years, but significant increase of

514

survival rate of Group A was also observed in n(-)ps(-) group of protocol II at 7 years (Table 4). From these results it may be concluded that the advantage of the addition of tegafur to MMC induction therapy as an adjunct to gastrectomy was definitely demonstrated in stage II of protocol I and in the advanced stages of III or IV in protocol II. Also it may be emphasized that adjuvant chemotherapy was not necessary or sometimes more harmful in the cases with early gastric cancer of stage I. It was obvious that the survival rates were generally better in protocol II than in protocol I. Even in the cases with stage II of protocol I where significant difference was observed between Groups B to A at 7 years, the survival rate of Group B was still lower than that of Group A or B in protocol II. The difference between protocol I and II is dependent only upon the administration method of MMC. In protocol I, MMC was administered intermittently in a moderate dosage and in protocol II MMC was administered in the highest tolerable dosage just after operation. The total dosage of MMC was greater in protocol I but the results were superior in protocol II. Therefore, MMC administration in protocol II can be regarded as standard induction therapy as an adjunct to gastrectomy, at least for the advanced stage III or IV gastric cancer.

From the results of the first study the question arises whether the induction therapy with MMC may be

dispensable. Since the radical gastrectomy itself can
be regarded as an induction therapy, especially in cases
of curatively resected gastric cancer, the long-term
administration of tegafur alone as postoperative
adjuvant therapy may be sufficient. In order to clarify
this respect, the second study was planned.

TABLE 3   Actuarial survival rate of the first study by
the Cooperative Study Group of Surgical
Adjuvant Chemotherapy for Gastric Cancer
(1975-1976): In relation with stages

	Protocol I		Protocol II	
	A	B	A	B
5-year survival rate %	%	%	%	%
Stage I	83.1	91.2	91.7	85.9
II	51.9	65.4	66.9	72.2
III	37.3	32.8	39.2	47.9*
IV	17.8	15.3	14.4	21.5
All cases	46.0	47.5	54.4	55.8
7-year survival rate				
Stage I	83.1	91.2	88.4	81.5
II	47.9	60.3*	64.3	63.0
III	30.3	29.7	35.5	42.8*
IV	16.4	13.7	13.1	20.2
All cases	42.7	43.4	51.6	50.7

*Significant difference between Groups A and B (p < 0.05)

TABLE 4   Actuarial survival rate of the first study by
           the Cooperative Study Group of Surgical
           Adjuvnat Chemotherapy for Gastric Cancer
           (1975-1976): In relation with n- and ps- factors

	Protocol I		Protocol II	
	A	B	A	B
5-year survival rate %	%	%	%	%
n(-)ps(-)	82.5	92.3	90.8	83.0
n(+)ps(-)	48.9	60.3	67.6	68.6
n(-)ps(+)	57.9	47.0	62.9	74.1
n(+)ps(+)	23.4	22.0	27.3	36.0*
7-year survival rate				
n(-)ps(-)	81.7	84.2	88.7	75.3*
n(+)ps(-)	45.7	57.1	61.7	63.9
n(-)ps(+)	52.8	34.4	58.6	71.6
n(+)ps(+)	20.0	20.9	25.4	31.5

*Significant difference between Groups A and B ($p < 0.05$)

2.   THE SECOND STUDY OF THE COOPERATIVE STUDY GROUP

The second study was performed from 1977 to 1979 and the preliminary results were reported in 1981 (7). In this study patients were allocatd at random into three groups after gastrectomy as shown in Fig. 2. In Group A, MMC was administered in a large-dose on the day of operation and on the next day as in protocol II of the first study. In Group C, only tegafur was administered in a daily dosage of 600 mg starting two weeks after operation without MMC induction therapy. In Group B, both MMC and tegafur were given in the same manner as in Group A or C.

Group A

MMC (i.v.) 20mg: the day of gastrectomy
(i.v.) 10mg: the next day

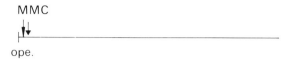

Group B

Futraful (p.o.) 600mg/day for one year

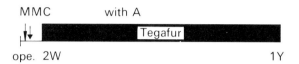

Group C

Futraful (p.o.) 600mg/day for one year

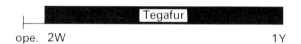

FIGURE 2 Treatment schedule of the second study by the Cooperative Study Group of Surgical Adjuvant Chemotherapy for Gastric Cancer (1977-1979).

A total of 4707 patients were entered and 3033 cases were finally analyzed for efficacy. Clinical backgrounds were indicated in Table 5 and no differences were observed between three groups. At present, the 4-year survival rates can be calculated as shown in Table 6. The interim results obtained so far suggests that the combined usage of MMC induction therapy and tegafur maintenance (Group B) shows the best result and especially in patients with stage III or n(+)ps(+) the survival rates of Group A are significantly higher than those of Group A (p < 0.01) or Group C (p < 0.05).

TABLE 5   Clinical background of the cases entered
(the second study)

Group	A		B		C	
Entered	1534	%	1525	%	1648	%
Excluded	552	(35)	521	(34)	601	(36)
Analyzed	982		1004		1047	
Curability		%		%		%
curative	704	(72)	714	(71)	767	(73)
noncurative	278	(28)	290	(29)	280	(27)
Stage						
I	259	(26)	213	(21)	253	(24)
II	258	(26)	277	(28)	282	(27)
III	243	(25)	262	(26)	255	(24)
IV	222	(23)	252	(25)	257	(25)
n,ps*						
n(-)ps(-)	262	(27)	219	(22)	259	(25)
n(+)ps(-)	181	(18)	187	(19)	191	(18)
n(-)ps(+)	120	(12)	130	(13)	160	(15)
n(+)ps(+)	415	(43)	468	(46)	437	(42)

*n: histological lymphnode metastasis
ps: histological serosal invasion

3.   STUDY   ON   ADJUVANT   IMMUNOCHEMOTHERAPY   AFTER GASTRECTOMY

In the next step the research of preoperative therapy for gastric cancer was directed to the combined usage of immunostimulants and chemotherapy. Various pilot studies on the use of OK-432, PS-K or levamisole based on the chemotherapy with MMC and tegafur after surgery for gastric cancer have been reported in Japan (8,9,10). OK-432 is the preparation of Staphylococcus and PS-K is the extract from the mycelium of Coriolous versicolor (Fr.) Quel, a protein-bound polysaccharide, and both of them were developed in Japan. Levamisole, a very simple chemical compound, was originally developed as an anthelmintic. OK-432 is used by intradermal injection and PS-K and levamisole by oral administration with few side toxicities.

TABLE 6 Actuarial 4-year survival rate of the second study by the Cooperative Study Group of Surgical Adjuvant Chemotherapy for Gastric Cancer in Japan (1977-1979)

Group		A	B	C
Stage		%	%	%
	I	87.9	93.3	91.9
	II	69.8	66.6	65.1
	III*1)	36.1	54.3	45.9
	IV	14.7	19.8	20.9
n,ps				
n(-)ps(-)		86.3	92.1	91.4
n(+)ps(-)		65.4	67.4	66.1
n(-)ps(+)		60.5	62.5	63.5
n(+)ps(+)*2)		25.9	35.5	28.1
All cases		53.9	57.3	56.1

*1) A vs B (p < 0.01), A vs C (p < 0.05)
 2) A vs B (p < 0.01), B vs C (p < 0.05)

In 1980, the Cooperative Study Group dissolved itself to be enlarged on a new authorized organization; the Japanese Foundation for Multidisciplinary Treatment of Cancer. The evaluation whether the combined use of immunopotentiators with chemotherapy is beneficial as a surgical adjuvant or not, was the first study planned by the Foundation. As shown in Fig. 3, the patients were assigned at random to either A, B, C or D Group after gastrectomy. In all patients 20 mg of MMC was

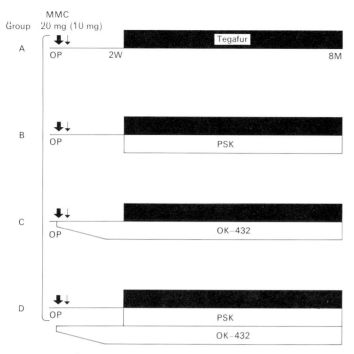

FIGURE 3 Treatment schedule of the cooperative multihospital study conducted by the Japanese Foundation for Multidisciplinary Treatment of Cancer.

Tegafur: 600 mg/day orally and 150 g in total.
PS-K : 3 g/day orally and 750 g in total.
OK-432 : Starting from 0.5 KE intradermally, increased upto 5 KE (maintenance dosage) and 100 KE in total.

administered on the day of gastrectomy and an additional 10 mg on the next day. In Group A, tegafur was administered orally in a daily dose of 600 mg, starting 2 weeks after operation and 150 g (for about 8 months) in total. In Group B, besides the same tegafur administration, oral PS-K was added in a daily dose of 3 g, starting 2 weeks after operation and 750 g (for 8 months) in total. In Group C, besides the same tegafur administration, intradermal injection of OK-432 was added from 0.5 KE, starting 2 weeks after operation and increasing upto 5 KE (maintenance dose) within 2 weeks and 100 KE in total. In Group D, oral tegafur, oral PS-K and intradermal OK-432 were combined in the same manner. This study is now ongoing and the favorable results are expected to be obtained in a few years.

REFERENCES

1. Kimura T. (1975) Chemotherapy as an adjuvant to surgery in gastric carcinoma. Jpn J Cancer Chemother 2: 391-405.

2. Imanaga H, Nakazato H. (1977) Results of surgery for gastric cancer and effect of adjuvant mitomycin-C on cancer recurrence. World J Surg 1: 213-221.

3. Hattori T, Mori A, Hirata K, et al. (1972) Five year survival rate of gastric cancer patients treated with gastrectomy, large dose of mitomycin-C and/or allogeneic bone marrow transplantation. Gann 63: 517-522.

4. Taguchi T, Hattori T, Inoue K, et al. (1979) Multihospital randomized study on adjuvant chemotherapy with mitomycin-C + futraful for gastric cancer; Three year survival rate. In: Adjuvant Therapy of Cancer II (eds) E Jones and SE Salmon. New York, Grune & Stratton, pp. 581-586.

5. Inokuchi K, Hattori T, Inoue K, et al. (1981) Multihospital randomized study on adjuvant chemotherapy with mitomycin-C + futraful for gastric cancer; Five year survival rate. 12th Int Cong Chemother, Florence.

6. Inokuchi K, Hattori T, Taguchi T, et al. (1983) Postoperative adjuvant chemotherapy for gastric carcinoma - analysis of data on 1805 patients followed 5 years. Cancer (in press).

7. Kasai Y, Inokuchi K, Hattori T, et al. (1981) A multihospital randomized study on adjuvant chemotherapy with mitomycin-C and futraful for gastric cancer; the second study. Two year survival rate. 18th General Meeting of Jpn Soc Gastroenterol Surg, Hiroshima.

8. Yasue M, Murakami N, Nakazato H, et al. (1981) A controlled study of maintenance chemoimmunotherapy vs immunotherapy alone immediately following palliative gastrectomy and induction chemoimmunotherapy for advanced gastric cancer. Cancer Chemother Pharmacol 7: 5-10.

9. Hattori T, Niimoto M, Koh T, et al. (1979) Postoperative long-term adjuvant immunochemotherapy with mitomycin-C, PS-K and FT-207 in gastric cancer patients. Jpn J Surg 9: 110-117.

10. Niimoto M, Hattori T, Itoh I, et al. (1982) Effects of levamisole in adjuvant immunochemotherapy of resectable stomach cancer. Jpn J Cancer Chemother 9: 2133-2147.

© 1984 Elsevier Science Publishers B.V.
Fluoropyrimidines in Cancer Therapy
K. Kimura, S. Fujii, M. Ogawa, G.P. Bodey, P. Alberto, eds.

SURGICAL ADJUVANT CHEMOTHERAPY OF COLORECTAL CANCER: GITSG STUDIES

Michael J. O'Connell

1.   INTRODUCTION

The Gastrointestinal Tumor Study Group (GITSG) is a collaborative research organization sponsored by the Division of Cancer Treatment of the National Cancer Institute (USA). In 1975 the GITSG initiated controlled, prospectively randomized trials of postoperative adjuvant therapy in selected patients with resectable carcinoma of the colon (protocol 6175) or rectum (protocol 7175). Patient entry into these trials was terminated in 1979 and 1980, respectively. The preliminary results of these studies have been published (1,2) and definitive manuscripts summarizing the current results are in preparation (3,4). Subsequently, second generation surgical adjuvant trials for patients with colon cancer and rectal cancer (protocol 6179 and protocol 7180) have been activated. This paper will present an overview of the current results of the completed studies and describe the study design of the trials in progress.

2.   COLON CANCER TRIALS

A.   Protocol 6175

Although surgical resection may be curative in many patients with early stage carcinoma of the colon, 50-75% recurrence rates have been reported following resection of tumors which have invaded the serosa or have spread to the regional lymph nodes. Since most recurrences tend to occur in distant sites (e.g. liver, lung, peritoneum), systemic therapy following surgery to destroy microscopic residual malignant disease is a rational strategy. Unfortunately, previous controlled trials of adjuvant 5-FU have not demonstrated any significant survival advantage. The present study was designed to test the value of 5-FU plus MeCCNU (FMe) in the surgical adjuvant setting, based on superior objective response rates observed with FMe combination chemotherapy compared to 5-FU alone in patients with advanced metastatic colon cancer in early randomized trials (5-7), in addition to studies in transplantable murine colon tumors which suggested FMe was a highly effective adjuvant therapy (8). The non-specific immunostimulant methanol extraction residue of bacillus calmette-guerin (MER) was chosen for study based on reports of immunostimulation in cancer patients and occasional observations of temporary tumor regressions in patients with advanced gastrointestinal cancer (9).

Patients entered into this trial had undergone curative surgical resection of a primary adenocarcinoma of the colon characterized by one of the following modified Dukes' stages: B2 (serosal penetration, no positive

nodes); Cl (one to four positive nodes); or C2 (five or
more positive nodes). Following stratification by Dukes'
stage and anatomic location of tumor (ascending colon,
transverse colon, descending and sigmoid colon) patients
were randomly assigned to one of the following treatments:
1. Control (no adjuvant therapy) 2. FMe chemotherapy
3. MER immunotherapy 4. Combined therapy with FMe +
MER. Treatment was begun within seven weeks of surgery
and continued for 70 weeks.

MeCCNU was given in a dose of 130 mg/m^2 by mouth
every ten weeks on the first day of alternate courses of
5-FU. 5-FU was given in a dose of 325 mg/m^2 intravenously
daily for five days every ten weeks in conjunction with
MeCCNU, and in a dose of 375 mg/m^2 for five consecutive
days every ten weeks beginning five weeks after the first
course of 5-FU with MeCCNU. MER was given intradermally
into five sites on the back in a total dose of 1.0 mg
initially, followed by 0.5 mg every five weeks for five
doses, then every 15 weeks.

Six hundred twenty-one patients were randomized into
the study and 572 (92%) were analyzable (49 patients
either did not begin treatment or were found to be ineligible). Dukes' stage, tumor location, age, sex and
presence of organ invasion were well balanced between
treatment arms. Median follow-up is 65 months from
surgery.

One hundred ninty-two (34%) have had documented
disease recurrence. The percentage of patients recurring
varies from 29-37% with no statistically significant
differences between treatments.

Two hundred thirty-seven patients (41%) have died.
No differences in distributions of survival time were
found (see Figure 1).

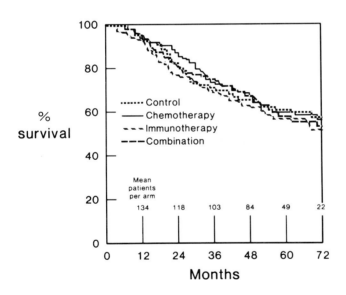

FIGURE 1   Survival according to adjuvant treatment in
patients with carcinoma of the colon.

Acute toxicity in patients receiving FMe consisted
of significant leukopenia (WBC < 2,000) or thrombocytopenia (platelet count < 50,000) in 30% and severe vomiting in 12%. Severe skin reactions (ulceration and necrosis) were seen in 65% of patients receiving MER. One
death due to sepsis associated with bone marrow depression following treatment with FMe was observed, and six
additional patients receiving FMe have developed leukemia.

Adjuvant therapy in this study was not associated
with any apparent clinical benefit and resulted in substantial immediate and delayed side effects. The importance of a randomized study design including a control arm
was demonstrated, since survival within Dukes' stages
for all treatment groups was superior to historical
series and may have led to an erroneous conclusion that
adjuvant treatment was of value if a randomized group of
patients treated with surgery alone were not available
for comparison.

B.   Protocol 6179

The current adjuvant study for colon cancer is a
randomized comparison of surgery alone (no adjuvant therapy) versus combination therapy consisting of hepatic
irradiation plus 5-FU chemotherapy given in conjunction
with radiation and in two five-day courses following the
completion of radiation.

3.   RECTAL CANCER TRIALS

A.   Protocol 7175

Carcinomas taking origin in the rectum have a much higher propensity to recur locally following surgical resection compared to tumors arising in the colon above the peritoneal reflection.   Thus, regional adjuvant therapy with pelvic radiation has been used in conjunction with surgical resection in an attempt to reduce the local recurrence rates.   This prospective clinical trial was designed to determine the value of postoperative radiation therapy (XRT) following curative resection of a rectal carcinoma.   In addition, the potential value of FMe chemotherapy given alone or in conjunction with XRT was studied to determine its effect in controlling systemic tumor recurrences.

Entry into this trial required curative resection of a modified Dukes' stage B2, C1, or C2 adenocarcinoma arising in the rectum ≤ 12 cm from the anal verge. Patients were stratified according to type of surgery (anterior or abdominoperineal resection), Dukes' stage, and interval from operation to first adjuvant treatment. Patients were then randomly assigned to one of the following treatments: 1.   Control (no adjuvant therapy)   2. Pelvic XRT alone   3.   FMe chemotherapy alone   4.   Combined pelvic XRT + FMe.   Treatment began within 60 days of surgery and continued for 18 months.

529

XRT was given at a dose of either 4000 rads or 4800 rads at a rate of 180-200 rads/day five days a week to parallel opposing anterior-posterior fields to include the entire pelvis to the top of the fifth lumbar vertebra using supervoltage radiation. FMe chemotherapy was given as described above. When chemotherapy and XRT were combined, 5-FU was given in a dose of 500 mg/m^2 intravenously during the first three days and last three days of XRT, followed five weeks later by the FMe regimen.

Two hundred twenty-seven patients entered this study and 203 (89%) were available for analysis. Prognostic variables were distributed evenly among the treatment groups. Median postoperative follow-up is 61 months.

Eighty-seven patients (42%) have experienced disease recurrence. There are statistically significant differences in time to recurrence among the four treatments using the generalized Wilcoxon test, and pairwise comparisons indicate a significant superiority for FMe + XRT compared to control. Local or regional recurrences at the time of initial tumor progression were significantly reduced in patients receiving XRT (15%) compared to patients not receiving XRT (23%). Disease-free survival is illustrated in figure 2.

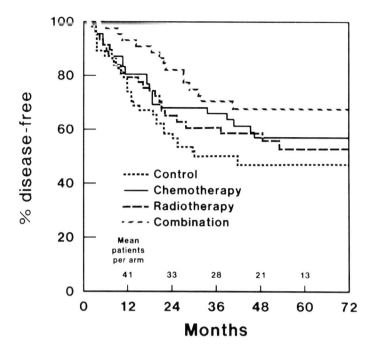

FIGURE 2   Disease-free survival according to adjuvant treatment in patients with carcinoma of the rectum.

Ninty-nine patients (49%) have died, including 55% of control patients and 41% of patients receiving XRT + FMe. However, there is currently no statistically significant difference in survival between treatment groups.

Hematologic toxicity consisting of severe leukopenia (WBC < 2,000) or thrombocytopenia (platelets < 50,000) was seen in about 15% of patients receiving FMe and 30% of patients receiving XRT + FMe. Seventeen percent of XRT + FMe patients had severe diarrhea, two patients receiving combined therapy died of complications related to radiation enteritis, and one patient died of acute leukemia.

This study has demonstrated a reduction in local

tumor recurrences in rectal cancer patients who received postoperative adjuvant XRT, and an improvement in disease-free survival for patients receiving XRT + FMe. Whether these findings will result in superior long term survival will require further follow-up. Toxicity from combined therapy was significant.

B. Protocol 7180

The current adjuvant study for rectal cancer randomly assigns patients to receive either: 1. XRT + FMe as previously given in protocol 7175 2. The same XRT combined with 5-FU alone (MeCCNU deleted from the chemo-therapy regimen).

REFERENCES

1. Killen JY Jr, Holyoke ED, Mittleman A, et al. (1981) Adjuvant therapy of adenocarcinoma of the colon following clinically curative resection: an interim report from the Gastrointestinal Tumor Study Group (GITSG). In: Adjuvant Therapy of Cancer III (eds) Salmon SE and Jones SE. New York, Grune & Stratton, pp. 527-538.

2. Mittleman A, Holyoke E, Thomas PRM, et al. (1981) Adjuvant chemotherapy and radiotherapy following rectal surgery: an interim report from the Gastro-intestinal Tumor Study Group (GITSG). In: Adjuvant Therapy of Cancer III (eds) Salmon SE and Jones SE. New York, Grune & Stratton, pp. 547-557.

3. Gastrointestinal Tumor Study Group. Adjuvant therapy of colon cancer. (submitted for publication).

4. Gastrointestinal Tumor Study Group. Adjuvant therapy of surgically operable rectal carcinoma, stages B_2 and C. (manuscript in preparation).

5. Moertel CG, Schutt AJ, Hahn RG, et al. (1975) Therapy of advanced colorectal cancer with a combination of 5-fluorouracil, methyl-1-3-cis(2-chlorethyl)-1-nitrosourea, and vincristine. J Natl Cancer Inst 54: 69-71.

6. Baker LH, Talley RW, Matter R, et al. (1976) Phase
   III comparison of the treatment of advanced gastrointestinal cancer with bolus weekly 5-FU versus
   methyl-CCNU, plus bolus weekly 5-FU, A Southwest
   Oncology Group Study. Cancer 38: 1-7.

7. Falkson G, Falkson HC. (1976) Fluorouracil, methyl-
   CCNU, and vincristine in cancer of the colon. Cancer
   38: 1468-1470.

8. Corbett TH, Griswold DP Jr, Roberts BJ, et al. (1975)
   A mouse colon-tumor model for experimental therapy.
   Cancer Chemother Rep 5: 169-186.

9. Moertel CG, Ritts, RE Jr, Schutt AJ, et al. (1975)
   Clinical studies of methanol extraction residue
   fraction of BCG as an immunostimulant in patients
   with advanced cancer. Cancer Res 35: 3075-3083.

© 1984 Elsevier Science Publishers B.V.
Fluoropyrimidines in Cancer Therapy
K. Kimura, S. Fujii, M. Ogawa, G.P. Bodey, P. Alberto, eds.

ADJUVANT LIVER PERFUSION WITH 5-FLUOROURACIL AND MITOMYCIN C FOLLOWING CURATIVE LARGE BOWEL CANCER SURGERY

Urs F. Metzger, Bernadette Mermillod, Peter Aeberhard
Rudolf Egeli, Urban Laffer, Sebastiano Martinoli, Rudolf Schroeder
and The Swiss Group for Clinical Cancer Research

1. INTRODUCTION

Colorectal carcinoma afflicts more patients then any other malignant disease occurring in the United States and in Western Europe. Colorectal cancer is second only to lung cancer as a cause of cancer death in women and men. Despite of advances in surgical technic and efforts at early case finding, survival rates following curative resection for colorectal cancer has not substantively improved over the past quarter century. Hepatic metastases have been well established as one of the leading causes of failure after surgical treatment of colorectal cancer. Of 583 patients with histologically proven metastatic carcinoma of largebowel, the liver was the site of metastasis in 353 patients or 61 % (14). It is presumed that hepatic metastasis occur primarily via the portal vein and that blood supply of the metastatic lesions, at least during the early phases of growth, is obtained from the portal vein.

Surgical adjuvant attempts for colorectal cancer using the alkylating agents or the fluorinated pyrimidines by varying routes and schedules have been grossly unsuccess-

534

ful. Survival advantage has been claimed for subsets of patient populations within some clinical trials, but none of the controlled trials have demonstrated a statistically significant advantage for the entire treated patient group in comparison to the entire control group (6, 9, 10, 13).

Following an encouraging report of a British study (19), the Swiss Group for Clinical Cancer Research initiated in 1981 a prospective randomized trial of adjuvant cytotoxic liver perfusion during the first seven postoperative days in an attempt to reduce the subsequent development of macroscopic liver metastases. This is an interim analysis at two years after the start of the trial. The results of an initial pilot study have been published previously (11).

2. PATIENTS AND METHODS

191 patients have been entered from 7 participating institutions with primary adenocarcinoma of either colon or rectum. By preoperative randomization the patients were assigned to liver perfusion through the portal vein with 5-Fluorouracil (500 mg/m2 daily x 7 continuous infusion during the first 7 postoperative days and Mitomycin C (10 mg/m2, 24 hrs. postoperatively as a two hour-infusion) or to no adjuvant treatment. Portal venous catether was placed through any side-branch of the mesenteric venous system during laparotomy. All patients (age below 75 years)

had normal blood counts and normal renal/liver function tests before surgery. In the majority of cases a preoperative liver scan or ultrasound scanning was carried out. 34 patients were randomized but were subsequently excluded from the study owing to the discovery of unexpect liver metastases at operation in 15, to incomplete resection in 6, to catheter-related problems in 4, and to various reasons in 9 patients. 24 patients are too early for a valid evaluation, leaving a total of 133 patients (67 perfusions and 66 controls) for analysis of peri- and postoperative morbidity, mortality and initial follow-up.

Standard surgical techniques of resection were adhered to, the actual procedure to be performed being left to the discretion of the surgeon. Postoperative blood counts and liver function tests were performed on day 1, 3, 5, 7, 10, 14, 28 and 42 whenever possible. A portal venogram was performed during operation to ensure, that the catheter was well positioned and was perfusing equally both main portal branches. If not, the catheter was manipulated under the image intensifier until adequate perfusion was achieved.

The operative specimens were histologically examined and classified according to Dukes (Astler-Coller modification) categorization. The degree of differentiation was also noted.

All patients were followed at 3-monthly intervals for 1 year, then at 6-monthly intervals by the participating institutions. Again, blood counts, liver/renal function tests, liver scan or liver ultrasound, chest X-rays and colonoscopic examination was done according to the proto-col.

3. RESULTS

3.1 Age and sex

The mean age of the patients in the control group was 62,6 (36 – 75) years and that of patients in the perfusion group was 60,6 (31 – 75) years. There were 42 males in the control group and 38 in the perfusion group.

3.2 Site and stage

The site and stage of each tumor are shown in Table 1. There are no statistically significant differences bet-ween the Dukes categorization and the degree of differen-tiation of the tumors in each group.

3.3 Postoperative morbidity

16 out of 67 (24 %) in the perfusion group and 12 out of 66 (18 %) patients in the control group experienced a moderate of more severe complication using the WHO-code. The complications are listed in Table 2. The mean post-operative hospital stay was $18,2 \pm 8,5$ days in the per-fusion group and $19,4 \pm 10,1$ days in the control group. These differences were not statistically significant.

3.4 Postoperative mortality

In the immediate 30 day – postoperative period, there were three deaths : two in the control and one in the per-

TABLE 1

SITE, STAGE AND DEGREE OF DIFFERENTIATION
(SAKK 40/81)

STAGE	CONTROL			PERFUSION		
	A	B	C	A	B	C
Right Colon	1	9	9	1	11	8
Transverse Colon	-	2	3	-	2	2
Left Colon	1	9	4	2	11	3
Rectum	2	20	4	2	18	7
TOTAL	4	40	20	5	42	20
Degree of differentiation						
Well		36			35	
Moderately		28			31	
Poorly / Anaplastic		2			1	

TABLE 2

POSTOPERATIVE MORBIDITY
(SAKK 40/81)

	CONTROL (N= 66)	PERFUSION (N= 67)
INFECTIOUS COMPLICATIONS	6 (1✝)	4 (1✝)
- WOUND INFECTION	4	2
- SEPTICEMIA	1	1
- PNEUMONIA	1	3
- URINARY INFECTION	2	-
ANASTOMOTIC DEHISCENCE	2	3
PERSISTENT PERINEAL SINUS	0	2
SMALL BOWEL OBSTRUCTION	2	3
POSTOPERATIVE HEMORRHAGE	1	1
THROMBOSIS / EMBOLISM	1	1
NEUROLOGIC DISORDERS	-	2
TOTAL (PATIENTS)	12 (18 %)	16 (24 %)
MEAN HOSPITAL STAY (D$^{\pm}$ S.D.)	19,4$^{\pm}$10,1	18,2$^{\pm}$8,5

fusion group.

One patient died of irreversible cardiac arrest during surgery, the two others died of therapy-resistent gram-negative septicemia at day 15 and day 21. It was considered, that the cytotoxic perfusion was a contributary factor in one of these patients. This 72 year old diabetic male had a persistent purulent secretion following rigth hemicolectomy. On the eleventh postoperative day he developed necrotizing fasciitis of the abdominal wall with bronchopneumonia and irreversible gram-negative septi-cemia. At this time, he had marked leucopenia of 2.200/mm3.

3.5 Hematologic toxicity

6 patients developed transient leucopenia (below 3.000/mm3) during perfusion. The white cell count was statistically significantly lower at day 7 and 10 in the perfusion group compared with the control group (Fig. 1). With one exception (see above), the values returned to-wards normal on completion of hospitalisation.

There were only two thrombocytopenia of 56.000 and 71.000/mm3 in the perfusion group, but the mean thrombo-cyte count was statistically significantly lower on day 28 in the perfusion group compared to the control group. These values returned to normal at the first follow-up examination.

Bilirubin and other liver function tests (SGOT, SGPT, alkaline phosphatase) were not significantly influenced

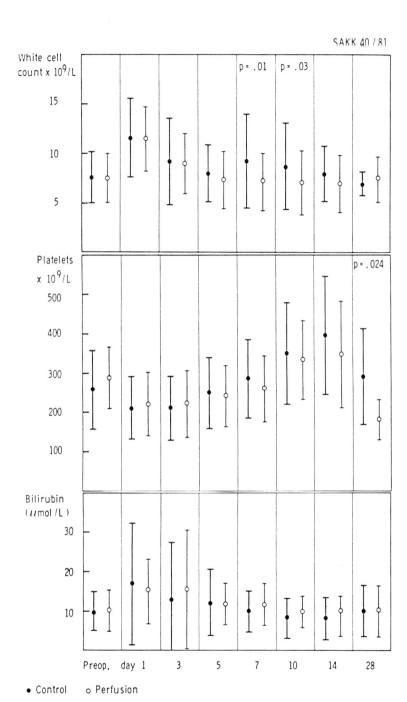

SAKK 40 / 81

FIGURE 1   Hematologic toxicity

541

by the perfusion treatment.

3.6 Follow-up data

18 recurrences have been observed so far in the follow-up period, 12 in the control group, 6 in the perfusion group. There were 5 and 4 local failures in these groups, 7 distant failures in the control group and 2 in the perfusion group. 5 patients of the control group already developed liver metastases, wereas two patients of the perfusion group had liver involvement.

There were 6 deaths in the control group, 4 due to recurrence, 1 to myocardial infarction, 1 to small bowel obstruction, compared to 3 deaths in the perfusion group, one to myocardial infarction, one to local recurrent cancer, and one to disseminated malignant disease.

DISCUSSION

Liver metastases are present at initial diagnosis of large bowel cancer in 25-30 % of the patients (2). After curative resection of colorectal primary, the liver again is the most frequent site of relapse in 40-50 % (4, 18). Once liver metastases have developed, the prognosis is poor with an expected median survival time of 6 - 8 months (2, 14).

A great deal of work has been done to determine the factors, that influence development of liver metastases. There is evidence, that tumor cells embolize into the portal venous system via the invaded mesenteric veins and enter the liver. In 1957, Dukes (7) found evidence of venous spread in 17 % of operative rectal cancer specimens. Fisher and Turnbull (8) discovered tumor cells in the mesenteric venous blood of 32 % of colorectal carcinoma patients at surgery. They suggested that manipulation of the tumor may force malignant cells into the circulation and they initiated the so-called "no touch - isolation" technique. This led to a significant reduction of the incidence of liver metastases (21, 22). However, not all circulating cancer cells give rise to metastases. Several reports have shown that patients with malignant cells in the venous blood fare no worse than those without (15, 17). Metachronous liver metastases may originate from microscopic deposits not visible at surgery for the primary tumor.

These micrometastases are the most important target for adjuvant systemic therapy (5, 16). Since systemic chemotherapy is of limited value in largebowel cancer, numerous studies have approached the issue of hepatic artery or portal venous infusion of fluorinated pyrimidines. Almersjö et al. (1) have shown the safety of portal venous infusion in man. They found that during continuous portal infusion of 15 mg 5 FU/kg for 24 hours, systemic serum concentrations were generally below 100 μg/ml and no side effects were noticed. It is generally accepted that adjuvant therapy should be started as soon as possible after surgery when the tumor burden is minimal (3, 16). Morales et al. (12) advocated intra-portal injection of cytotoxic agents at the time of surgery for colorectal cancer in an attempt to prevent liver metastases by diminishing the number of circulating tumor cells.

In this study, the primary aim was to confirm the results of Taylor et al. (19, 20) and to assess the possible benefit of the 5-FU/Mitomycin-C combination.

The actual method of liver perfusion through any side branch of mesenteric veins was easy to perform, cannulation proved technically impossible in two patients only, which seems to be superior to a 10 % failure rate in cannulating the umbilical vein (19). Using the transabdominal route, there has been no direct catheter-related complication with therapeutic consequences.

Despite a large cumulative dose of 5-FU given during the immediate postoperative period, the systemic side effects were minimal and morbidity of large bowel surgery was not significantly increased nor was the hospital stay prolonged by the adjuvant perfusion.

Interestingly, the overall operative mortality rate in this study is considerably lower than reported by previous multicenter trials. This indicates a possible advance in surgical technique and pre-/postoperative patient management in this type of elective surgery. One insulin-dependent diabetic male patient developed postoperative wound infection, necrotizing fasciitis and gramnegative septicemia. He died of therapy-resistent septicemia with leucopenia and it is considered that cytotoxic perfusion contributed to his death and accordingly patients with insulin-dependent diabetes are no longer included in the study.

Apart from this single patient, the results of adjuvant liver perfusion in colorectal cancer appear encouraging and tend to support the data of Taylor (20). During the period of follow-up, 6 patients have died in the control group, compared with 3 in the perfusion group, 5 of the control patients have developed multiple liver metastases compared with 2 patients in the perfusion group. Although the results are superficially promising, the period of follow-up is too short for accurate statistical conclusions. Since the study is still ungoing with the same patient entry rate, it is hoped, that a total number of 400 patients will be entered into the trial within another two years.

CONCLUSION

1. Surgical catheter placement into the portal vein is easily feasible through any side branch of the mesenteric veins.

2. This type of adjuvant therapy does not significantly increase surgical morbidity, mortality or duration of hospitalisation.

3. Initial results are superficially promising, further

patient entry and prolonged follow-up is needed.

Liver metastases of colorectal origin develop by malignant cells entering the portal venous circulation. A prospective randomized clinical trial was initiated in 1981 to assess the value of adjuvant portal venous perfusion with 5-Fluorouracil and Mitomycin C following curative large bowel cancer surgery.

170 patients without macroscopic liver secondaries have so far entered the trial. 133 patients (67 perfusions and 66 controls) are completely evaluable for peri- and postoperative morbidity and for initial follow-up. Patient and tumor characteristics are evenly distributed among the 2 random arms and there is no statistically significant difference in postoperative complications or hospital stay (18,2 $\pm$ 8,5 days in perfusion and 19,4 $\pm$ 10,1 days in control group).

So far, 12 recurrences have been observed in the control group and 6 in the perfusion group. Liver metastases were present in 5 control patients and in 2 perfusion patients. 4 patients in the control group and 2 patients in the perfusion group died of recurrent disease.

These results show an encouraging trend and suggest that adjuvant cytotoxic liver perfusion may reduce the indicence of liver metastases without significantly increased morbidity and mortality in large bowel cancer surgery.

REFERENCES

1. Almersjö O, Brandberg A, Gustavsson B. (1975) Concentration of biologically active 5-fluorouracil in general circulation during continuous portal infusion in man. Cancer Letters 1: 113-118.

2. Bengmark S, Hafström L. (1969) The natural history of primary and secondary malignant tumours of the liver. 1. The prognosis for patients with hepatic metastases from colonic and rectal carcinoma by laparotomy. Cancer 23: 198-202.

3. Burchenal JH. (1976) Adjuvant therapy – theory, practice, and potential. The James Ewing Lecture. Cancer 37: 46-57.

4. Cedermark BJ, Schultz SS, Bakshi S, et al. (1977) The value of liver scan in the follow-up study of patients with adenocarcinoma of the colon and rectum. Surg Gynecol Obstet 144: 745-748.

5. DeVita VT. (1983) The relationship between tumor mass and resistance to chemotherapy. Implications for surgical adjuvant treatment of cancer. The James Ewing Lecture. Cancer 51: 1209-1220.

6. Dwight RW, Humphrey WE, Higgins GA, Keehn RJ. (1973) FUDR as an adjuvant to surgery in cancer of the large bowel. J Surg Oncol 5: 243-249.

7. Dukes CE. (1957) Discussion on major surgery in carcinoma of the rectum, with or without colostomy, excluding the anal canal and including the rectosigmoid. Proc R Soc Med 50: 1031-1052.

8. Fisher ER, Turnbull RB. (1955) The cytological demonstration and significance of tumor cells in the mesenteric venous blood in patients with colorectal cancer. Surg Gynecol Obstet 100: 102-106.

9. Higgins GA, Humphrey WE, Juler GL, et al. (1976) Adjuvant chemotherapy in the surgical treatment of large bowel cancer. Cancer 38: 1461-1467.

10. Lawrence W, Terz JJ, Horsley S, et al. (1975) Chemotherapy as an adjuvant to surgery for colorectal cancer. Ann Surg 181: 616-623.

11. Metzger U, Aeberhard P, Egeli R, et al. (1982) Adjuvante portale Leberperfusion beim kolorektalen Karzinom. Helv Chir Acta 49: 175-178.

12. Morales F, Bell M, McDonald GD, et al. (1957) The prophylactic treatment of cancer at the time of operation. Ann Surg 146: 588-595.

13. Moertel CG, Killen JY, Holyoke ED, et al. (1981) Adjuvant therapy of adenocarcinoma of the colon following clinically curative resection: an interim report from the GITSG. In: Adjuvant Therapy of Cancer III (eds) E Jones and SE Salmon. Grune & Stratton, New York, pp 527-538.

14. Pestana C, Reitemeier RJ, Moertel CG, et al. (1964) The natural history of carcinoma of the colon and rectum. Am J Surg 108: 826-829.

15. Roberts S, Jonasson O, Long L, et al. (1961) Clinical significance of cancer cells in the circulating blood Two- to five-year survivals. Ann Surg 154: 362-371.

16. Schabel FM. Concepts for systemic treatment of micrometastases. Cancer 35: 15-24, 1975.

17. Sellwood RA, Kapper SW, Burn JI, et al. (1965) Circulating cancer cells: the influence of surgical operations. Br J Surg 52: 69-72.

18. Swinton NW, Legg MA, Lewis FG. (1964) Metastasis of cancer of the rectum and sigmoid flexure. Dis Colon Rectum 7: 273-277.

19. Taylor I, Rowling JT, West C. (1979) Adjuvant cytotoxic liver perfusion for colorectal cancer. Br J Surg 66: 833-837.

20. Taylor I, West C, Rowling J. (1980) Can colorectal liver metastases be prevented ? In: Progress and Perspectives in the Treatment of Gastrointestinal Tumors (ed) A Gerard. Pergamon Press, Oxford, pp. 89-92.

21. Turnbull RB. (1970) Cancer of the colon: 5-10 year survival rates following resection utilizing the isolation technique. Ann R Coll Surg Engl 46: 243-250.

22. Wiggers T, Arends JW, Jeekel J, et al. (1983) The no-touch isolation technique in colon cancer. A prospective controlled trial. J Exp Clin Cancer Res 2: 37.

© 1984 Elsevier Science Publishers B.V.
Fluoropyrimidines in Cancer Therapy
K. Kimura, S. Fujii, M. Ogawa, G.P. Bodey, P. Alberto, eds.

ADJUVANT CHEMOTHERAPY FOR RECTAL CARCINOMA

Kimiyuki Kato and Tomoyuki Kato

1. INTRODUCTION

The incidence of rectal cancer has become high in Japan. Vital statistics indicate that the number of deaths from rectal cancer and their proportion among all kinds of malignacies and diseases have increased during the past two decades. The most effective treat-

TABLE 1   Number of deaths from rectal cancer by year (from Vital Statistics)

Year	No. of Deaths from Rectal Ca.	No. of Deaths from Rectal Ca. / No. of Deaths from All Malig.	No. of Deaths from Rectal Ca. / Total No. of Deaths
1965	3,796	3.4%	0.5%
1966	3,840	3.3	0.6
1967	4,124	3.5	0.6
1968	4,394	3.6	0.6
1969	4,582	3.8	0.7
1970	4,717	3.8	0.7
1971	4,966	3.9	0.7
1972	5,066	3.8	0.7
1973	5,506	4.0	0.8
1974	5,917	4.4	0.8
1975	5,904	4.1	0.8
1976	6,018	4.1	0.9
1977	6,273	4.1	0.9
1978	6,402	4.1%	0.9%
1979	6,908	4.2	1.0
1980	6,917	4.4	1.0
1981	7,279	4.4	1.0

ment at present for rectal cancer is surgery, so it is important to improve surgical results for rectal cancer in order to further decrease such mortality. The rationale for combining chemotherapeutic agents with curative operative attempts for "solid tumor" has had great appeal as an potential means of imporving end result of cancer surgery. Despite a great deal of interest in this approach there have not yet been any clinical studies conclusively demonstrating the benefits from surgical adjuvant chemotherapy for any of the common adult cancers.

The present study covers our experience with "adjuvant chemotherapy for rectal carcinoma."

2. DESCRIPTION OF STUDY

From January, 1971 through May, 1982, 224 acceptable study patients have been evaluated. All of these patients underwent curative resection for adenocarcinoma of the rectum. Criteria for exclusion of patients were: patients more than seventy years old, patients considered to be a poor risk for chemotherapy because of nutritional, cardiopulmonary, hepatic, renal or hematologic problems; patients with a history of previous or concomitant malignancy, patients with a white blood cell count less than 4,000 cells/mm^3; and patients in whom surgical resection was not performed.

2.1. First trial

From January, 1971 through May, 1975, 65 acceptable study patients were evaluated. These patients were allocated to the two treatment groups: (A)mitomycin C (MMC) 0.1 mg/kg and 5-FU 10 mg/kg into the superior rectal artery at the time of operation, then post-operatively MMC 0.04 mg/kg and 5-FU 10 mg/kg intravenously twice weekly for 8 times; or (B) surgery alone.

Regimen of the Ist Trial

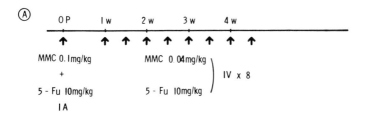

FIGURE 1   Regimen for first trial

2.2. Second trial

From June, 1975 through October, 1979, 111 patients were evaluated. These patients were randomized to three groups: (A) MMC 0.2 mg/kg into the superior rectal artery during operation, then postoperatively MMC 0.08 mg/kg intravenously twice weekly for 4 time and Tegafur 800 mg/d per os for 3 months; (B) postoperatively MMC O 0.08 mg/kg twice weekly for 6 times and Tegafur 800 mg/d per os for 3 months; or (C) surgery alone.

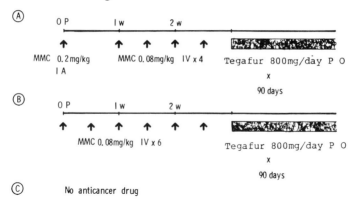

Regimen of the 2nd Trial

FIGURE 2   Regimen for second trial

2.3.   Third trial

From October, 1979 through May, 1982, 57 patients
were evaluated. These patients were given either:
(A) MMC 0.2 mg/kg intravenously on the previous day of
operation, adriamycin (ADR) 0.4 mg/kg intravenously on
the 7th postoperative day and again 0.2 mg/kg of ADR
intravenously on the 21st postoperative day and con-
comitantly 800 mg/d of Tegafur per os for 6 months after
operation; (B) the same regimen of (A) and 5.0 KE/w of
OK-432 intracutaneously for 6 months; or (C) surgery alone.

All study patients, whether receiving drug therapy
or not, were followed at periodic intervals every three
months to check for evidence of recurrence of disease.
The periodic examination included a brief interim
history, a physical examination, chest x-ray, and certain
laboratory studies, including a hemoglobin, white blood
cell count, platelet count, CEA and liver function
studies.

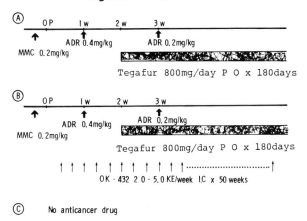

Regimen of the 3rd Trial

FIGURE 3   Regimen for third trial

3.   RESULTS

3.1.   First trial

Of the 65 patients who underwent a curative resection
35 received MMC and 5-FU, and 30 were controls. There
have been no signs of hematologic or other toxicity in
the early postoperative period in the treatment group.
The actual data and visual graph of these results reveal
no significant difference.   The MMC and 5-FU adjuvant
treatment groups have fewer positive lymph node cases
than the control group.   A selected subgroup of the
whole, negative lymph node were examined separately
despite the small number of patients concerned.   There
was some suggestion of benefit from therapy but no
significant difference.

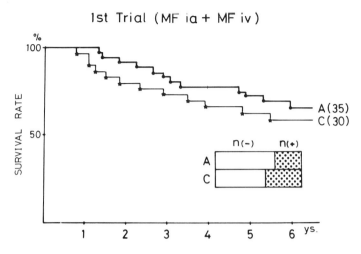

FIGURE 4 Survival curves for first trial (MF IA +MF IV).

3.2. Second trial

Of the 111 patients who underwent a curative resection 74 received   MMC   and Tegafur, and 37 were controls. There were no significant differences between adjuvant and control groups.

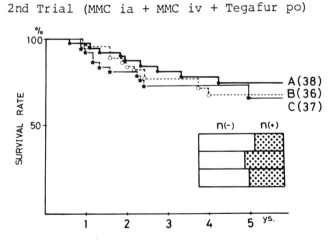

FIGURE 5 Survival curves for second trial (MMC IV + Tegafur PO).

554

3.3.   Third trial

Of the 57 patients who underwent a curative resection, 30 received ADR, MMC and Tegafur.   It was too short a follow-up period to determine drug benefits.

TABLE 2   Recurrence observed in the third trial (MMC iv +ADR IV + Tegafur PO)

66 group		
A	1 / 16	(6.3%)
B	1 / 14	(7.1%)
C	4 / 17	(23.5%)

2nd Trial (MMC ia + MMC iv + Tegafur po)

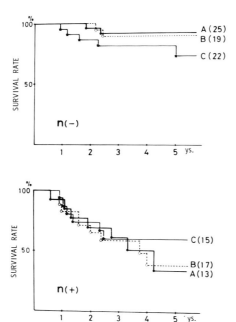

FIGURE 6   Survival curves for second trial (MMC IV + Tegafur PO) by lymph node involvement.

4. COMMENTS

The data, although showing a slight but consistent benefit in the treatment groups, do not make a convincing argument for the effect of MMC and 5-FU as an adjuvant to the surgical treatment of rectal cancer. These studies appear to indicate slight but consistent benefits in the treatment group, but they were not statistically significant in most catagories examined. But on the second trial, in patients without lymph node involvement there were significant differences between treated groups and controls.

It has been suggested that adjuvant chemotherapy should not be pushed to the point of toxicity to minimize the risk to patients who have a reasonable chance for permanent control of their disease.

It is of considerable interest and has certain implications for future trials that adjuvant studies in rectal carcinoma, using prospectively randomized simultaneous controls, reveal either little or no treatment benefit in the chemotherapy group of patients. This is in contrast to studies in which historical controls were used and adjuvant therapy appeared to confer a significant treatment advantage. Use of historical controls substantially diminishes the impact of such studies.

REFERENCES

1. Holden WD, et al. (1967) The use of triethylene-
    thiophosphoramide as an adjuvant to the surgical
    treatment of colorectal carcinoma. Ann Surg 164:
    481.

2. Higgins GA, et al. (1976) Adjuvant chemotherapy in
    the surgical treatment of large bowel cancer.
    Cancer 38: 1461.

3. Lawrence W et al. (1975) Chemotherapy as an adjuvant
    to surgery for colorectal cancer. Ann Surg 117: 616.

4. Grossi CE, et al. (1979) Intraluminal fluorourasil
    chemotherapy adjuvant to surgical procedure for
    resectable carcinoma of the colon and rectum. S G O
    145: 549.

5. Grage TB, et al. (1977) Adjuvant chemotherapy with
    5-fluorourasil after surgical resection of colo-
    rectal carcinoma. Amer J Surg 133: 59.

6. Kaplan EL, Meier P. (1958) Nonparametric estimation
    from incomplete observation. J Am Stat Assoc 53: 457.

7. Gehan EA. (1965) A generalized Wilcozon test for
    comparing arbitrarily singly-censored samples.
    Biometrika 52: 203.

© 1984 Elsevier Science Publishers B.V.
Fluoropyrimidines in Cancer Therapy
K. Kimura, S. Fujii, M. Ogawa, G.P. Bodey, P. Alberto, eds.

DISCUSSION

Holyoke: I have a general question. You excluded some patients because they did not receive a complete dose. Do you follow them along to see what happens? Is that usual procedure - that a patient who does not receive a full course of chemotherapy is not tallied?

Abe: We did exclude those patients who did not receive the dose designated in the regimen. I don't know if this is the right way to assess or not, but in any event those patients who couldn't tolerate the whole course of the dosage (7.2%) because of gastrointestinal toxicity were dropped.

Sadée: This is just a brief comment concerning positive and negative estrogen receptors. Are any attempts made to differentiate those, for example, by measuring the translocation of the receptor into the nucleus as a measure of activity with binding of an estrogen antagonist?

Arafah: Not in this particular study. The action of estrogen receptors appears to be difficult to evaluate with translocation studies. As you know, the progesterone receptor is under estrogen control, primarily through the estrogen receptor mechanism. That is the whole idea behind measuring the progesterone receptor. This indicates at least that the estrogen receptor in a particular tumor is functional. I don't want to jump to the conclusion that this indicates that once the estrogen receptor is functional in terms of its action on the progesterone receptor it means that it is functional in terms of tumor growth, because the two may be totally different.

Tattersall: Apart from the survival difference in the ER positive and ER negative tumors, is there any other survival difference between the various treatment arms you have compared?

Arafah: Apart from the fact that they were positive or negative, no.

Tattersall: That wasn't treatment related, was it?

Arafah: No, it was not, but there is no survival difference according to treatment.

Taguchi: Did you observe any side effect with tamoxifen?

Arafah: The side effects were really minimal, and at no time did we have to stop the treatment because of side effects.

Ogawa: I understand that methyl-CCNU is carcinogenic; therefore, I would like to know the incidence of second malignancies in patients treated by methyl-CCNU plus 5-FU. The drug is also known to have some chronic toxicity such as nephrotoxicity. Would you comment on this?

Holyoke: The nephrotoxicity seems under control with the maximum 1 gram dose, but you are quite correct.

Ogawa: How about other secondary tumors?

Holyoke: We have looked, but the problem appears to be mainly hematological; that is quite definite.

O'Connell: I would like to congratulate both Dr. Hattori and Dr. Nakajima for their excellent presentations. I am impressed with the tremendous volume of material that is available for surgical adjuvant studies in gastric cancer. As I understand it, the primary treatment effects that have been seen in these studies have been in certain subgroups of patients, particularly the stage III patients or those with positive nodes or serosal penetration. I have one question of clarification: have any of these trials demonstrated a statistically significant advantage for treatment compared to surgical controls when all patients are considered for analysis, not just the subgroups? Secondly, since the treatment effect seems to be most predominant in specific subsets, have you considered in your current trials limiting the study of the adjuvant therapy to the subsets where there is some apparent benefit?

Taguchi: Perhaps Dr. Nakajima can answer that. He has a control group that has undergone operation alone.

Nakajima: Taken as a whole, we could find no statistically significant difference between the treated and control groups. It is mainly due to the insufficient number of cases accumulated in this trial. If we had accumulated more cases, the p value would have been less than 0.05. In our trials, of stage II and stage II plus stage III subsets, we found a quite significant difference between treated and control groups. Thus, I concluded that mitomycin C plus 5-FU adjuvant chemotherapy is effective for locally advanced groups.

O'Connell: Are you limiting your case accrual in your current studies to that particular patient subgroup at this point, or are you still treating all patients with gastric cancer with chemotherapy?

Nakajima: Recently, we exclusively select stage II and stage III patients.

Taguchi: I would like to ask the audience and the speakers what regimen they recommend for adjuvant chemotherapy.

Holyoke: My recommendation is 5-FU with radiation in selected circumstances. If I were looking into the problem in
the laboratory, I would look to see what happened to the
various levels of appropriate enzymes in radiated tissue.
The colon studies of GITSG and a Pancreas Study indicate
this may be an important combination. In my mind it is
probable that 5-FU has a small effect. It is so small
against background that it usually cannot be demonstrated,
and I believe a surgery alone control group is still
justified. Obviously, another way to potentiate it is
through the addition of appropriate drugs and, as far as
I can see, that is open for discussion.

Taguchi: Dr. O'Connell, what kind of regimen do you recommend for stomach cancer?

O'Connell: That is a difficult question to give a definitive answer to, but I do have several comments. I would agree
with Dr. Holyoke that postoperative adjuvant radiation
therapy is a rational concept. Approximately one-third of
patients subjected to second-look surgical procedures at
the University of Minnesota following gastrectomy were
found to have recurrences limited to the tumor bed and
regional lymphatics or localized peritoneal recurrences.
Therefore, since there seems to be a substantial proportion
of patients that recur locally, a local modality makes some
sense. I would also combine this with at least 5-FU because
of the apparent potentiating effects. I must emphasize,
though, that if such a trial were to be undertaken, that
we would still include a surgery-alone group for comparison.
The second approach that we are currently studying at the
Mayo Clinic and the North-Central Cancer Treatment Group
is 5-FU-adriamycin combination without methyl-CCNU to try
to determine whether there is any adjuvant effect. Hopefully, this combination will avoid the leukemogenic potential of methyl-CCNU. And we are comparing 5-FU-adriamycin
to surgery-alone control.

Taguchi: Dr. Woolley, do you recommend FAM?

Woolley: I agree with everybody who has said that there
are no firm recommendations that can be made at this point.
Dr. Holyoke has not really dwelt upon the stratification
of the GI Tumor Study Group study as far as nodal status.
The effect in node-positive patients was greater than the
effect in node-negative patients. The major contribution
to the adjuvant effect in all patients was in node-positive
patients.

There have been a great number of well-designed studies
that are negative. I think that there are two active
studies with the FAM regimen. There is an international
study that is looking at FAM versus observation only. There
is a Southwest Oncology Group study which is presently
positive, but the numbers are fluctuating and the people
who are closest to that study are unwilling to say that the

study is going to remain positive. I am concerned about
the use of leukemogenic drugs in patients who have a good
prognosis. So I am very interested in trials that look at
combinations that don't use either methyl-CCNU or mitomycin
C. I am concerned about the long-term effects, not necessarily leukemogenic, of mitomycin C as well. We have been
studying hemolytic-uremic syndrome, thrombocytopenic
purpura syndrome quite intensively. We are in a stage of
evolution with adjuvant studies. We just don't know what
the results with FAM will be. I will be very interested in
the NCCTG Group study of 5-FU-adriamycin. The 5-FU-adria-
mycin-BCNU combination will also be very interesting as
well. I am afraid it will be three or four years before we
have really solid information.

Holyoke: I would just like to make one comment. After Dr.
Hattori's talk, it seems to me that mitomycin C and 5-FU
or tegafur quite possibly has an effect. Even though we
don't see the effect overall, we see it in subsets; and we
are looking forward to the stage III study, and it may
certainly be on a par with all the others.

Kimura: I have one question for the three speakers. Have
you had any results in terms of any relationship with staging and the Borrmann classification?

Holyoke: I have not thought that through, although I should
have. In the Gastrointestinal Tumor Study Group, it appears
that the drug effects cut across and overcome the effects
of node and/or location of tumor and is seen in all subgroups.

Hattori: We have no data showing a positive relationship
with Borrmann classification. I would like to emphasize
that a more important factor may be the timing of the start
of adjuvant chemotherapy after surgery. According to my
understanding, most American protocols begin about one
month or so after surgery. In Japan, they usually start
from the day of operation. Dr. Holyoke reported today, in
his first study, that it started from perhaps ten days
after operation, and that the results were very good. So I
would like to emphasize this timing of the starting of
chemotherapy.

Holyoke: I didn't make myself clear. We didn't actually
start that early. But we have some information that if the
chemotherapy is delayed in patients with local residual
disease, it may be that shorter survival is due to that
fact. Therefore, if I were doing a combined radiation study,
I would be inclined to give a dose of drug immediately. I
agree with you that we are too slow. It may make a difference.

Nakajima: In our trials, MFC plus 5-FU was effective for
the Borrmann type 3 and some of Borrmann 4 types with a
diameter of less than 8 cm.

O'Connell: I would like to make a comment and as a question concerning the portal vein infusion program that Dr. Metzger described. We are also conducting a controlled study of portal vein infusion at the Mayo Clinic comparing the regimens Dr. Taylor initially described (500 mg/m^2 of 5-FU daily times seven) versus surgery alone as a control. We have currently entered about 90 patients into this program, and although we have no therapeutic results to report at this time, I would like to agree with Dr. Metzger that this is a safe and clinically tolerable method of administration of 5-FU. The question I would like to address to Dr. Metzger is: are you aware of any follow-up data from the original report by Dr. Taylor, which was published in 1979 and suggested a significant reduction in hepatic metastases and improvement in survival in patients who received portal vein 5-FU?

Metzger: Unfortunately, I do not have any follow-up data from Dr. Taylor. Duke's B patients do better than the Duke's C patients in the perfusion group. But I wouldn't say that we can draw any conclusion yet. I hope we may get further information on his trial in the near future. When we started our perfusion trial, we decided to add mitomycin C to the perfusate. I am not sure whether that works any better than 5-FU alone, but it was the advice of our medical colleagues to do so. We, as well as Dr. Taylor, added heparin to the perfusate, and there is at least basic scientific evidence that heparin alone may have some beneficial effect. That is the reason why EORTC is currently conducting a three-arm study with the third arm using heparin alone.

Holyoke: I would like to ask Dr. O'Connell more about the methyl-CCNU. We have one death from leukemia, but I think we ought to discuss about how many patients have some change - either preleukemic or leukemic change - who are still alive of that hundred or two hundred patients.

O'Connell: In the rectal surgical adjuvant study, I am only aware of one case of acute leukemia patient who died. There were six confirmed cases to date in the colon surgical adjuvant study, for a total of seven cases in the two studies. That would involve approximately seven cases among 450 patients who received 5-FU-methyl-CCNU in the two studies. With the delayed occurrence of the leukemia, this may be an underestimate of the eventual leukemic risk.

Holyoke: It is still occurring. On the other hand, do you have any thoughts as to why gastric and rectal studies didn't see similar number? Perhaps we have to include a larger denominator, and it may or may not be a problem in defence of methyl-CCNU.

O'Connell: Yes, I agree with that statement. We do not yet have an accurate estimate of the risk of leukemia following treatment with methyl-CCNU.

Holyoke: Many of us have been waiting for many years to have a repeat of Dr. Taylor's work, and I think that infusion study is really fascinating. We have had trouble getting surgeons to do it. You have one operation and it is placed, and then it is just removed after seven days, and that's it.